"For anyone in the prison of depression, this workbook might help you get out. It's both scholarly and practical, and leaves no stone unturned in laying out self-help strategies for helping deal with this widespread problem."

> —Frank Farley, PhD, L. H. Carnell Professor at Temple University in Philadelphia, PA, and former president of the American Psychological Association

"William Knaus has been a leading practitioner and teacher of cognitive behavior therapy for over four decades. In *The Cognitive Behavioral Workbook for Depression*, he draws from his vast store of experience to provide people who struggle with depression practical, usable strategies they can put to immediate use to not only feel better, but to get better. Written in an engaging, accessible manner, the book is chock full of powerful tools that, when compiled into a personal action plan, can both defeat depression and build a happy, productive life. I think this is a substantial book anyone, not just the depressive, will find valuable, and I highly endorse it for both the lay public and the clinical community alike. I know that I will keep it handy for my own personal reference and repeatedly encourage my clients to purchase it."

> —Russell Grieger, PhD, clinical psychologist in private practice, organizational consultant, and adjunct professor at The University of Virginia

"I have waited for this book my entire career! With compassion, flexibility, and scientifically sound earnestness, Knaus helps the depressed reader navigate the wide variety of cognitive behavioral treatments to choose the package that is right for him or her. Second editions often contain few, if any, theoretical concepts and clinical exercises that are significantly different from those in the first edition. Not so with this volume! It is full of fresh ideas and therapeutic assignments that help the motivated depressed individual finally crawl out of self-defeating misery."

> —Barry Lubetkin, PhD, ABPP, founder and director of the Institute for Behavior Therapy in New York, NY

"There are many self-help books on the market, but many are somewhere between vague and incomprehensible. Not this one. Knaus is a true teacher in the mold of Socrates, an instructor who takes you by the hand and leads you step-by-step to a successful outcome. Depression has become virtually viral during the last few years, and this is a book that promises to relieve the distress and delivers on its promise. And you don't need an advanced degree in psychology to understand the Knaus message. Anyone who can follow the plans to build a model airplane or follow recipe directions can use this book to conquer depression. It is so readable that you'll think Knaus is standing beside you. Without question, he is the country's leading expert on the cognitive-behavioral approach."

> —Richard C. Sprinthall, PhD, professor emeritus at American International College and licensed clinical psychologist

"In this second edition of *The Cognitive Behavioral Workbook for Depression*, Knaus eloquently and compassionately converts a three-pronged truth about depression—that it is a time-limited state of mind that can be remedied through activity—into a set of incredibly powerful cognitive behavioral tools for defeating depression. Helping you to identify and refute irrational thoughts that may be keeping you depressed, Knaus gently guides you to take action. Read this book, do the exercises, and don't just find out how to conquer your depression—actually do it!

—Elliot D. Cohen, PhD, author of *The Dutiful Worrier*


"Knaus has again produced a handbook that is filled with useful ideas and practical exercises to help people overcome a wide variety of challenges. He takes a simple approach with explanations and examples that give people confidence that they can get started without great difficulty. The handbook includes lots of ways to track progress and document the results of exercises, and employs a graduated approach by beginning with simple, less challenging exercises and progressively building to much more challenging issues. Knaus' book should prove very helpful to anyone wanting to improve their handling of many of life's challenges."

—James W. Thompson, PhD, business psychologist


"Knaus's *The Cognitive Behavioral Workbook for Depression* provides depressed individuals with all the psychological 'workouts' that are needed to pull them out of that state. A great resource for professionals, as well."

—Edward J. Garcia, MA, CSW


"'Simplify and clarify' seems to be the credo of Knaus. He has distilled his own experience and a thorough perusal of the germane literature into an accessible and succinct series of explanations and exercises that will make profound change in thinking seem facile and, if not effortless, then at least possible."

—Joseph Gerstein, MD, FACP, founding president of SMART Recovery Self-Help Network and assistant clinical professor of medicine at Harvard Medical School (retired)


"Whether you are solving the problem of depression through medication, professional therapy, or doing it yourself, this book will be of tremendous help. *The Cognitive Behavioral Workbook for Depression* is chock-full of the ready-to-use strategies you will need to help you feel good again."

—Jon Carlson, PsyD, EdD, Distinguished Professor at Governors State University

"This is an excellent second edition of Knaus's workbook for overcoming depression. It contains a clear explanation of the complete range of cognitive behavior therapy techniques for managing depressive episodes and preventing relapse. It includes plans and worksheets one can readily use to keep you on track. I recommend it without reservation."

—Anthony Kidman, AM, PhD, clinical psychologist and director of the health psychology unit of the University of Technology, Sydney

"Knaus is one of the world's leading authorities on depression. The second edition of *The Cognitive Behavioral Workbook for Depression* will be an invaluable tool for the understanding, treatment, and elimination of this complex emotion. If you, a family member, or a friend suffers from depression, you need look no further. The knowledge contained in this workbook can guide you out of a debilitating haze that often leads to a chronic dissatisfaction in life. I cannot recommend it more highly."

—Vincent E. Parr, PhD, clinical psychologist at the Institute for Advanced Study MRL

"One of the best, most highly readable manuals on overcoming depression I've ever seen. It provides explicit methods for identifying and countering the negative thought patterns that underlie depression—but that is just a start. This workbook details a compendium of the best of the empirically proven techniques for mastering depression's major accompaniments, including self-blame, perfectionism, worthlessness, anxiety, and low frustration tolerance. Knaus then guides readers to set goals and strategies for achieving them in order to move from being enervated to being energized. Most strikingly, this book's self-help exercises don't pull the reader into further frustration; they are clear and doable."

—Janet L. Wolfe, PhD, former executive director of the Albert Ellis Institute and staff psychologist for over thirty-five years

# PRAISE FOR THE FIRST EDITION

# The Cognitive Behavioral Workbook *for* Depression

## SECOND EDITION

**A STEP-BY-STEP PROGRAM**

## WILLIAM J. KNAUS, EdD

New Harbinger Publications, Inc.

Distributed in Canada by Raincoast Books

Copyright © 2012 by William J. Knaus
New Harbinger Publications, Inc.
5674 Shattuck Avenue
Oakland, CA 94609
www.newharbinger.com

Acquired by Jess O'Brien; Cover design by Amy Shoup; Edited by Brady Kahn; Text design by Tracy Carlson

---

### Library of Congress Cataloging-in-Publication Data

Knaus, William J.
  The cognitive behavioral workbook for depression, second edition : a step-by-step program / Bill Knaus, foreword by Albert Ellis.
    p. cm.
  Summary: "This revised new edition of The Cognitive Behavioral Workbook for Depression draws on the most current evidence-based and empirically supported techniques from cognitive therapy and rational emotive behavior therapy for defeating the symptoms of depression"-- Provided by publisher.
  Includes bibliographical references.
  ISBN 978-1-60882-380-2 (pbk.) -- ISBN 978-1-60882-381-9 (pdf e-book) -- ISBN 978-1-60882-382-6 (epub)
  1. Depression, Mental. 2. Cognitive therapy. I. Title.
  RC537.K57 2012
  616.85'27--dc23

                    2012003622

Printed in the United States of America

17  16  15
15  14  13  12  11  10  9  8  7

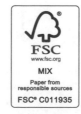
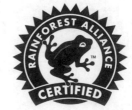

# Dedication

I dedicate this book to the memory of Albert Ellis, PhD, the founder of rational emotive behavioral therapy, who died in his ninety-third year. Throughout his career, he showed an amazing clarity of thought and continued to be productive and to contribute until the last month of his life. To the amazement of his physicians, he left this world with a rational acceptance of his mortality. He lived what he taught others to do. Al's thoughts live on and have great relevance today, as they will continue to have in the future.

Starting in the mid-1950s, Ellis pioneered a revolution in the field of psychotherapy when he boldly asserted that people feel the way that they think. By this he meant that evocative events, such as a job loss or a depressive change in biochemistry, are the tip of the iceberg. Because most of these events filter through our belief systems, the way we define, interpret, and judge activating situations stimulates what we feel and guides what we do.

Our beliefs, attitudes, and related cognitive processes are the deep base of an iceberg that is more massive than what is seen at its tip.

Some environmental, psychological, social, and biochemical events can activate self-harming thoughts and beliefs. Ellis saw that by recognizing, examining, and purging these harmful, irrational beliefs and other forms of unrealistic thinking, our surplus suffering and misery could go the way of the dinosaur. Over the past fifty years, a continuing line of research has demonstrated the validity of this position.

Albert Ellis brilliantly helped change the psychotherapeutic landscape by tirelessly working for over sixty years, often for over fifteen to eighteen hours a day, directly helping thousands through his counseling and millions more through his books and the network of counselors and psychotherapists that he helped train. The rational emotive behavior therapy (REBT) system he pioneered inspired the evolution of numerous complementary systems, such as psychiatrist Aaron Beck's evidence-based cognitive therapy and the generic and popular cognitive behavioral therapy approach. REBT is the bedrock system for this area.

In honor of his magnificent achievements and his enormous, tireless contributions to the emotional health and welfare of others, I dedicate this book to my longtime friend and colleague, Albert Ellis.

# Contents

## PART 1
## Basic Techniques to Defeat Depression

## PART 2
## Recognizing and Defeating Depressive Thinking

PART 3
Building Emotional Resilience

# PART 4
## Special Strategies to Anchor Positive Changes

# Foreword

Dr. Bill Knaus's *The Cognitive Behavioral Workbook for Depression* is not exactly a wonderful book, because, as Alfred Korzybski showed in *Science and Sanity*, to say it is wonderful is to overgeneralize and to imply that it is 100 percent filled with wonderful things. Inevitably, this book has omissions as do all books on depression, including outstanding ones like those of Aaron Beck, David Burns, and my own *Guide to Rational Living*. Be that as it may, *The Cognitive Behavioral Workbook for Depression* is wonderfully thorough and, if consistently followed, is exceptionally helpful.

Bill Knaus, whom I helped train in rational emotive behavior therapy (REBT) in the late 1960s, used REBT particularly well in dealing with human problems and then became an authority on overcoming procrastination. Our 1977 book by that title is still a best seller, as are other books of Bill's.

Not content with helping his readers with their fears of failure and low frustration tolerances, Bill decided to tackle the extremely prevalent and serious problem of depression. He has done so with a vengeance. He has thoroughly investigated and therapeutically dealt with its many related issues of hopelessness, blame, perfectionism, and emotional stresses. He shows readers how to deal with the most important aspects of depression, and he has covered it beautifully.

In his excellent chapters, Bill Knaus has researched and cited scores of studies on depression and shown how these findings can be used by readers who are in various depressed states. In many of his chapters, he emphasizes the use of the well-known ABCs of REBT. He shows how to look for and apply the ABCDE technique to depressive thoughts, feelings, and actions. *A* stands for the activating event, such as an imperfect performance. *B* stands for your rational beliefs ("I acted stupidly, and I'd prefer to do better next time") and your irrational beliefs ("I should have done better, and I am a stupid person"). *C* stands for your emotional and behavioral consequences. This includes healthy feelings, such as regret, and the emotional results of unhealthy thinking, such as self-downing. *D* stands for disputing your irrational beliefs by questioning them and taking problem-solving actions ("Where is it written that I absolutely must behave flawlessly?"). *E* stands for an effective new philosophy (you may be dissatisfied with certain performances and accept yourself despite them).

Bill Knaus also shows you how to change your basic self-defeating, depressive philosophies to help achieve the REBT choice of unconditional self-acceptance, unconditional acceptance of others, and unconditional life acceptance. Then you will rarely depress yourself about anything!

Simple, isn't it? Yes, but as Bill Knaus shows, it takes much work and practice: thinking, feeling, and behavioral homework. Apply his many methods and strategies to your depressiveness. Don't wait. Get going.

—Albert Ellis, 2006

# Acknowledgments

I'd like to acknowledge the following people who contributed tips and ideas for this book: Edward Garcia, MA, Atlanta; Dr. Nancy Knaus, Spofford, New Hampshire; Dr. Dom DiMattia, Goshen, Connecticut; Dr. Diana Richman, New York City; Dr. Robert Heller, Boca Raton, Florida; Dr. Robert Moore, Clearwater, Florida; Dr. Arnold Lazarus, Princeton, New Jersey; Dr. Russell Grieger, Charlottesville, Virginia; Dr. George Morelli, San Diego, California; Dr. James Byrne, Hebden Bridge and Halifax, England; Dr. Nando Pelusi, New York City; Dr. Clifford Lazarus, Skillman, New Jersey; Dr. Jack Shannon, Matawan, New Jersey; Dr. Judith Beck, Philadelphia; Dr. Barry Lubetkin, New York City; Dr. John Hudesman, New York City; Dr. Irwin Altrows, Kingston, Ontario; Dr. Robert Zettle, Wichita, Kansas; Dr. Bruce McEwen, New York City; Dr. Nosheen K. Rahman, Lahore, Pakistan; William J. Knaus II, MD, Dallas, Texas; Dr. Jeffrey Rudolph, New York City and Ridgewood, New Jersey; and Diana Cleary and Dale Jarvis, who worked with me to create original jointly written poetry for this book.

# Introduction

Depression is nothing to mess with. If serious enough, depression can have a devastating effect on your relationships, work, health, and the general quality of your life. The good news is that depression is not forever. You can act now to stop feeling depressed and to avert future episodes.

If you begin this book not knowing what to do to defeat your depression, you are like many others. Depression has baffled people for thousands of years. But there are many tried-and-true ways, as well as new innovations, for defeating this ancient nemesis.

Activity is a classic psychological remedy for depression. This workbook offers a crash course on depression with dozens of activities to do better, get better, and feel better, using a wide range of activity remedies, from changing depressive thinking habits to normalizing your daily routine. You'll discover how to manage relationships, get your biology into balance, take tested steps to changing, and avoid procrastinating. You'll learn many ways to address this psychosocial biological process we call depression.

Look through the table of contents. Flip the pages. I'm confident that you will find promising ideas that will work for you.

It's important to concentrate on exercises that are likely to do you the most good. In chapter 2, you'll find a depression test that can help you uncover depression hot spots that merit special attention.

This book maps key areas that apply to curbing depression. However, there is no one book, program, or system that perfectly fits everybody's situation. Your challenge is to master approaches that help you. As a bonus, you'll find many hot tips from top experts who donated some of their best ideas for this book to help free you from depression.

## COGNITIVE BEHAVIORAL THERAPY FOR DEPRESSION

This workbook delivers cognitive, emotive, and behavioral ways to overcome depression and many of the psychological conditions that commonly accompany this condition. Here is a preview of what I'll share that you can use to help yourself:

- *Understanding negative thinking and cognitive solutions.* You'll normally have depressive thinking when you feel depressed. Hopelessness, powerlessness, worthlessness, and blame can elevate your misery. Depressive thinking can be challenged and defeated. You can use cognitive approaches to change this thinking, gain relief, and prevent relapses. For example, if you believe that you are helpless to address depression, you are suffering from depressive thinking. How can you be helpless? If you were truly helpless, you wouldn't be reading this book.

■ *Understanding negative emotions and emotive solutions.* A melancholic mood weaves through all depression. When this gloom seems impenetrable, you are likely to draw into yourself and feel worse. To help yourself break this pattern, you can accept that a depressed mood is both painful and temporary. Acceptance can feel liberating. Anxiety, anger, and other negative affects commonly weave through depression. You can simultaneously address these coexisting conditions with the same methods you use for defusing depression.

■ *Understanding negative behavioral habits and behavioral solutions.* Behavioral methods, such as activity scheduling, have top change potential (see chapter 17). Procrastination technology is an activation approach that applies to depression. You'll learn how to use this technology to get right to the issue of curbing depression (see chapter 5).

## The Science Behind the System

Over four hundred clinical outcome studies confirm the effectiveness of cognitive behavioral therapy methods. A meta-analysis of sixteen rigorous meta-analyses of cognitive behavioral therapy shows that cognitive behavioral therapy is effective for correcting a wide range of disabling conditions (Butler et al. 2006). A meta-analysis is a statistical study of the results of related studies.

The Butler meta-analysis amply shows that the cognitive behavioral approach is a significantly more effective means of curbing depression than a medication approach. So, if medication has not worked for you, try this comprehensive approach.

## Changing through Reading

*Bibliotherapy*, or what is known as healing through reading, compares favorably to individual psychotherapy (Gregory et al. 2004). The books that have greater promise are theme-centered books on topics such as depression written by doctoral-level mental health specialists (Redding et al. 2008). This book meets that standard.

A self-help manual for depression is helpful for some but not for all. Some of my depressed and nondepressed clients have read and continue to use the ideas contained here. Some report going back over highlighted sections in order to keep perspective. Other clients have no interest in reading and will politely take resource materials that I offer and place them in a corner, where they lie fallow.

By working to defeat depression, you develop coping skills that you can use over a lifetime.

If you count yourself among those who believe that if they had the tools to defeat depression, they'd use them, you may put wind in the sails of your self-help efforts if you follow a written approach. An interactive reading approach is effective for defeating mild and moderate forms of depression (Wampold et al. 2002; Newman et al. 2011). A cognitive behavioral self-help approach can be used by some to overcome the more severe forms of depression (Cuijpers 1998). Here's why:

- A well-designed self-help book on depression can flesh out key issues within a shorter time span than the therapeutic setting can provide.

- Self-help books with evidence-based information on depression prescribe steps for addressing and overcoming depression.

- You don't have to rely on memory. You can return, as many times as you choose, to review a section of the book that you once found helpful.

- You can pace yourself, study an idea or exercise in greater depth, and test and modify what you are learning.

- Although self-help readings and individual counseling represent different ways to get to the same result, they can be used in combination with each other.

If you believe that you can gain from hands-on written prescriptions, you are likely to benefit from using a cognitive behavioral self-help manual (Mahalik and Kivlighan 1988). This approach can be especially useful for people who think that they can address their own depression if they have the tools (Burns and Nolen-Hoeksema 1991). However, in applying self-help methods, persistence is important to a successful outcome (Gould and Clum 1993).

## Building a Psychological Skill Set

This book addresses psychological and natural ways to alleviate depression and prevent it from coming back. Thus, the benefits and side effects of antidepressant medication and electric convulsive therapy are the subject of someone else's book.

The literature on depression is vast—and rapidly growing—such that no one book can cover all the bases. Nevertheless, I think you'll find this revised edition of *The Cognitive Behavioral Workbook for Depression* much more comprehensive than other psychology self-help books on overcoming depression.

You get a bonus. The psychological principles you learn here to address depression will also apply to other life challenges. You can reapply what you learned, again and again, to gain greater satisfaction in living.

Here is how to take advantage of the self-help methods described in this workbook:

- Emphasize and complete the exercises that you think are most relevant for overcoming your depression. If it is hopelessness thinking, concentrate on that first.

- Force yourself to follow through on meaningful exercises that you feel tempted to put off because you tell yourself that you are too depressed to try. These may be the exercises most worth pursuing.

- Refuse to listen to your own excuses. If you think something could be helpful to do, but you want to feel comfortable first, do it anyway. Take a moment to think about the many important things you've accomplished that included discomfort and frustration. I'll bet you'll see a link between allowing yourself to feel tension and your greatest accomplishments.

- Practice tested ways to question the validity of depressive thinking. Build upon this knowledge. This process can lead to defeating depression and preventing it from coming back.

- At the end of each chapter, you'll find a section called "End Depression Plan" where you can record key ideas and action steps you found most valuable. This gives you a record that you can draw from to overcome and prevent depression.

If you believe that you can take steps to defeat depression, read on. Even if you don't think you can help yourself, read on. If you are in this latter group, you'll discover ways to address depressive thinking and unrealistic pessimism. You may change your mind.

## A Toolbox for Change

The alphabet has twenty-six letters. You can use these letters to write millions of words and blend them into infinite phrases, sentences, and paragraphs. In a similar sense, you can take basic self-help strategies and find many ways to build these ideas into your life. You can start defeating depression at any time. It doesn't matter if you are nine or ninety.

Defeating depression is a trek. Your toolbox of coping methods can help speed your journey. You'll find the following tools in this book:

- Lists of ideas to curb depression.

- Practice exercises to counter and debunk depressive thinking and strengthen coping skills.

- Sidebars and text boxes that highlight key ideas.

- Reinforcement of key ideas. If you miss a point, you'll likely find a related one later.

- Optional ways to counteract depressive thinking.

- Guiding principles.

- Metaphors, similes, analogies, fables, and parables to make important ideas memorable.

- Stories of people who faced depression and prevailed, and how they did it.

- Encouragement.

- Standard and new technologies for defeating depression.

- Creative ways to view and address depression.

- Tips from top depression experts who submitted ideas specifically for this book.

You'll also find information about and techniques to respond to conditions that commonly accompany depression. We'll explore the many nooks and crannies of depression and methods you can use to stop feeling depressed. Perfectionism increases the risk for depression (Hewitt et al. 1998). People plagued by this form of stressful thinking can find help in chapter 19. When depressed, you may put off addressing depression until you feel better. Chapter 5 shows how to break a procrastination connection. When you are depressed, your relationships may suffer. You'll find help for managing your relationships in chapter 20.

There is no perfect solution for depression. Developing and following a highly structured routine can make a positive difference for some. Antidepressant medication works for others. Changing depressive thinking is helpful for most. Perhaps, as with a good spaghetti sauce, you must combine several quality ingredients to achieve results. But whatever approach you choose to take, give it a fair trial.

> The early twentieth century French educator and philosopher Jules Payot (1909) observed that once you establish a goal, information will flow in from many sources.

## BRIDGING THE GAP BETWEEN DEPRESSION AND FEELING GOOD

In the early phases of cognitive therapy, you may feel an uplifting sense of relief. Psychologist Albert Ellis (1971) was among the first to observe this rapid-change phenomenon. I've called this initial uplift a *preview experience* (Knaus 1982), but it seems as if this rapid shift can be more than a preview. It can have durability. Research has shown that for people who follow a cognitive approach to quell depression, rapid gains tend to stick (Tang et al. 2007).

In the early phases of this therapy, you do get insight into the positive effects of countering negative thinking and of having a new perspective on your depression. This shows you that your depression is not indelibly written into your future. That's a good start. But you will likely need to finish other steps in this process to feel better longer and to buffer yourself against lapsing into another depression.

Indeed, for most people, the gap between feeling depressed and sensing relief takes time to bridge. Although you can learn about how to defeat depressive thinking within hours or days, applying the principles can take weeks or months. That's because it is one thing to know what to do and another to put to use what you know. You can, for example, read about how to drive an automobile, but learning how to drive requires getting behind the wheel and practicing. In a similar sense, you can learn to become an expert in defeating depression only by working at defeating depression. As with developing any new skill, learning how to defeat depression will take time.

You may want this to happen quickly. The parts of your brain where depression lives will probably change at a slower pace than you'd prefer. However, as you work to defeat depressive thinking, your brain is creating structures that encode the counterdepression skills that you develop. Thus, the gap between knowing and doing closes with practice.

## READY YOURSELF FOR POSITIVE CHANGE

Ending depression is like building a wall. By putting the pieces together, step by step, you erect the structure.

This book describes not only what you can do to address depression but also how to go about this business in a step-by-step manner. This approach provides a way for you to organize your thinking, expand upon what you learn, and progressively master the methods that defeat depression.

If you find yourself having difficulty concentrating on an idea, this is normal when you feel depressed. You can mark the page and come back to the idea later. You'll naturally move at your own pace. But it is important to work at a pace that will eventually lead to a progressive mastery over methods for curbing depression.

# HOW FAR CAN YOU GO ON YOUR OWN?

This workbook is for those who feel mildly to moderately depressed, as well as for others with more severe depression who believe they can chip away at their depressive thoughts, mood, sensations, and behaviors. How do you know if you are in the subgroup of people who can potentially benefit from self-help measures? You can ask yourself this question: if you had the tools, do you think you could take steps to defeat depression? If your answer is yes, then cognitive, emotive, and behavioral approaches merit your consideration.

What is a reasonable amount of time to engage in self-help work to defeat depression? This question has no simple answer. How far to take self-help will depend on a variety of factors. Tolerances for depressive symptoms vary. A lot depends on how stoic you are about your depression. Depression comes in different forms. Causes differ. Depression follows different courses. Depression is often a blend of biological, psychological, and social factors that complicate any well-intended process of change. Biological factors that can trigger depression vary across depressive conditions. Still, it may be useful to establish time boundaries.

> It is not your fault if you got depressed any more than it's your fault if you get the common cold more often than your neighbor. But it is your responsibility to do better if you intend to take charge of yourself and of the controllable events that take place around you.

Past experiences with depression can be used to predict the probable course of your depression. If you are new to the challenge of defeating depression, applying tested techniques can tell you what you can do on your own. If you have severe depression, this book may augment your work with a cognitively oriented therapist. Cognitive approaches appear effective for people with severe depressions (Driessen et al. 2010).

The more you do on your own, the more credit you can give yourself for your progress. Still, you need not follow the trek of a lone traveler. You may profit from professional help, and you can use the information in this book to support your progress. Your friends, family members, or a support group can help you follow through on your antidepression program, as well as lend timely encouragement and calmly help you adjust your perspective if you exaggerate your plight.

Whenever possible, weigh the evidence to see what is right for you to do. Separate fictions from facts. For example, realistic optimism is a belief that you can find a way to self-improve. If someone tells you—or you tell yourself—that realistic optimism is impossible for people who are depressed, question that assumption. If the assumption was true, any action to overcome depression would be futile. As you will see, breaking free from depressive negativity is not only possible but likely. That's realistic optimism!

# WHEN TO SEEK PROFESSIONAL HELP

If, after a reasonable time of testing self-help methods, you find yourself treading water, you may want to consider working with a counselor. Depending on your situation, a reasonable time may be anywhere from a few days to three months. You should consider talking with a professional now if you are at risk of losing your job or a vital relationship, or are facing a significant crisis that relates to your depression.

When you're depressed, you might feel so bad at times that you want to die. If you are seriously contemplating suicide, you should immediately seek professional help. Suicide is preventable. This is not a time to procrastinate. Establish an alliance with a professional with a specialty in depression who can assess your situation, help you gain clarity on what is happening, and work with you as you recover from this potentially disabling but highly correctable condition.

## PART 1

# Basic Techniques to Defeat Depression

Learn how the ancients successfully fought depression.

Discover famous people with depression, just like you.

Recognize the different masks of depression.

See how to separate sadness from depression.

Take a test and discover your depression hot spots.

Use start-up techniques to get going with your antidepression program.

Learn twelve proven steps to end depression.

Develop self-observant skills to address your depression thinking, feelings, and habits.

Follow six self-guidance steps to address depression and to add quality to your life.

Use five phases of change to propel yourself forward.

Learn how to overcome a procrastination-depression connection with a three-step cycle of change process.

# CHAPTER 1

# Depression Is Not Your Life

What is behind depression? Here is depression's point of view: "I am depression. Cold like an arctic mist, I dampen your spirit and your soul. I fill your thoughts with gloom. When I am with you, you are but a withered leaf beneath wet snow with nowhere to go. Still, I can do much more. I can fill your mind with dismal thoughts. I can drive laughter into the shadows. I drain all pleasure from your life. I fatigue you as I rob you of your ambition. I can overwhelm you with thoughts of helplessness and hopelessness. For when you are in my web, I have the power to trap you with all my threads."

Depression is not in charge of your life. Throughout this book you will find many evidence-based and clinically tested approaches that you can apply. By design, you can use the coping skills you learn to defeat depression and become a more effective, resilient, nondepressed you.

## YOU ARE NOT ALONE

Depression can affect anyone. Abraham Lincoln suffered from depression. So did Winston Churchill. Other well-known people who suffered from depression include the founder of American psychology, William James; the poets Edgar Allan Poe, Walt Whitman, and Emily Dickinson; comedian Rodney Dangerfield; *60 Minutes* commentator Mike Wallace; television entrepreneur Ted Turner; talk show host Dick Cavett; and actress Catherine Zeta-Jones. Each found ways to continue contributing despite a depressed mood that was sometimes paralyzing.

Since the early 1900s, the prevalence of depression has steadily risen. It doubled in the United States between 1991 and 2002 (Compton et al. 2006). The rate of depression among British youth doubled between 1986 and 2006 (Collishaw et al. 2010). Whether or not this research correctly tracks the trend, most experts agree that the rate of depression is increasing.

The national comorbidity replication study projected that 20.8 percent of the US population will suffer from significant depression over the course of their lives (Kessler et al. 2005). A 2009 study estimated that about 19.7 percent of the US population suffered from a

Depression comes from the Latin *depressio*, to press down and make lower.

mild to severe depression over a seven-year period, and the lifetime prevalence is likely to go higher (Patten 2009).

Furthermore, compared to surveys in the 1980s and 1990s, we see an important shift taking place. The risk for depression has shifted from young adults to middle-aged adults (Hasin et al. 2005).

Even the so-called minor depressions often have a profoundly negative impact in multiple areas of life (Kessler et al. 1997). When you feel depressed, it may seem like no one cares or that nothing matters. But you are not alone. The World Health Organization (WHO) estimates that 340 million people currently suffer from depression. By the year 2020, WHO predicts depression will rank second among the most serious health conditions behind ischemic heart disease (Murray and Lopez 1996; World Health Organization 2001; Ustun et al. 2004; Prince et al. 2007). The mortality rate for untreated depression may exceed that of cigarette smoking (Mykletun et al. 2009). Depression is already the number one disability for women.

In your struggle to end depression, you join hands with hundreds of millions who face a similar challenge. However, dealing with depression comes down to an individual effort. No one can do this for you. Fortunately, there are many great ways to defeat depression and prevent recurrences.

# DEPRESSION THROUGH THE AGES

People have struggled with depression since ancient times, and we have much useful information about depression that has been passed on since the beginning of recorded history. By sifting through the history of depression, you can get a feel for how people in bygone times viewed this ancient affliction and learn about some nifty corrective actions that have stood the test of time. Here is a brief excursion into our past.

Depression is at least as old as civilization. Over five thousand years ago, depression appeared in the hieroglyphics, paintings, and statues of pharaonic Egypt (Okasha and Okasha 2000). At that time, people with depression were not stigmatized (Okasha 2001). That was a big plus. You are more likely to address depression if you view it as a natural but interruptive phase of living rather than as something shameful. The Egyptian remedies included sleep, journey, and dance.

In ancient Greece, Hippocrates—also known as the father of medicine—found that depression had many symptoms, such as nameless fears, irritability, loss of appetite, despondency, and sleeplessness (Radden 2000; Simon 1978). He thought that you're born with a vulnerability for depression and that stressful circumstances evoke it. Your biology can influence your thoughts and behavior, and your emotions affect the course of a disease. By modern standards, many of his observations seem on target. He prescribed diet and exercise as the first line of treatment against depression.

The eleventh century Arabian physician Avicenna connected depression to physical and psychological causes (Radden 2000). He was among the first to say that you can think your way into depression and think your way out.

California psychologist and archpriest George Morelli (pers. comm.) discovered that the Desert Fathers of the Eastern Orthodox Church saw depression as despondency. This state was triggered by inappropriate thoughts (*logismi*), which lead to missing the mark (*amartia*), which was corrected by right thinking (*diakresis*).

In the plays of Shakespeare, many well-known characters, such as Hamlet, Macbeth, and Henry VI, suffered from depression.

The seventeenth-century British scholar Robert Burton (2001) saw depression as either a disposition or a habit. As a disposition, depression arises with each mental discontent.

Burton saw depression as both a biological and psychological state that can exist without obvious cause or that can go beyond the reason of a cause. He theorized that depression can be ignited by an expansive imagination, such as making something heinous out of something that is not that way at all. Burton advocated easing depression through diet, exercise, and changes in thinking.

This scholar deserves special recognition in the history of depression. *The Anatomy of Depression* was a most comprehensive study on depression and the first legitimate self-help book on this topic in his day. The book contained important insights on the relationship between psychological, biological, and social processes and depression that remain relevant today.

# CAUSES OF DEPRESSION

The modern version of Hippocrates's theory is *diathesis-stress theory* (Sullivan, Nealee, and Kendler 2000). This is a core principle in Aaron Beck's theory of depression. You have to have both vulnerability for depression (diathesis) and a triggering situation (stress). The diathesis can be a neurochemical event, negative early experience, or something else. Stress can come from a job loss, divorce, the death of a mate, living for years in a moribund marriage, or an accumulation of hassles. Depression may be secondary to a specific medical condition, such as diabetes, coronary heart disease, pneumonia, irritable bowel syndrome, and anemia.

In most instances, there will be a triggering event or series of events that precedes depression, including insomnia. You may have a habit of thinking negatively and magnifying events. This can trigger depression. A generalized anxiety often comes before depression.

Depression may seem to come out of the blue, without any clearly identifiable stressful event. Sylvia Plath (1972), author of *The Bell Jar*, tells us she had it made. She had an adoring, handsome boyfriend and a career she loved. Then, as if a bell jar had descended over her head, she felt enclosed by depression. *The Bell Jar* describes Plath's feelings of hopelessness, suffering, and sense of worthlessness connected to a bipolar form of depression.

Depression has many causes. Early pubescence is linked with depression. Sedentary lifestyles, being out of work for sustained periods, rapid social changes, and a host of other psychological, social, and biological factors can presage depression. Although it is useful to understand why depression is increasing, it is crucial to take corrective actions to overcome your own depression and to learn to buffer yourself against social adversities.

# WHEN DEPRESSION IS SERIOUS

Most people label moods rather loosely as "depression." At the least, depression reflects a dark and unrelenting mood, but with some periodic reprieves.

A melancholic mood that lasts for several days or weeks is not necessarily a cause for alarm. This can be part of the normal ups and downs of life. You may pin a false label of depression on yourself, believing that you are depressed when you get bummed out, feel sad, have a bad day, or feel moody. You fight with your mate and you say you feel depressed, but how does this differ from hurt or anger? You get a flat tire on the highway, and your jack is missing. You say you feel depressed. But how does this differ from frustration? You don't get selected for a promotion. You say you feel depressed. But how does this differ from disappointment? Your best

## Factors That Correlate with Depression

- Depression tends to run in families.

- Alcohol and drug abuse are associated with depression.

- Preoccupations with unrealistic expectations, worry, anxiety, feelings of failure, and anger increase the risk for depression.

- Dispositions toward perfectionism, lack of assertiveness, and withdrawal are associated with depression.

- Major life changes connect with depression, whether they are the death of a mate or multiple life-changing events, such as marriage, the birth of a child, or moving into a new home. Such events can be stressful and connect with depression.

- For women, chemical or hormonal imbalance following childbirth or during menopause is associated with elevated risks for depression.

- For both sexes, chemical imbalances, such as a decreased efficiency in the neurochemical serotonin, are associated with depression.

- Traumatic experiences associated with an elevated risk for depression include a near-death experience and physical, sexual, or psychological abuse.

- Life circumstances that correlate with an elevated risk for depression include poverty, dangerous environments, and chronic illness.

friend moves out of the country. You say you feel depressed. But how is this different from feeling sad? These ups and downs of life can get confused with depression.

Depression is beyond the limits of the normal sense of disappointment, loss, bereavement, sadness, bad days, holiday blues, or even down moods. Disappointment can pass within hours. Bereavement diminishes over time. Depression grinds on from day to day and is difficult to bear. It can feel like the life is sucked out of you. It can linger on for weeks, months, and sometimes years. This is not the kind of situation where you just pull yourself up by your bootstraps and get on with your life. Like a broken leg that takes time to heal, depression ordinarily takes time to defeat.

The cognitive and behavioral skills you develop through applying what you read in this book will open opportunities for you to gain control over the manageable parts of depression, such as depression thinking. These methods are corrective. Use them to build resilience by taking on meaningful challenges that can benefit you and others. Use them to prevent depression in the future by applying them when you feel like you are sliding into a downward spiral.

# THE MANY FACES OF DEPRESSION

Depression is not a simple, uniform condition with the same causes and symptoms for everyone. Beyond a depressed mood, most people have special features in their depression that include some that are atypical. This complex condition has different causes and comes in different forms. Depression exists on a continuum from mild to very severe. Even when depression falls below the diagnostic standards, this condition is highly disruptive and burdensome.

You may have some or many of the experiences classified under depression. However, you are more than the label "depression." You are a complex thinking, feeling, doing, pluralistic person with countless attributes who happens to feel depressed now. That means that depression is not you.

Knowing the type of depression you face does make a difference. Structuring your daily activities can make a difference, especially if you suffer from bipolar depression. Exercise seems effective for people with major depression. However, regardless of the type of depression you experience, depressive thinking, your emotional reaction to depression, and depressive behavior habits cut across categories, and you can beneficially address these three major dimensions of depression.

Once a problem is known, it is no longer mysterious. There are solutions. However, as practically everyone who has experienced depression can testify, knowing about depression, while helpful, doesn't substitute for taking corrective actions.

## Major Depression

Everyone periodically feels down in the dumps. This is not true depression. Major depression is different. A depressed mood and loss of interest or pleasure in nearly all activities are core features of major depression (Kennedy 2008). Major (unipolar or clinical) depression has a variety of unpleasant symptoms, such as several or more of the following:

- depressive thinking

- reductions in frustration tolerance

- sleep disturbances

- appetite disturbances

- difficulties paying attention and concentrating

- diminished sense of personal worth, self-doubts, and indecisiveness

- loss of ambition and enthusiasm

- loss of sexual desire

- sluggish movements

- fatigue

- suicidal thoughts

Experiencing these symptoms for two or more weeks is the current professional standard for you to qualify for a major depression (American Psychiatric Association 2000). However, this time line is arbitrary, and adjustments are currently underway to refine the definitions of the various forms of depression and to add and delete some categories. If you've been through depression before, you may want to start to address a recurrence of depression before two weeks have passed.

Major depressions can follow a normal bereavement, a catastrophic loss, or any condition you perceive as traumatic. Depression can start after a pattern of worry leading to general anxiety. Recurring patterns of negative self-talk that evoke negative emotions can set the stage for depression and aggravate an already depressed mood. It may just seem to come out of the blue.

> When you need a diagnosis for depression, consult a professional.

## *Dysthymic Depression/Chronic Depressive Disorder*

A dysthymic depression is a persistent, mild depression that lingers, or goes on for two years or more (American Psychiatric Association 2000). Dysthymic depression is viewed as mild depression. Try telling people who are suffering from this condition that it's mild.

Before I get into a more optimistic perspective on dysthymic depression, here are some prevailing views on this form of depression. You can spend 70 percent of your life feeling down (Klein et al. 2000). People with dysthymic conditions tend to have low productivity and a lower quality of life (Hellerstein et al. 2010). When you are in this correctable state, you find little pleasure in life. You may feel cranky, irritable, and testy. You may take for granted that life will continue this way. Dousing your troubles with alcohol can seem like an appealing solution, but alcohol or drug abuse only aggravates an already festering condition.

Along with a down mood, restlessness, and a sense of going through the motions of living, anxiety often accompanies this depressed state. Procrastination is common and, from the looks of things, rarely noted in the research. However, here is an interesting opportunity. You can effectively address both dysthymic depression and procrastination (see chapter 5).

Dysthymic depression often precedes major depression. Dysthymia can also follow major depression. This combination is called double depression. By recognizing and addressing dysthymic depression early, you can reduce the risk of double depression.

### IS CHRONIC A MISNOMER?

Dysthymic depression may undergo a name change to "chronic depressive disorder" in the next version of the American Psychiatric Association's diagnostic manual. The word "chronic" may be misleading, however. Over the past forty-five years that I've worked with people with depression, a significant number have had ongoing dysthymic depression, which in some cases extended over decades. Most of these people made positive changes in the form of an improved mood that appears to have stuck.

Calling this depressive state "chronic" could be harmful in two ways:

- Professionals who help people with so-called chronic depression are at risk of showing complacency with their clients, for there is no reason to expect much in the way of change.

- If you are a person with ongoing depression, you have enough of a challenge without additionally labeling your condition as chronic. If you already think that you are helpless to change, then this label can add a layer of discouragement and pessimism to an already negative situation.

Instead of putting yourself into a chronic category, it may be wiser to look at the correctable aspects of this and other forms of depression and see how far you can go.

- You can change negative thinking and lighten your psychological load.

- You can increase emotional resilience, avoid feeling whipsawed by down moods, and feel better more often.

- You can engage in and reinforce behaviors that lead to better results than you are used to experiencing. This change can be a confidence builder for doing more of what works to lift your mood and produce positive results.

You also have to be realistic. Some forms of depression are more tenacious than others. So you may have to consider lifestyle changes and specific activities to ameliorate physical symptoms of depression; you can regularize your daily routine, get more physical exercise, and identify and disqualify negative thinking before it cascades out of control.

Rather than seeing your situation as chronic, why not see yourself as chronically coping? In that sense, you commit to a lifetime of development and growth through applying a growing body of psychological knowledge to meet the challenges you meet along the path of life.

> Depression has different causes, occurs in different forms, varies in degree, and how long it lasts will depend on the person and situation. As a knowledgeable person on depression, you can choose what to do that best fits your abilities and circumstances, and know when professional advice is warranted.

## Adjustment Disorder with Depression

A significant and unwanted change, such as divorce, job loss, property loss (theft, hurricane, flood, tornado, and fire), coronary bypass surgery, stock market loss, or betrayal can precipitate an adjustment disorder with depression.

Your mood is down. You feel preoccupied with and strained by negative thoughts about the troubling situation. This lingering mood is deepened by depressive thinking and by mentally magnifying stressful sensations and emotions. Nevertheless, you continue to have ample resources available that you can use in making an adjustment to the situation. There are periods when you feel fine.

What makes adjustment disorder different from major depression? It has a lesser intensity and a shorter duration. There are greater mood fluctuations during the course of a day. But this presumed minor form of depression also is not minor! It may extend into major depression.

## Postpartum Depression

About 13 percent of women are at increased risk of depression following childbirth (O'Hara and Swain 1996). Sometimes called "baby blues," this euphemism can detract from the significant importance of a condition that affects both mother and child.

Postpartum depression shares features with other forms of depression:

- depressed mood
- dating difficulties (being overweight or experiencing excessive loss of weight)
- difficulties sleeping
- loss of interest, including sexual interest
- headaches, backaches, and other unpleasant aches and pains
- difficulties paying attention, focusing, and remembering things to do
- overanxiety about the baby or fear of hurting the baby or yourself

- depressive thoughts, such as helplessness, hopelessness, worthlessness, shame, or guilt

- anger

- blame

Postpartum depression can be prevented through education and brief psychotherapy. If you suffer from postpartum depression, you can take corrective actions using methods you find in this book.

## Seasonal Affective Disorder

When winter looms in northern climates, we experience shorter days, cold, snow, slush, and cloudiness. For many, this is a dreary time of the year. Life can seem oppressive compared with the balmy days of summer.

With the changes in temperature, a shorter day, and a sense of being cooped up, some feel a negative mood change. The technical term for this form of depression is *seasonal affective disorder* (SAD). This malaise starts around late fall in areas with distinct seasons, and lingers until spring.

SAD seems regional. You rarely hear of SAD cases in Southern California and Florida. SAD is primarily concentrated in northern latitudes. This winter doldrums syndrome is serious for about 10 percent of people living in northern winter climates and affects many more in lesser ways (Westrin and Lam 2007).

In a SAD state of mind and body, you might plant yourself with glazed eyes fixed on the TV. You might get testy with mates and friends. You might worry excessively about the future.

With longer days and exposure to light, SAD wanes. If you suffer from SAD, chapter 18 describes how to get a lift during the winter months.

## Atypical Depression

*Atypical depression* is actually one of the more typical forms of depression. Depression is labeled "atypical" when its symptoms vary from those typically associated with major depression. Whereas with major depression, you probably will have insomnia, with atypical depression you are likely to sleep excessively. You are likely to lose weight with major depression and gain weight with atypical depression. While in both major and atypical depression, you may be sensitive to rejection, with atypical depression you are more likely to be oversensitive to real or imagined rejection.

Where even a surprise visit from a good friend has no mood-changing effect for someone suffering from major depression, any positive change can temporarily lift the mood of someone who is atypically depressed.

Some forms of depression are misdiagnosed, and those afflicted get the wrong medications from their primary care physicians (Kessler et al. 2006).

The founder of American psychology, William James, may have suffered from atypical depression. He described instances when he was unable to move because of the heaviness of his depression. Then a bird might fly by his window and his mood would lift.

As with other forms of depression, you can effectively address atypical depression with cognitive and behavioral forms of intervention.

## Bipolar Depression

The second-century Greek physician Aretaeus was the first to see that the radical mood swings between depression and elation were part of the same condition, which is now called *bipolar disorder*. He also saw this condition as existing on a continuum.

Bipolar disorders fall into two general groupings. Bipolar I is characterized by major mood swings between high levels of elation, or mania, and depression. It's critical to control the manic phase, and drugs, such as lithium carbonate, are effective for this purpose.

Bipolar II is similar to bipolar I except that the highs don't reach a manic level. These less intense "ups" are called *hypomanic* episodes.

In milder forms of manic euphoria, you may have thoughts racing through your head, talk faster than usual, have a greater interest in sex than usual, and spend much more money than usual. These elevated times are relatively brief compared to depressive cycles that tend to include lingering melancholic feelings, anxiety, guilt, anger, and hopelessness.

People with bipolar depression often spend up to 33 percent of their adult lives in depression. They may languish in depression for months or even years without seeking help (Kupfer et al. 2002). Antidepressants, such as the SSRIs, can worsen bipolar depression. A cognitive-behavioral bibliotherapy program, such as the one in this book, promotes improved functioning (Veltro et al. 2008).

Bipolar disorder is often associated with noteworthy accomplishments. Composer Ludwig van Beethoven, the humorist Mark Twain, and Clifford Beers, the founder of the mental health movement in the United States, all suffered from bipolar disorder. So does the actor Catherine Zeta-Jones.

If you've been diagnosed with bipolar disorder, you'll want to start by educating yourself about it and accepting that bipolar disorder is a lifetime condition that needs to be managed. There are many positive stories of people who've accepted that they had bipolar depression. They accept it as they would accept a diabetic condition. They do what is necessary to contain and rise above it.

Managing a bipolar condition takes a special effort—much like sustaining a desired weight loss takes effort. Defusing depressive thinking and following a predictable schedule helps you lead a more normal life.

---

Your depression merits attention if you've had a depressed mood and any two or more of these conditions that linger:

- You've lost interest and pleasure in life.

- You have no desire for sex when you previously had desire.

- Your depressed mood seems out of proportion with your life situation.

- Depression significantly interferes with your day-to-day functioning.

- You have persistent sleep and appetite problems.

- You feel apathetic, lethargic, and dull.

- You have thoughts of hopelessness, helplessness, and worthlessness.

- You have trouble paying attention and concentrating.

- You have a low tolerance for discomfort.

- You've thought about suicide.

> When depression clouds you in darkness, it's time to look for a flashlight.

## Masked Depression

Although this is not a conventional diagnostic category, masked depression is worth noting. Some depressions may be masked by anger, alcohol, or drugs, or by putting on a happy face. In Ruggero Leoncavallo's opera *Pagliacci*, we are introduced to a smiling face of sadness. The smiling Pagliacci clown hid his tears. In "The Tears of a Clown," Smokey Robinson sang of crying when no one was around to hear. Putting on a happy face to disguise a sense of being alone in your sorrow applies to other forms of depression as well.

# DEPRESSION AND BUM DECISIONS

### Remembrances from a Gravestone in Hinsdale, New Hampshire

*Miss Meranda Stebbins, daughter of Lieutenant Elihu and Mrs. Leucretia Stebbins*

*Died Feb the 3rd 1803 in the 16th year of her age*

*What tho her days on earth were few*

*Sharp pangs of guilt she never knew and never would*

*For here in this deep Grave her mortal parts,*

*Secure from Guilt and Grief and Smart*

*Will reft from year to year*

*Until that all important Day when death yields up all his Prey*

*And from this putrid tomb*

*Meranda all refined Shall rise*

*A spotless Maid adorn the Skies*

*Clothed in immortal bloom.*

To break free from depression, some people impulsively make changes to escape the mood: they quit their jobs, move to a new location, or go on a spending spree and buy items they don't need or won't use. Some impulsively file for divorce. These impulse-driven changes can have highly negative consequences, and moving from a coastal city to a Southwest farmhouse brings no guarantee that you'll escape depression.

When you are depressed is normally not the time to change mates, quit your job, or sell your house. This is not the time to seek refuge in a cabin deep in the woods. It also is not the time to give up on yourself.

Most depression authorities suggest postponing major life changes during periods when you feel significantly depressed. Your judgment is likely to be fogged. However, there are practically always exceptions to this guideline. For example, if you live in a high-crime area and you were recently assaulted, moving to a safer area (if possible) can help eliminate a prime cause for depression that is linked to a stressful environment.

# SEPARATING DEPRESSION FROM SADNESS

If you could experience sadness safely, you might seek it. Sad movies are popular. People read sad novels to get in touch with the feeling of sadness. It isn't the feeling of sadness that people dread. What people dread is the personal significance of a loss that leads to sadness.

Sadness is a bittersweet memory. An uncontrollable feeling of loss, a welling of tears, a memory of what once was and that will never again be—this is sadness or a natural response to a loss of something or someone you value. Sadness is more than a thought. It is a profound awareness that comes deeply from within. It is a solemn emotion. It can be brief. It can linger.

Loss is inevitable. Sadness is inevitable. It is because we form attachments with people, with animals, and with ideals and places that sadness becomes part of our lives. The size of the loss doesn't matter. A child who experiences the death of a cherished pet hamster weeps at a loss that others might find trivial. But it's not trivial. This loss is as real as any other.

Losses come in different ways at different times. The loss of a tradition can be a shock to your psychological system. Children leaving home to live on their own are missed. The death of a friend leaves a feeling of emptiness, perhaps for years thereafter. All sad. All inevitable.

When my childhood friend Al's daughter Erin died, I saw my six-foot-five, 350-pound friend collapse in despair. He asked, "How will I ever get through this?" There was no answer. There was only time. All I could do was to be there. I wrote a poem in her memory. At that moment, I wished I could have done more.

Within the year of his daughter's death, Al died from cancer. I felt a great loss. Sadness still awakens within me when I think of memorable times from our boyhood until his death. When I visit his grave, I bury an old coin in the ground. Silly? Perhaps. Al loved to collect old coins.

When my dog Apollo died, I wept uncontrollably. I felt his absence and a profound sense of loneliness. For fifteen years, Apollo was my companion, as I was his. Now, when I look around to see him, he is no longer there. I hear a noise. I look up, expecting to see him. I see movement in a bush outside, but he is not there. Loss and loneliness are part of sadness.

Still, the feeling of loss brings to me a sense of meaning. My new dog, Cider, helped mute the loss. Life goes on. Walking along a country road one day, my wife and I spotted a graveyard from the US Revolutionary War era. A tombstone inscription grabbed our attention. It reminded us that across time and space, people have expressed sadness over loss. The sidebar on the facing page is the inscription from the tombstone.

If there were no meaning to our relationships, there would be no sad feelings. There are sad times because there were once happy times, cherished times, and valued attachments. Sadness reminds us that we are human. It is part of our biology and our heritage. If you accept that reality, you may find that you don't go through phases of denial, anger, and resignation following a major loss. Acceptance of sadness is enough. Meanwhile, write poetry. Organize a march to raise money for a cause. Paint. Walk. Solve a problem. As sadness ebbs, life continues.

Loss. Sadness. Time to grieve. Time to heal. Time. Time. Time. It can go so slowly. There is acceptance. There is allowance. There is working through the process of loss. But in situations where the loss came from a tragedy that is followed by depression, it can take considerable time and work to come to grips with the experience.

Bob's fiancée, Jane, died hours before their wedding. It was a tragic automobile accident. Bob was shocked, numbed, and grief stricken. Three years after this tragic event, Bob continued to feel great guilt. He told himself, "If only I had phoned Jane before she left, she would have gone through the intersection at another time." He told himself, "I can't live without her." He believed, "I will never find anyone like Jane." As long as depression cloaked Bob's

People with depression universally experience a down mood, but depression is typically more complex than that. Ninety percent of those with major depression have sleep problems. Sixty percent of the time, people with depression have a history of anxiety. Fifty percent of people experience coexisting anger. Some experience practically all the common conditions associated with depression but in different degrees.

reality, he no longer did what he enjoyed. Once an avid tennis player, Bob let his racquet gather dust. There were no more dinners with his friends. He withdrew from his family. Previously a successful accountant, Bob quit his job. Thereafter, he mostly did odd jobs, such as buffing automobiles at an auto-detailing shop.

Bob felt overwhelmed by the details of daily living. His mood was despondent. He awakened in the middle of the night with a frightening image of the accident that took Jane's life. But the tragedy of this loss was compounded by his sense of defeatism, pessimism, and self-loathing. As he learned to defuse the negativity in his thoughts and accept his lack of control over Jane's tragic death, Bob's inner turmoil softened to sadness. Months later he resumed his accounting career. At the time of this writing, he is happily married with three children. His family is a source of great joy. Jane lives on as a cherished memory.

> You can be free of depression and still feel sad.

Sadness is very different from depression. Sadness has meaning. Significant depressions are disabilities. Sadness is a reflection of what once was. Depression haunts the mind with negative thoughts, such as helplessness and hopelessness. Sadness is a feeling reflected in the meaning of the loss. Depression is a drawing inward that can erupt in uncontrollable anger. In sadness, there is depth in experience.

But depression and sadness can coexist. Sadness, you accept. You deal with depression.

# HOW WILL YOU CARRY YOUR SORROW?

Robert Zettle, Wichita State University professor of psychology and author of *ACT for Depression* (2007), contributed a tip on sorrow (pers. comm.):

> Sorrow is a natural and healthy emotional reaction to personal loss and life's disappointments. There is as much value in tears of sorrow as in tears of joy. Check and see if it isn't the case that the very same things in life that have given it so much meaning and pleasure—such as your relationships with friends and loved ones—have also been the source of your deepest suffering. However, this is no reason to become a hermit; rather it is a reason to value those who are closest to you who also value you.
>
> Consider the possibility that what is problematic about sadness is not the feeling itself. The problem is that of becoming disconnected from life when trying to squelch this natural emotion. You may attempt to minimize existing suffering by trying to convince yourself that you no longer care about what was once so important to you. Or you may seek to prevent any additional sorrow by leading your life in a confining way that avoids any further disappointments. Even if these efforts have kept a lid on sorrow, haven't they also precluded joy?
>
> What if the power you have in your relationship with suffering is not to be found in minimizing or preventing sorrow, but in choosing how to carry it through life? Imagine that the sorrow you've been struggling with could be placed in a trash can. As much as you would like to leave it behind, doesn't your experience tell you that this is not possible? If you move, it goes with you. One way of carrying your sorrow is to hold it as far away from you as possible and perhaps even out of your eyesight. Try carrying a five-to-ten-pound object like a metal trash can or sack of potatoes around like that. Compare that to carrying the same object cuddled up to your chest as you might a baby. Which do you choose?

# TWELVE STEPS TO POSITIVE CHANGE

When you are depressed, it can be hard to think of positive steps to take. You may feel that you lack energy. Pessimism may cloud your judgment. This section discusses the best natural and psychological steps that I know of to use. I developed them for myself when I was once depressed. Even psychologists are not exempt from depression.

Thirty-five years ago, I went through a moderately severe major depression. I definitely experienced a seriously depressed mood. My physical symptoms included early morning awakening (arising early and not being able to fall back asleep), irritability, appetite problems, fatigue, and difficulties concentrating. I often felt like I was wading through a knee-deep tar pit with a lodestone on my back.

My depression evolved slowly. It was connected to major life changes and long workdays. This depression crept up on me. First, there were signs of an approaching storm. Then I felt swamped. If I'd known what was happening, I'd have taken corrective steps at the early phases. But I didn't expect to get depressed.

I knew that it was important to deal with depression and that it was important to take steps—even small steps—to counteract this process. Three thoughts helped:

- Depression is time limited.

- Activity is a remedy for depression.

- Depressive thinking is a state of mind, not a concrete reality.

I was not under any illusion that I could quickly fix myself. I also knew that this was a condition that I could not afford to let fester.

I recognized the signs of depression, so I knew what I was up against. I'd also had success helping others deal with their depression. That knowledge and experience gave me a unique advantage. If the techniques I'd used were helpful with my clients, they were good enough to use on myself.

Fortunately, I knew the *cognitive signatures* of depression. These are distinctive thought patterns that commonly coexist with depression. They include helplessness and hopelessness thinking. Knowing that certain thoughts are normally present with depression made it simpler to accept their existence. I took them as a symptom of a depressed mood. In my case, they were not a cause but a reflection of the mood. When I caught the ideas weaving through my mind, I acted quickly to adjust my thinking to regain a realistic perspective.

I admit that I was not always on top of this process. Nevertheless, by making a special effort to overcome depressive thoughts, I did myself considerable good. I'm convinced that this shortened the duration of my depression. Throughout this workbook, I'll share how to meet the challenge of defeating depressive thinking.

The following are the twelve steps I used for alleviating depression. I would recommend them to my family and friends. They can help you.

1. Avoid depressive-thinking traps.

2. Exercise.

3. Eat healthily.

4. Get adequate rest and sleep.

5. Use downtime constructively.

6. Maintain positive relations.

7. Resolve conflicts quickly.

8. Get fresh air and sunshine.

9. Stick to priorities.

10. Each day, do something novel.

11. Make a daily change in routine.

12. Persist.

These twelve steps normally apply, in one degree or other, to all forms of depression. Today I'd add an activity-scheduling step. You'll find this method in chapter 17.

Here's how I followed the twelve steps:

**Avoid depressive-thinking traps.** I made sure that I immediately avoided mental traps associated with depressive thinking. I monitored my self-talk and identified and contested depressive thinking.

**Exercise.** I joined a health club and set aside time to exercise. I worked out five times a week. I often had to force myself to go to the gym. This helped me overcome fatigue, improve my concentration, and break the depressive cycle I was in at that time.

**Eat healthily.** Despite a poor appetite, I ate regular meals.

**Get adequate rest and sleep.** I did not concern myself over interrupted sleep. Rather, I used a relaxation technique when I couldn't fall back to sleep. I found that this had restorative value.

**Use downtime constructively.** I turned my early morning awakening to good advantage. Between 4:00 and 9:00 a.m., I wrote a book titled *Do It Now*. I found this writing tedious. I persisted. The book was published. After 9:00 a.m. I started seeing clients. I had no other reasonable choice. A lot of people depended on me.

**Maintain positive relations.** I acted to maintain good relationships with people and to seek opportunities to be with people. During those times, I refused to complain about how I felt. Instead, I encouraged people to speak more about themselves. Since most people like to hear themselves talk, this worked well.

**Resolve conflicts quickly.** I pushed myself to resolve conflicts and to overcome difficulties as they arose. That eliminated festering issues.

**Get fresh air and sunshine.** I made sure I got out in the sun and walked for about a half hour a day. I did this around noon.

**Stick to priorities.** I tried not to overtax myself at low-energy periods. I drastically cut back on low priorities and stuck to my main priorities.

**Each day, do something novel.** Each day, I tried to find something I hadn't seen before. During my walk, I'd look for things to discover, such as a gargoyle below the roofline of a building, a bird's nest in a tree, or an interesting-looking person. This helped shift my focus from my depressed mood onto events that were novel. Seeking novelty served as a productive distraction from depression.

**Make a daily change in routine.** Every day I planned one change in my routine. The change required an action initiative. I thought about this initiative the day before I executed it. I walked myself through the mental paces. Then, when the anointed hour arrived, I walked myself through the actual paces. These new activities were normally of low impact, such as eating breakfast at a new restaurant or walking around a block the opposite way. However, I'd sometimes act like an extrovert, and found that doing so created feelings that fit that form of expression.

**Persist.** I maintained a high level of trust and confidence in my plan, and I persisted with it. This is easier said than done. I practically always had to push myself to start and keep going. This became easier as I got into the habit of taking positive steps even when I didn't feel like it, and indeed, I felt a strong resistance to taking corrective steps.

Although I did not follow the twelve steps like clockwork, I managed to follow through in a pretty reasonable way. My depression lasted about four months, but I had pretty much waded out of the worst part of the muck within two months. Since that time, I've been fairly consistent in maintaining the twelve-point routine. I've rarely felt depressed since. Those times did not last more than a day or two.

# END DEPRESSION PLAN

If you had a photographic memory, you could remember this entire book and immediately go to the sections that apply to you. Few have perfect memories. You don't have to know and use everything known about depression to start doing something about it and get better. Selectivity is often the better answer.

A *depression log* is a classic way to keep track of important ideas and to gain traction in your campaign to overcome depression. At the end of each chapter, you'll find space to log notes about the key ideas and exercises that you found most useful, what you did to test them, and what resulted. By actively using what you find helpful, you can promote positive change sooner than later. Try it and see!

**Key ideas** (What three ideas did you find most helpful in this chapter? Write them down.):

1.

2.

3.

**Action steps** (What three steps can you take to move closer to your goal of overcoming depression?):

1.

2.

3.

**Execution** (How did you execute the steps?):

1.

2.

3.

**Results** (What did you learn that you can use?):

1.

2.

3.

# CHAPTER 2

# Your Depression Test and Action Guide

From time to time, people will take inventory of their lives to see what is going well, what is not, what to drop, what to continue doing, and what to do next.

To help you fill in the blanks, this chapter provides a depression test. Taking the test will help you target key areas to work on and change. After the test, I'll describe some creative techniques for moving forward against your depression.

> "The unexamined life is not worth living."
>
> —Socrates

## HOW TO TAKE A DEPRESSION TEST

Depression can range from a major inconvenience to a hindrance to a disabling condition. The following depression test won't tell you where you stand in this range. It's not attempting to diagnose your depression. That's not the goal. Instead, this test will help you examine your changeable depression thinking, emotions, behaviors, and related conditions. The test identifies common problem areas and the chapters in this book where you can address your particular issues.

## YOUR DEPRESSION TEST

Read each statement that follows and decide whether it is "not you," "somewhat like you" or "like you." Place a check mark in the column that best describes how you feel, using the past two weeks as your reference point. Use the last column to refer to the chapters in this book that address these subjects.

| Depressed Statements | Not you 0 | Somewhat like you 1 | Like you 2 | Chapters where this book addresses these subjects |
|---|---|---|---|---|
| 1. "My mood is depressed." | | | | 1, 3, 13, 17–19, 21 |
| 2. "I can't set priorities." | | | | 3, 5, 16–17 |
| 3. "I can't change." | | | | 4, 6, 7, 14, 18, 22 |
| 4. "I have trouble following through." | | | | 5, 7, 17–19, 21, 22 |
| 5. "I have reasons why I can't do better." | | | | 5, 12, 16, 18 |
| 6. "I will never recover." | | | | 6, 8, 17–18 |
| 7. "My thinking is negative." | | | | 6, 13–14, 21 |
| 8. "My life is going from bad to worse." | | | | 5–6, 14 |
| 9. "I'm stuck in negative thoughts." | | | | 7–8, 22 |
| 10. "I keep blaming myself." | | | | 8, 12, 15, 19–20 |
| 11. "I feel helpless." | | | | 1–22 |
| 12. "I feel worthless." | | | | 6, 9, 19 |
| 13. "My future looks dismal." | | | | 11, 17 |
| 14. "I feel awful." | | | | 13, 21 |
| 15. "I don't want to live." | | | | 1–22 |
| 16. "I have many unexplained illnesses, aches, and pains." | | | | 13 |
| 17. "I feel fatigued." | | | | 13, 21 |
| 18. "I feel nervous and tense." | | | | 14, 21–22 |
| 19. "I have sudden intense fears." | | | | 14 |
| 20. "I can't escape past traumas." | | | | 14 |
| 21. "I feel irritable and angry." | | | | 15, 20 |
| 22. "I can't stop feeling guilty." | | | | 15 |
| 23. "I feel ashamed of myself." | | | | 15, 21 |
| 24. "I become easily frustrated." | | | | 16, 21 |
| 25. "I'm easily distracted." | | | | 16 |

| | | | | |
|---|---|---|---|---|
| 26. "I smoke or use drugs to calm down." | · | | | 16, 21 |
| 27. "I don't get enough exercise." | | | | 18 |
| 28. "I have appetite problems." | | | | 18 |
| 29. "I have trouble sleeping." | | | | 18 |
| 30. "I don't do what I should do." | | | | 5, 19 |
| 31. "I have troubled relationships." | | | | 20 |
| 32. "I have a poor sex life." | | | | 20 |
| 33. "I feel lonely." | | | | 20 |
| 34. "I'm afraid of getting depressed again." | | | | 21 |
| 35. "I'm depressed about feeling depressed." | | | | 22 |

Give yourself one point for each "somewhat like you" answer and two points for each "like you" answer. Then total your points.

## How to Interpret Your Depression Test

When you feel depressed, your total score is likely to be high; if your score is 70, the maximum number of points, this means that you can use most of the action strategies presented in this book. If your score is 30 or higher, you are certainly reading the right book. But below that doesn't mean you are home free. If you have only one "like you" (2) score, that area can be a bane of life worthy of addressing. Furthermore, lots of 1 scores suggest that you may be depressed even if you don't have any 2 scores.

Regardless of your actual score, you now have a lot of useful information about yourself and what to target. First, you will want to home in on the statements that you believe warrant the most attention, or statements that you gave a "like you" (2) score. To do this, you will want to refer to the chapters that address these subjects (see the last column in the test). Note that if you feel tempted to put off addressing certain issues, chapter 5 shows how to get past this procrastination barrier.

"Somewhat like you" suggests an opportunity to take action so that later on, you can say that this issue is no longer yours. It's important to address those issues to prevent them from becoming worse.

Your depression will probably lift eventually, even if you take no formal action to end it. However, waiting out depression is like sitting naked in a swamp on a cold winter day.

> When depressed, you can feel so miserable about your present life and pessimistic about your future that you may think that any light at the end of the tunnel is from a freight train heading your way.

Note that even if you marked a statement in the test as "not you," this is a positive sign that's worth paying attention to. Is there something you can take from it that you can apply to help yourself defeat depression? For example, you may have many depressive thoughts, but if you marked "0" for statement 11, then you believe you are not helpless. If this is the case, you're in a position to start making positive changes sooner rather than later.

Statement 15 is also noteworthy. At one time or another, most people who experience significant depression will wish they were dead. Although the topic of suicide prevention goes beyond the scope of this self-help book, there are many things you can do to feel better about life. If you regularly have suicidal thoughts, you should contact a licensed mental health depression specialist right away.

This test also gives you a baseline for comparing future measures of your depression. Once you make progress in some of these areas, you can continue to use the test to isolate areas where you still have work to do. Retake it every two weeks to track your progress. Once you are past your depressed mood, retaking the test every two months can act as an early alert system.

Depression prevention is easier than stopping a depression cycle, and chapter 22 describes prevention interventions.

# ACTIVITY AS A REMEDY FOR DEPRESSION

Activity is a remedy for depression. The question is what activities are right for you? Here are some guidelines.

## Follow Meaningful Pursuits

Life is so much more than trying to negate negatives, such as depression. The more time you spend in meaningful pursuits, the less time you'll spend absorbed in depressive thoughts, feelings, and behavioral habits.

It is never too early in the process of curbing depression to think about engaging in a positive or passionate pursuit. A passionate pursuit is more than a planned disruption of depression, such as watching a butterfly in flight. It may be the study of butterflies and searching for them in their natural habitat.

Reengaging in a pursuit that you enjoyed in the past may reactivate your interest.

## Engage in Positive Activities

Positive activities can distract you from negative thoughts and bring about a change of mood. Make a list of brief activities you'd ordinarily like to do if you did not feel depressed. They may include soaking in a tub of warm water, putting up a bird feeder, or listening to a favorite song. Do a favorite activity each day.

# POSITIVE ACTIVITY LIST

Use this activity list to note former pleasures. Then do the activity again, even if you don't feel like it.

1.

2.

3.

4.

## *Attend to Sensory Experiences*

When you feel drawn into a world of depression, your senses may feel dulled but are still available.
Atlanta psychotherapist Ed Garcia (per. comm.) suggests charting the use of each of your five senses once a day. For the sense of smell, pay attention to something you find pleasant, such as the aroma of a rose. Touch comes into play when you move your hands over a tree trunk. You may enjoy the sounds of birds chirping in the morning.

# FIVE-BY-FIVE SENSORY EXPERIENCE

Use the following chart to list how you plan to experience your senses over the next five days. The first column gives some examples:

| Sense | Day 1 | Day 2 | Day 3 | Day 4 | Day 5 |
|-------|-------|-------|-------|-------|-------|
| Touch | Run fingers over velvet. | | | | |
| Taste | Lick honey from the surface of a cracker. | | | | |
| Smell | Sniff the aroma of fresh coffee. | | | | |
| Sight | Watch a bird in flight. | | | | |
| Sound | Listen to the sound of a brook running over rocks. | | | | |

## *Encourage the Right Side of Your Brain*

One of the most consistent findings in brain research on depression is that depression is associated with less activity in the right frontal lobes (Heller and Nitschke 1997). By creating positive metaphors, using simile, and writing poetry, you can put this right side of your brain to constructive use.

### USING METAPHORS

Metaphor is a figurative comparison, such as "life is a cornucopia." Winston Churchill said his depressed mood was a black dog that followed him. "A prison beneath jimsonweed" calls forth another depressing image. "Trapped in a tomb" captures another.

Metaphors can point to exits from depression. Adjust your sails toward safe harbors when the winds of depression descend upon you. Bats of depression fly in the night and can be dispatched by the light. Now, find an action that gets you to the harbor and the bats ducking for cover.

# FIND A POSITIVE METAPHOR

Use the space below to create a positive action metaphor that contrasts with a depression metaphor.

- Your depression metaphor:

- Your antidepression metaphor:

## USING SIMILES

A simile draws a comparison between two things, such as in the expression "dark as depression" or "depression is like a chilling cold." Reverse them. If depression is like darkness, concentrate on "enlightenment as a light." If depression is like a chilling cold, imagine a warm ray of light cloaking your body in warmth.

# FIND A POSITIVE SIMILE

Contrast your depression simile with its reverse:

- Your depression simile:

- Your antidepression simile:

## USING POETRY

You could portray your depression through poetry. The rhymes would describe misery. You could also write a poem that shows how to move away from depression. The following two collaboratively written poems illustrate this contrast.

The negative stories we tell ourselves about our lives can be a staging ground for depression (Dalgleish et al. 2011). Developing a broader perspective is associated with less narrative negativity (Schartau, Dalgleish, and Dunn 2009). To broaden your perspective, rewrite old scripts to show how you're a survivor.

The Cognitive Behavioral Workbook for Depression

| A Shadow World | A World of Disengagement |
|---|---|
| *Into a mirror I see* | *On the trail of life one day* |
| *A world of shadows following me* | *I met depression on the way* |
| *As life faintly echoes through the hollow* | *Although the burden sank me low* |
| *The shadows cloak the path I follow* | *I decided to let depression go* |
| *Like a dog that hunts in darkness* | *Now that the challenge is set* |
| *With no scent or sight* | *It's up to me to see it met* |
| *It experiences a dulling fright* | *Perhaps the dog will get the scent* |
| *As it climbs a lightless height* | *Through action, I'll see depression relent* |
| *Reflecting* | *Farewell to my familiar guard* |
| *Detecting* | *Who kept me sheltered within my nest* |
| *Suspecting* | *I'll consider you a friend who protected me* |
| *Why has this struggle chosen me?* | *When my heart wasn't ready to solo this quest.* |
| —Bill Knaus, Dale Jarvis, Diana Cleary | —Bill Knaus, Diana Cleary |

The philosopher Aristotle said about 2,500 years ago that life and events have a beginning, a middle, and an end. So does depression: by learning what to do and applying what you know, you can bring it to its end sooner. Use your imagination as constructively as you can. Taking the tiniest step signals that you have started the process of making positive personal changes and disentangling yourself from the web of depression: a complex, sticky place where few would voluntarily choose to go or to stay.

In the remaining chapters, you'll find may ways to do the same thing, which is to end feeling depressed, feel good again, and prevent another depressive episode.

# END DEPRESSION PLAN

**Key ideas** (What three ideas did you find most helpful in this chapter?):

1.

2.

3.

**Action steps** (What three steps can you take to move closer to your goal of overcoming depression?):

1.

2.

3.

**Execution** (How did you execute the steps?):

1.

2.

3.

**Results** (What did you learn that you can use?):

1.

2.

3.

# A Master Plan to Defeat Depression

To quote Walt Kelly, creator of the famous *Pogo* comic strip, "We have met the enemy and he is us." You can be your own worst enemy when you are depressed. But you are also more knowledgeable about yourself than anyone else can be. When it is well channeled, this knowledge is a source of power.

This chapter invites you on a journey to explore how to use objective self-knowledge to change direction from a self-absorbing cycle of depression to a sense of realistic optimism.

## DEVELOP YOUR SELF-OBSERVATION SKILLS

In a melancholic mind, you feel drawn into your tensions as you filter reality through your darker thoughts. In this visceral vice, you clamp onto how rotten you feel. You fixate on your sufferings, disappointments, losses, and desperations. You think about events that plague you. Pessimism is pervasive.

Your interpretations of reality are affected by your expectations and mood, however. When you are in a grim mood, most things will look bleak. Too much of this inner reflection will give you a warped sense of yourself. Your sense of identity, or what makes you different or special, gets absorbed in your depressed mood as you dwell on your worries and troubles. It doesn't have to be that way. In a radical shift to an objective self-observant way of thinking and knowing, you can break from the vise. This objective self-observant way of knowing is where you think about your thinking and separate depressive thinking from facts. You see your depressed mood for what it is, a depressed mood. You accept the value in acting to gain traction in a productive direction of freedom from depression.

How can self-observation be objective? The test would be if a disinterested party would be likely to agree that your observation is fair-minded and relatively free from bias and prejudice; you would normally be able to confirm your observation about yourself. Through the lens of this mental perspective, you can examine the validity of your depressing thinking. You teach yourself to accept—not necessarily like—the tensions of depression. You take seriously the concept of activity as a remedy for depression by putting one foot in front of the other to show yourself that you can take charge of what you do to address depression.

Objective self-observation involves probing your depressive expectations. Here's an example: "If I think I will stay miserable forever, how is this view likely to affect how I feel and what I do? Are there plausible alternative views? How might these alternative views affect my emotions and behavior?"

The French chemist Louis Pasteur, who discovered that germs cause disease, said that "in the field of observation, chance only favors the prepared mind." When you've objectively thought about your depressive thinking, you may unexpectedly discover opportunities to get unstuck from your negative thought themes, emotional despondency, and depressive behavioral habits, such as withdrawing.

> Self-Study is a never-ending process.

# SIX SELF-GUIDANCE STEPS

The degree to which you can profit from self-observation largely depends upon the accuracy—or inaccuracy—of your observations. If you were to play guitar and practice using false feedback, you'd likely get better at playing sour notes. If you use the negative emotions from negative thinking as proof that your life is going downhill, then you'll have more sour notes in the form of negative thinking and stressful, depressive feelings. However, you can make adjustments.

Psychologist John Dollard (1942) thought that people could monitor their thoughts and connect them to their emotions and actions. He called this process "self-study." Later, psychologist John Flavell (1979) coined the term *metacognitive* to describe a self-monitoring approach that involves thinking about thinking and connecting knowledge, beliefs, and strategies to achieve desired results. Metacognition is a form of self-study.

Here is framework for a metacognitive self-guidance plan for taking an organized approach to defeating depression:

1. By setting a mission, you give yourself a direction.

2. Through establishing goals, you identify steps to achieve the mission.

3. Your action plan provides a design for achieving your goals.

4. By executing the plan, you move forward and test its validity.

5. By evaluating the results of your plan, you identify its strengths and where you need to improve.

6. Using your evaluation, you revise your plan.

## *Establishing a Self-Development Mission*

It's important to articulate a mission statement that describes your long-term direction for change, for this will help to direct your actions.

Indian independence leader Mahatma Gandhi's mission was to free India for self-rule. Missions also can represent a special purpose, such as to develop your personal resources to contribute to the welfare of those who can't care for themselves. An example of a counterdepression mission would be to defeat depressive thinking to free your mind from depressive strain.

Your mission will act like a beacon to illuminate a future where you no longer feel depressed. President Abraham Lincoln had a beacon. He continued on despite depression because of a cause that he believed was greater than himself. He saw the Civil War as a just undertaking to keep the nation together. He further recognized that his personal happiness was his own responsibility. With that form of beacon thinking, he illuminated the path that he forged.

Think of a mission as your organizing principle and as a platform for constructive actions. If one doesn't come to you right away, let your thoughts incubate. Meanwhile, consider overcoming depression both a mission and a beacon.

## YOUR MISSION STATEMENT

Describe your antidepression mission in the space below:

_____

_____

_____

_____

_____

## Setting Goals

The next step is to set goals that will help you achieve your mission. A goal is definable, meaningful, measurable, and attainable. Goals may be open ended, such as a goal to deepen your understanding of the mechanisms behind depression. Or you may have a specific goal, such as lowering your score on the depression test.

Whatever you choose to do, setting goals is one of the most important steps that you can take in an ongoing process of ridding yourself of depression. Note that you are better off setting goals that fit with your values and interests than what you think others may want from you.

At first it may be helpful to set short-term goals that are easy to accomplish. When the goal is accessible, you may get to it sooner (Webb and Sheeran 2008). For example, if your goal is to log your depressive thoughts, that goal is accessible and achievable.

Longer-term goals may often take multiple steps to accomplish, such as addressing depression hot spots in your depression test. A goal for effectively dealing with depressive thinking can involve recording depressive thoughts in a notebook and evaluating the validity of this thinking that you record. A goal to boost your activity level can be to identify the single most important activity to accomplish during the day. A walk in the park thirty minutes a day is a physical exercise goal.

# SETTING GOALS TO COUNTER DEPRESSION

What are your counterdepression goals?

Goal: _____

_____

_____

Goal: _____

_____

_____

## CONVERTING NEGATIVITY INTO POSITIVE GOALS

When you are thinking pessimistically, missions and goals may sound good for the other guy. You may see yourself as too depressed to care or too listless to act. You may find yourself in a pool of negativity where you feel so discouraged that you don't know where to begin to shift from self-absorbing thinking to an objective self-observant approach. In fact, this is an ideal opportunity for you to identify and address some of your self-defeating thoughts and beliefs and convert your negativity into something positive. One depressive thought tends to trigger another: "I am lost." "No one appreciates me." "I can't get through this." "I can't stand how I feel." "I am useless." Although such pessimistic thoughts sound bleak, you can convert them into positive statements that can function as counterdepression goals.

| Depressive Pessimistic Thought | Positive Alternative Goal |
|---|---|
| "I am lost." | "Find a bearing." |
| "No one appreciates me." | "Find exceptions to this statement." |
| "I'll never get over feeling depressed." | "Question hopeless-thinking assumptions." |
| "I can't stand how I feel." | "Learn to tolerate what I don't like." |
| "I'm useless." | "Question uselessness assumption." |

Use the space provided to translate your own negative thinking into positive goals. In the left-hand column, record some of your pessimistic thoughts. Then, on the right, convert them into positive statements of what you can do to change.

| Depressive Pessimistic Thought | Positive Alternative Goal |
|---|---|
|  |  |
|  |  |
|  |  |
|  |  |
|  |  |

## Planning to Meet Your Goals

Missions give you a general direction. Goals describe where you'll focus efforts to accomplish your mission. The next step is to make a plan to turn these ideas into actions.

The planning phase starts with a two-part question: "What do I need to know, and what do I need to do to achieve my goals?"

In the planning phase, you set priorities. The priorities determine the how, where, when, and who part of planning. Your plan also defines what you will do first, second, and so forth.

Suppose your mission is to engage in planned activities to regularize your life as a means for curbing depression. One of your goals is to build a routine into your early morning activities. Your plan is to set your alarm to wake you at 6:55 a.m. each morning, shower at 7:00 a.m., and be out to a local breakfast nook at 8:00 a.m.

At other times, scheduling is unnecessary. Here's an open-ended plan where your goal would be to defeat depressive thinking whenever you catch yourself in these thoughts:

- "I'll record depressive thinking in a notebook."

- "I'll organize this thinking according to logical categories."

- "I'll look at how these thoughts affect how I feel."

- "I'll use objective self-awareness methods to create alternative explanations."

# YOUR ANTIDEPRESSION ACTION PLAN

What is your plan? Use the following space to design your plan:

_____

_____

_____

_____

_____

_____

_____

_____

_____

_____

Depression can get in the way of the best-articulated goals. But even when you are not depressed, you can stall on achieving your goals. For example, every year people make New Year's resolutions. Common resolutions include losing weight, getting physical exercise, finding a better job, and having less stress. Few achieve their goals. That is because most people have vague plans or no plans at all. A goal without a plan has a good chance of fizzling.

Articulating your plans can seem like taking an unnecessary step. After all, if you have goals, why not just achieve them? The fact is that goals without plans are often fated to fail (Gollwitzer 1999). Goal attainment increases when you design how, where, and when to take action (Gollwitzer and Oettingen 2011). Your mood is likely to improve when you make progress in meeting your goals (Koestner et al. 2002).

> Accept stress, but the right kind. Tension that arises from overcoming obstacles is a propellant, or healthy stress.

## Implementing the Plan

Executing a plan involves commanding your muscles to move. It can involve assertions of will at a time when will is in short supply. It can involve getting past impediments such as pessimistic thinking.

Depressive pessimism is often fatalistic in tone and content. It can be a form of prophesying as if your future were already written. Depressive pessimism can be a self-fulfilling prophecy, but you can counter this kind of thinking.

Here is a thought on pessimism. If you could accurately foretell your future, you might conclude that your life is predetermined. You have no freedom. You must abide by what will be. However, if you believe that you can influence your future by what you do today, this guided self-help book can help you along the way.

## Evaluating Your Progress

Few self-guidance plans are flawless from the start. For example, you may experience strong inner opposition if you plan to regularize your daily routine. If you tend to wake up early, you may be up well before 5:00 a.m. If your plan is to shower regularly when you wake up, you may find showering at 7:00 a.m. less workable than showering at 5:30 a.m. Or you may need to fill the time between 5:00 a.m and 7:00 a.m. with a few productive activities, such as writing songs about depression where you put yourself in control.

Your self-guidance evaluation starts with these questions:

- "Did I give myself workable instructions to implement the plan?"

- "Did I follow the process that I set for myself?"

- "If I accurately followed the plan, what did I learn?"

- "What unexpected conditions came into play?"

- "If I avoided the plan, where did the breakdown occur?"

## YOUR EVALUATION

What did you learn through this evaluative process? Use the following space to describe what you learned:

_____

_____

_____

_____

_____

_____

_____

## *Revising the Plan*

Accomplishments are often preceded by revisions. You don't get to be a skilled accountant by just reading a job description. You have to learn the trade. Accomplishment is often found by engaging in the process of making positive changes. A potential by-product is decreasing depression.

Here are two key questions: What have you learned through this process of engagement? What modifications or revisions would improve your plan?

## YOUR REVISIONS

Use this space to modify and improve your plan:

_____

_____

_____

_____

_____

A metacognitive self-guidance approach takes more than an afternoon of reflection to master. People develop this skill over several weeks or months. But this is not a footrace. You can continue to refine this skill over your lifetime.

# REALISTIC OPTIMISM

Optimism is a state of mind in which you are hopeful that things will turn out well. However, when you have or exert no control over an outcome, your optimism is not grounded in anything real. Such a false sense of optimism supports procrastination, when you sit on your hands waiting for something good to happen.

Realistic optimism is different. This is a perspective grounded in reality, or what is. You filter your experiences by seeing opportunities and challenges. If you come to a dead end, you try a different way. However, as a realistic optimist, you know when you are up against an immovable wall.

Realistic optimism may start with questions: "How do I apply my talents to learn new ways to make a radical shift from self-absorbing thinking to objective self-awareness?" "How do I organize, regulate, and direct my actions to meet my most basic antidepression goal(s)?" Start thinking about what you can do to defeat depression, and you open the portal to realistic optimism.

# END DEPRESSION PLAN

**Key ideas** (What three ideas did you find most helpful in this chapter?):

1.

2.

3.

**Action steps** (What three steps can you take to move closer to your goal of overcoming depression?):

1.

2.

3.

**Execution** (How did you execute the steps?):

1.

2.

3.

**Results** (What did you learn that you can use?):

1.

2.

3.

# CHAPTER 4

# How to Make Changes That Stick

In 1976, I introduced a blueprint for personal change to help my clients meet their self-development goals. Following this approach, you engage in five phases of change: awareness, action, accommodation, acceptance, and actualization. These five phases blend and overlap, and their order depends upon your unique situation. This chapter will show you how to use this blueprint.

## AWARENESS

When depressed, you can experience yourself marinating in mental misery. This is a kind of depressive awareness, but you come to know less and less about yourself as you concentrate on how rotten you feel. An enlightened self-awareness grows from objective self-observation. This is the mirror opposite of depressive awareness. This self-awareness includes a growing body of factual self-knowledge and perspectives.

## AWARENESS EXERCISE

Use the following checklist to see where you stand on objective self-observant awareness. Respond to each statement with yes or no.

| Level of Self-Awareness | Yes | No |
|---|---|---|
| "I'm aware of my depressive thoughts." | | |
| "I'm aware of how negative thoughts affect how I feel and what I do." | | |
| "I'm aware that I can accept depressive thoughts and still contest them." | | |

| Level of Self-Awareness | Yes | No |
|---|---|---|
| "I'm aware that my worth does not depend on ridding myself of depressive thoughts." | | |
| "I'm aware that I still have the ability to adapt even when I feel depressed." | | |

This awareness exercise is both a check on where you stand on depression self-awareness and a progress measure. The more you check yes, the higher your level of enlightened self-awareness. You can use this exercise again later to see how much your self-awareness has increased.

## Levels of Awareness

Enlightened self-awareness can occur at practical, empirical, and core levels. When you act at one level, you can influence the other two for the better.

### MAKING PRACTICAL CHANGES

At a *practical level*, you test practical solutions for depression. These are specific things that you can do, such as logging your thoughts when you feel depressed. This practical logging exercise helps make depressive thinking visible and subject to your conscious review and rebuttal. Because you can now interrupt a depressive-thinking cycle, you climb a step on the ladder to higher levels of enlightened awareness.

### MAKING EMPIRICAL CHANGES

At an *empirical level*, you wear a scientist's hat. For example, you treat depressive thinking as hypotheses to test. If you've been thinking that you'll stay depressed forever, you recognize that this thought is only a hypothesis, which is not a statement of truth but rather a testable proposition. Your goal is to learn what works and what doesn't. You are testing solutions and not your "self."

If you feel stuck in a depressive line of thought, you can reframe the issue from depressive dogma to a hypothesis.

## CONVERTING YOUR DEPRESSIVE THOUGHTS

Use the following framework to transform your depressive thoughts into fluid hypotheses. Two examples are given at the beginning. Fill in the remaining blanks with your own thoughts and hypotheses.

| Depressing Thought | Conversion to a Hypothesis |
|---|---|
| Example: "I can't do anything right." | "I hypothesize that whatever I undertake will turn out badly." |

| Example: "I will never stop feeling depressed." | "I hypothesize that depression will last forever." |
| --- | --- |
| | |
| | |
| | |

Now you are in a good position to compare your hypotheses to actual outcomes. Give yourself credit for taking another step up the enlightened awareness ladder.

### MAKING CORE CHANGES

At a *core level* of change, you connect the dots between, say, depression and inner ideas you hold about yourself. Say that you feel insecure and vulnerable. You identify with this insecure self. You feel fragile. You fear a loss of self if you change in any way. So you avoid activities that threaten your sense of self.

Core-level change includes working through insecurities. You can take another awareness step by recognizing your strengths. You can accept your strengths and test them. This activity both develops your sense of objective self-awareness and counters core depressive beliefs. Take this step, and give yourself credit for moving up another level on the enlightened self-awareness ladder.

Practical, empirical, and core awareness often flow together like sugar, cream, and coffee. Each part can exist separately and still complement the others.

# ACTION

Action is doing something, such as lifting a book, working out a problem, or executing a plan. When depressed, you may believe that you don't have the will or energy to act. Oh, but you do! Free will is choosing one direction when you could have chosen another. Willpower occurs in degree. It is possible to push yourself to do some things ahead of others, even if you don't feel like it, such as educating yourself about depression.

## *How to Take Action*

Thinking of doing is easier than doing. You can use one of the two techniques offered here—the Kelly role technique and the simple activity technique—to speed the process of getting yourself into action.

## KELLY ROLE TECHNIQUE

George Kelly (1955), the founder of the psychology of personal constructs, predicts that people can change their thinking as a by-product of changing their behavior. The idea is that role-playing will encourage positive changes in your thinking. By stepping out of character, you may come closer to the sometimes-elusive goal of self-awareness and understanding.

We play many roles in life. At first, we are a child playing the role of a son or daughter, student, or friend. Later, we assume the role of parent, specialist, club member, writer, investigator, negotiator, chauffeur, gardener, or any number of other identities. Some roles are self-defined, such as the protector, gadfly, or martyr. If your self-assigned role ceases to make sense, you can define and teach yourself to take on other roles that benefit you and others.

> Aristotle saw power as the ability to make things happen.

One of Kelly's techniques is to write a new script for yourself that addresses a specific area of your life that you think is in your enlightened interest to develop. The script can include new thinking that goes along with acting out a new role.

Sometimes adopting a title makes it easier to perform a job if the title defines the responsibilities inherent in the role. Here is a job description for a person who plays the role of *the questioner*.

- The questioner monitors and records depressive thinking.

- The questioner raises questions about depressive thoughts, perhaps following Socrates's prescription of first defining the terms, and then obtaining examples and exceptions.

- The questioner raises questions as to whether alternative, evidence-based or rational thoughts exist and what they might be.

- The questioner matches the depressive thoughts against their evidence-based counterparts. For example, by questioning and defusing depressive thinking, you eliminate the extra burden brought about by that thinking. How does this evidence-based view compare to a depressive thought such as "I can never get over feeling depressed?"

You can play many different roles with different scripts, such as one where you focus on developing empathy for others. Play out the script as though you were an actor playing the part. Test the script for a few weeks. Make modifications using your observed results. Based upon the results, quit the new role, modify it, accept some parts, or embrace it.

## THE SIMPLE ACTIVITY TECHNIQUE

Simple activities are those that you can do even when fatigued. They require little motivation and just a bit of persistence. Here are some examples:

- Do dishes the old-fashioned way; wash them by hand.

- Remove your stored groceries and reorganize them.

- Sand and refinish a piece of furniture.

- Walk in place for fifteen minutes while counting your steps.

- Join a dance or aerobics class.

# ACCOMMODATION

In "Song of Myself," the poet Walt Whitman says, "Do I contradict myself? Very well then, I contradict myself (I am large, I contain multitudes)." You'll surely have contrary views. You can think both rationally and irrationally. You can have many juxtaposed assumptions about the same event.

As a by-product of awareness and action exercises, you exercise accommodation. This is where you take in and adjust to ideas and actions that have a better fit with reality.

To promote positive accommodation thinking, you can intentionally create a paradox in your depressive thinking to dislodge depressive beliefs. For example, if depressive thinking deepens depression, then what happens when you intentionally think a depressing thought? As an exercise, deliberately try to convince yourself that you can't change. Deliberately declare yourself helpless. As you do so, do you find that these beliefs lose their emotional value and become hollow thoughts? If so, you've experienced a paradoxical effect.

## *Accommodation Paradoxes*

We have many paradoxes within us: we can be passive at times and active at others, both patient and impatient, cheerful and depressed. These well-known dualities don't occur simultaneously, however. An accommodation paradox is different. In this case, you believe one thing is true and discover an alternative reality that is closer to the truth.

You face a paradoxical situation when you tell yourself that you are completely useless, but this is contrary to your history, in which you did useful things. You can set the stage for an accommodation paradox by asking yourself, "How can I be only one way when I am also other ways?"

Or say you are someone who is great at the details. This helps you in your career, but you also get into minute detail in supporting a case against yourself that you are a "loser." Or say you have a creative and searching mind, so you do well at a job where you get paid for creative ideas. But in a depressed state, your creativity can flow along the darker channels. In both of these cases, one of your strengths is working against you when you are depressed.

An accommodation paradox lies in seeing this duality between reality and mind-fogging beliefs and fantasies. Resolving the paradox enables you to get back to the positive uses of your strengths. To get there, you look for flaws in the depressing details. You detail the flaws. You can then turn imaginary dark horizons into complex places where colors give light to the darkness. Now, you're back to using your strengths.

### Five Phases of Change

Awareness sets the stage for change.

Action makes it happen.

Accommodation allows for adjustments.

Acceptance eases the burden.

Actualization speeds you forward.

## *Accommodation Adjustments*

In the following exercise, you'll explore several paradoxes.

# PARADOX EXERCISE

Here is a challenge. Explore the paradox between the two positions expressed in each of the following sets of statements. In the spaces that follow, justify the first position and then answer the following reality-promoting question. Finally, decide which of these two responses makes the most sense, and explain why.

**Paradox 1:** The position "I'm helpless to change" versus the position "I'm to blame for all my troubles"

1. Justification for the position "I'm helpless to change": _____

2. How can you be helpless and still totally blameworthy? _____

   _____

3. Which position makes the most sense, and why? _____

**Paradox 2:** The position "I have no worth" versus the position "people are complex, with literally thousands of different traits, qualities, and characteristics"

1. Justification for "I have no worth" position: _____

2. How can you be worthless and still have thousands of traits and characteristics of different strengths and visibilities? _____

   _____

3. Which response makes the most sense, and why? _____

**Paradox 3:** The position "unless I'm perfect, I'm nothing" versus the position "none of us is infallible"

1. Justification for perfectionism position: _____

2. How can a fallible human ever reach perfection? _____

   _____

3. Which response makes the most sense, and why? _____

**Paradox 4:** The position "I can't do anything right" versus the position "such a generalization about millions of performances is an overgeneralization and can't be right"

1.  Justification for "I can't do anything right" position: _____

2.  How can such a single depressive idea define your life? _____

    _____

3.  Which response makes the most sense, and why? _____

By exploring opposing positions, you can give yourself a different way to understand the significance of inconsistencies, adjust your thinking, and resolve such paradoxes.

# ACCEPTANCE

Acceptance is where you integrate change on an emotional level. In a spirit of acceptance, you accept yourself regardless of whether or not you think depressively, or whether your plans succeed or fail. If you try to make a change and your plan proves premature or fruitless, you can try again or try a different way.

Acceptance has three overlapping dimensions. First, you are *nonjudgmental*, which means that you need never put yourself down, but you can judge and change your thinking and your actions if you are displeased with the process and the outcome. Second, you use *tolerance*, which involves the patience to put up with unpleasant realities but not to acquiesce to what most reasonable people would consider deplorable. When tolerant, you are likely to experience flexibility. The third part of the acceptance process is *allowance*. This is letting something happen that you don't like but can't immediately change. You have a negative thought. You let it be without magnifying it. It soon becomes like a whisper in the wind.

You won't be accepting with unwavering consistency. Indeed, I've never met anyone who was fully accepting. Thus, allowing imperfections in acceptance is part of the process of acceptance.

## *Working on Self-Acceptance*

Self-acceptance is a cognitive process. Your level of self-acceptance influences how you are likely to think, feel, and act.

The following exercise suggests that you can always accept yourself, even if you find some of what you do unacceptable and worth changing.

# COMPARING ACCEPTANCE THINKING WITH DEPRESSIVE THINKING

Compare each statement about depressive thinking on the left with its counterpart on the right, showing a more objective self-observant perspective. The comparison points to a choice.

| Depressive Thinking | Acceptance Thinking |
|---|---|
| Depressive thinking blinds us with a sense of bleakness. | Acceptance unleashes the idea that bad times pass and new, good times begin. |
| Depressive thinking forecloses on life as a miserable experience. | Acceptance partially involves acknowledging that life continues even when you face limitations; you can continue to participate—perhaps in a more limited than usual way—in your activities of daily living. |
| Depressive thinking magnifies the significance of a disturbing event or possibility and makes it the engine driving what you do. | Acceptance makes the most untoward experiences of life more tolerable without diminishing their significance. |
| Depressive thinking adds distress to an already sad or unfortunate condition. | Acceptance of unpleasant, unfortunate, and catastrophic experiences leaves us with a sense of sadness for what was, what is, or what can never be. |

The previous chart suggests a way to see through the shallowness of depressive thinking using a relabeling method that is softer in tone and stronger in logic.

# ACTUALIZATION

Actualization is where you integrate awareness, action, accommodation, and acceptance. At this stage, you typically experience yourself as grounded in what you think, feel, and do. You can expand from that platform.

Ridding yourself of depression normally involves doing something else first, such as stretching your resources to actualize specific abilities. This actualizing process involves making self-development efforts that include improving your communications, seeking positive opportunities, facing meaningful challenges, initiating ways to build more quality experiences into your life, and exercising choices that yield long-term advantages.

## Perfectionism vs. Actualization

By actualizing your efforts, you work to achieve quality. This involves persistence and acceptance of inevitable setbacks.

Actualization is a different path from that of striving for perfection. Actualization involves stretching to do well, whereas perfectionism means believing and acting as though you have to act flawlessly in whatever you do.

Although perfectionism and actualization can both involve high standards, and although it is true that perfectionist striving can lead to driven successes, more often perfectionism walks in the company of core conditions of self-doubt, fear of failure, anger, and procrastination.

## Psychological Stretch Exercise

The following stretch technique spotlights a way to actualize your abilities and other positive resources.

# STRETCHING YOUR RESOURCES

Use the space provided to record the following:

1.  Identify three personal resources that, when extended, have proven to be a positive expression of your capabilities. These resources could include such skills as problem solving, communicating well, being tolerant of others, having an active imagination, or anything that has sometimes served as a strength. Record these personal resources in the first column of the chart.

2.  Stretch these resources by putting your mind and muscles in motion to go through the paces of making a positive change. Write down what you plan to do and then execute the action. As a positive change, for example, you might draw your rendition of depression, what freedom from depression might look like, and the steps on a bridge between your image of depression and freedom for depression.

3.  Make a note of what you learned from the experience. What you learned can point to adjustments to make and where you choose to stretch next.

| Your Personal Resources | Stretch Actions | What You Learned |
|---|---|---|
| 1. | | |
| 2. | | |
| 3. | | |

# A DUAL THEORY OF CHANGE

When you effectively apply a five-phases-of-change cognitive, emotive, and behavioral approach to depressive thinking, why might positive changes take place?

- You have altered your thinking and no longer believe that your situation is hopeless.

- You have come to believe that you can do something to help yourself and, therefore, you can't be helpless to act.

- You come to see that you have the skills to make constructive behavioral changes.

- You rediscover your ability to solve your problems and view yourself as capable of exercising this ability.

- You start to believe in yourself again.

- You increasingly feel a sense of well-being.

- As you engage in positive, problem-solving actions, you will tend to strengthen and expand your positive resources.

- When you are in control of your actions, you are likely to have better command over your thoughts and emotions.

Your body simultaneously recalibrates itself in rhythm with psychological changes, thus reducing sensations that can activate depressive thinking. You are likely to feel energized and accomplish more with less strain and effort. This positive process feeds on itself. When your body is in a state of positive equilibrium, or when your thinking is clear, you are likely to feel free of distress. That's the gist of the dual theory of change.

## Changes through Adversity

Throughout this combined five-phase process, you will face many frustrations. Facing frustrations will boost your tolerance for frustration. Your ability to withstand discomfort and distress will predictably rise. With this resilience will come a greater sense of inner command and confidence and a decreasing tendency to think depressively. At different times through this process, your body will recalibrate itself to reflect clear thinking, a higher frustration tolerance, resiliency, and a "can do" mentality.

Exiting from depression involves patience. When you do all the right things to overcome this state of mind and body, you are likely to find that you can control your thoughts and actions more directly than you can your biology. The body has its own rhythms. It normally takes time to get back into sync. For example, flying from New York City to Honolulu leads to jet lag. Within several days, your sleep cycle will normally adjust to the change. Still, your adrenal hormones can take several weeks to reset to the new schedule. In a similar sense, it normally takes time for positive thoughts and actions to recalibrate and stabilize your biological processes.

> Personal change has no end point.

When you follow a self-help approach and your depression lifts, what does this say? Your outlook has changed for the better. You've come to believe that you can turn your life around. Then, where did the depressed ideas and sensations go?

## Brain Changes

You can't see depression in the same sense as you might a broken leg. But just as a cast or other suitable device will help a leg mend properly, you can do a lot on your own to help along the process of overcoming depression. And as you apply cognitive skills to a process of ridding yourself of depressive beliefs, the cognitive, emotive, and behavioral changes you make may be noted in brain-wave patterns (Deldin and Chiu 2005).

Through your antidepression efforts, you can make neurological changes that continue to strengthen over time. For example, reasoning and problem solving activate the prefrontal cortex, which is the part of the brain we associate with reason and logic (Keightley et al. 2003). Neural imaging devices, such as functional magnetic resonance imaging, show how these areas expand as your counterdepression reasoning skills improve (Goldapple et al. 2004).

# END DEPRESSION PLAN

**Key ideas** (What three ideas did you find most helpful in this chapter?):

1.

2.

3.

**Action steps** (What three steps can you take to move closer to your goal of overcoming depression?):

1.

2.

3.

**Execution** (How did you execute the steps?):

1.

2.

3.

**Results** (What did you learn that you can use?):

1.

2.

3.

# CHAPTER 5

# Break a Procrastination-Depression Connection

Procrastination is the invisible elephant in the room. It  can stand between you and the use of marvelous methods for stopping depression.

In its annual Stress in America survey, the American Psychological Association (2010) omitted procrastination as a factor explaining why people don't follow through on addressing their stresses. Yet if you know what to look for, the signs of procrastination are clear. Survey participants assert that a lack of willpower interferes with adopting healthy lifestyle changes. They also report that they could develop willpower if they had more energy and confidence. This excuse is a sign of the invisible procrastination elephant in the room.

Here's how it gets in the way: You set up a series of contingencies you deem necessary to follow through on healthy actions. First you have to have the will. But you can't develop the will without energy and confidence. And since you lack the energy and confidence, you are helpless and can do nothing. This may seem like a silly word game, but this line of thought is crippling.

In this chapter, you'll see how procrastination interferes with taking corrective actions and how to change direction by addressing procrastination and depression simultaneously. As a long-term bonus, you can apply what you learn about breaking the procrastination-depression connection to other areas of your life where procrastination interferes with progress, such as investing for your retirement or overcoming a harmful inhibition.

## DEFINING PROCRASTINATION

When most people think of procrastination, they think of putting off deadline obligations, such as filing tax forms. Deadline delays are the tip of the procrastination iceberg, however. Putting off personally relevant activities is the more serious form of procrastination. Practically everyone has at least one important life goal they've put off.

## The Tomorrow Illusion

When procrastination fogs your vision

Tomorrow comes with a hidden division.

Concealed within a twisted hope,

Blinders cloak the way to cope.

Procrastination pretends to be reality,

When we know with finality,

Tomorrow is on the run.

We smile, we laugh,

We greet strangers with our mask.

Long lost is our able nature.

Finding it is now the task.

—Bill Knaus, Diane Cleary, Dale Jarvis

Procrastination is a process, or a series of steps and actions, that is employed to delay facing a fear, avoid a boring situation, or maintain an illusion that you could do better, if you tried, at achieving a particular end result. When you can map what you do when you procrastinate, you can more carefully target your efforts to break the pattern.

To further define the process, procrastination is an automatic, problematic habit where you needlessly put off, postpone, or delay a timely and relevant activity until another day or time. This process is normally a by-product of avoiding an unpleasant feeling. You'll always substitute something less timely or relevant for a more pressing priority. You'll practically always engage in some form of procrastination thinking, such as "I'm too weak and tired to do anything to overcome my depression."

Procrastination can be a simple default reaction. You feel uncomfortable about an activity, so you avoid it. More often, procrastination is a complex process that coexists with distress conditions, such as anxiety and depression. You put off dealing with what you fear. You believe you are disabled by your mood. Uncertainty can trigger the discomfort-dodging feature of procrastination. If you view yourself as overwhelmed and unable to perform, you are likely to delay taking corrective actions. As a reaction to anxieties, a negative mood, uncertainty, and other unpleasant conditions, you do something different or nothing at all.

When depressed, you may additionally view getting started as impossible to do. After all, if you already feel burdened by depression, you may default to the thought "I can't do this."

Both procrastination and depression have overlapping, distinctive features. With the procrastination-depression connection operating, you do the following:

- Feel uncomfortable at the thought of taking a corrective action and duck the discomfort.

- Always detour into some diversionary activity, such as hand-wringing, dwelling on your depressive thoughts, or napping.

- Normally engage in self-fulfilling prophesies, such as "I can't succeed, so why try?"

Procrastination and depression go hand in hand, but you can become aware of when you are procrastinating and take steps to stop.

If you wait by the wayside for relief from depression, you are procrastinating.

# WHY BLAME WON'T WORK

If you feel depressed and simultaneously blame yourself for procrastinating, blaming yourself for this automatic habit won't help. Procrastination is rarely assuaged by ridicule, threat, guilt, or humor. Attempts to use blame to evoke social emotions (shame, guilt, embarrassment, humiliation) to curb procrastination typically flop.

It's better to stop blaming yourself and take a first step to follow through on what is presently useful for you to do.

Nineteenth-century procrastination books for children describe tragic tales about people whose procrastination led to death (Barr 1857), who brought failure and disgrace upon themselves (American Sunday School Union 1848), or who caused agonizing grief to self and others (Margaret 1852). On the lighter side, a more contemporary children's story series describes procrastination as a way that people can get themselves into a pickle (Reinach 1977).

Neither scary nor humorous stories have rid us of this behavior. Procrastination remains, and it can interfere with corrective action for depression. Luckily, this book offers some more-effective tools for overcoming procrastination.

> If you tell yourself that you have to feel inspired to start your antidepression plan, this is like paying a loan shark interest. You get a quick gain in the way of relief for your decision, but you take a long-term loss when you keep paying the same price.

# A COGNITIVE, EMOTIVE, AND BEHAVIORAL SYSTEM FOR CHANGE

If you stretch a bit to follow through on cognitive, emotive, and behavioral activities to curb depression, with practice you are likely to find that you can get past your tendency to procrastinate.

## Cognitive Changes

Procrastination normally involves a justification for delaying and a hope for a better tomorrow. You can call this false hope a *mañana* ploy because you are putting things off until later. The illusion is in thinking that, later on, circumstances will be better for doing the thing you are putting off. For example, you may tell yourself it's too much of a hassle to deal with your depressive thinking right now. You'll get to it later when you feel inspired. But what is ever inspiring about dealing with an oppressive condition of mind?

Nevertheless, you con yourself into thinking that what you put off today will be convenient or easier to do later. When procrastination coexists with depression, this false optimism is often replaced by a false pessimism, such as "I'll never be able to do this" or "I don't have the energy."

In this case, you want out of depression but have boxed yourself into a pessimistic perspective with no way out. If you take no action to defeat depression because you think you have no hope, you are using hopelessness as a reason to procrastinate. Yet as you procrastinate, and do nothing to eliminate depression, you will likely continue to feel a sense of hopelessness.

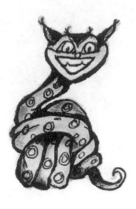

If you find yourself thinking something like "I don't have the energy to change" or "I can't succeed, so why try?" you're boxed into a procrastination-depression way of thinking. To break this procrastination-depression connection, look for weak points in the connection. For example, if you have the energy to think depressing thoughts, you have the energy to think proactive thoughts, such as, "I can slowly work my way up from under this malaise."

By getting specific with yourself, you can change your perspective. You can convert your defeatist thought into an action-minded goal: "I will write a check to pay my mortgage at 2:00 p.m." This action is definable, purposeful, measurable, and achievable. You also have a timeline that you can meet. By taking small, defined steps, you can stop procrastination thinking from driving your actions.

It helps to put a face on your inner procrastination voice. Let's give it the face of a Wheedler. Historically, this is a crafty creature skilled in subterfuge, beguilement, finagling, and conniving. I see the Wheedler as having a smiling, enticing, Cheshire cat's face. But watch out for the reptilian attitude behind this defeatist view.

## PROCRASTINATION FLIP TECHNIQUE

The procrastination *flip technique* is a device for reversing a form of primitive reasoning that, left unchecked, fuels procrastination. The flip technique is to do the opposite of what your Wheedler tells you. Here is an example of how to use the flip technique.

| Wheedler Thinking | Beat the Wheedler with the Flip Technique |
| --- | --- |
| Take a break before you start your antidepression program. Read the newspaper. Play solitaire. Get out that pool cue and start a game. | Work at your antidepression priority for an hour and take a ten-minute break by reading your favorite newspaper column. After the next hour of chipping away at your project, play ten minutes of solitaire. After the next hour, play a game of pool. |
| Don't think about going to the gym. Wait. You'll feel rested and ready. Perhaps you'll go in a day or so. Besides, exercise as a remedy for depression won't work if you're depressed. | Use the flip technique by putting one foot in front of the other and heading to the gym. |
| Get into a squabble with your mate. That will stimulate you more than setting antidepression priorities and goals. | Get started on setting goals and making plans. Get in front of the computer, boot up, and type the letters of the alphabet to break the inertia of inaction. Then continue with setting a meaningful, measurable, and attainable antidepression goal. |
| Activity remedies for depression, like house cleaning, are a pain and waste of time. You have better things to do, like watching your favorite soap opera. | Start cleaning the house while listening to the soap opera. Here you are doing two things at once: one activity that is passive, the other that is active. |

| You are behind on too many things. You're overwhelmed. It's better to hide in the shadows. Perhaps no one will see you and ask you to do more. | Bring your priorities to light. What is the most important thing to do now? What is your first step to start chipping away at the mound of pending actions? Start with the most pressing activity and begin that activity by taking the most basic step. Accept that you may move more slowly than when you don't feel depressed, but even a snail gets to its destination eventually. |
|---|---|

## Emotive Changes

At times your mood will affect whether you procrastinate or not. You've probably had days when you took on challenges that you'd normally put off and other days when you couldn't seem to get going. However, when depression persists, more things tend to get pushed aside.

Procrastination may pivot on your moods. Procrastination can start with a whisper of negative affect. When you are depressed, it's common to magnify what seems unpleasant, so this discomfort may grow even bigger.

A combination of normal discomfort-dodging and depression can be like a double whammy. It will help if you *accept* that this combination goes with the territory. You are then more likely to feel *tolerant* of discomfort and more willing to *allow* yourself to start. And even if you don't feel better after following up, your consolation is that you have one less hassle to contend with.

You are in a contingency mañana procrastination trap when you tell yourself that you will learn to use antidepression coping tools later, after you feel better. If you are in a depressed mood, how are you to feel better first? Instead of falsely making your activity conditional on feeling good, learn and apply coping tools first. You will feel better later as a by-product of the corrective steps that you take now.

> As you get better at diverting, you'll lose ground at coping.

## Behavioral Changes

When you procrastinate, you always substitute something less pressing for what you can gain the most from doing. Thus, behavioral diversions are a classic sign of procrastination. I call these behaviors *addictivities,* when you seem stuck with virtually worthless sidetracking behaviors. Bickering and quarreling can be an addictivity, as can stewing, napping, and watching TV. This gets complex when you are depressed. These activities can also extend from depression.

Activity may be a useful remedy for depression. An active procrastination pattern is an exception. You are reinforcing the wrong behavior. Procrastination can add to stress. The results of this needless delaying may prompt helplessness and hopelessness thinking for excusing putting off problem-solving actions. Let's look at how to change this pattern.

DIVERSION REDUCTION

When you procrastinate, you always sidetrack yourself from your priority. Instead of engaging in corrective actions against depression, you say you lack willpower. That's a diversion.

If you tend to engage in diversions, you can construct ways to change this pattern. The following diversion reduction chart shows how one client simultaneously addressed procrastination thinking, a double-trouble problem in which you layer an unnecessary problem onto your depression, and behavioral inertia.

# DIVERSION REDUCTION CHART

|  | Diversion | Action Plan | Results |
|---|---|---|---|
| **Cognitive** | Telling myself that change is impossible | Writing examples that show both positive and negative changes made when depressed and when feeling better. | This demonstrated that change is not only possible but inevitable. The choice lies in what action to take to prompt positive changes. |
| **Emotive** | Waiting to feel inspired to do something that normally isn't inspiring to do | Acceptance of double trouble as part of depression. My first trouble is the down mood of depression. My double trouble is creating more stress by telling myself something like, "I can't stand this mood," where dwelling on how bad I feel substitutes for taking corrective actions. | Acceptance seems to transform double trouble to a more peaceful state of mind. |
| **Behavioral** | Sitting in a darkened corner twirling my hair | Picking one small change activity each day (such as knitting, sanding a piece of furniture, calling a friend). Commit five minutes and start the activity at a specific time. | Started by procrastinating on the activity. Over two weeks, developed greater consistency in selecting activity and following through. |

# YOUR DIVERSION REDUCTION STRATEGY

Now, you can come up with your own strategy. In the first column, describe the cognitive, emotive, and behavioral elements of a diversion that you engage in. Construct an action plan for each one and write these plans in the second column. Record the results in the third column:

|  | Diversion | Action Plan | Results |
|---|---|---|---|
| **Cognitive** |  |  |  |
| **Emotive** |  |  |  |
| **Behavioral** |  |  |  |

# COMBINING AWARENESS WITH TAKING ACTION

Now that you are more aware of how procrastination keeps you from taking action to counter your depression, a solution is to identify the thoughts that get in the way, and then take action in spite of these thoughts. As with depression, procrastination can operate on cognitive, emotive, and behavioral levels, so here is an example of a cognitive-emotive-behavioral solution to break a procrastination-depression connection:

| | Depression | | Procrastination | |
|---|---|---|---|---|
| | **Awareness** | **Action** | **Awareness** | **Action** |
| **Cognitive** | "I can't change." | Identify areas where you have changed and still can change. | "I'm too depressed to take any corrective actions." | Change now to stop feeling down. |
| **Emotive** | "I feel too numbed and drained to move." | When depressed, you are likely to have a lot of pent-up energy. Imagine being in a room that has caught fire. I bet you'd move. | "I have to wait until I feel better." | Waiting to feel better is an excuse for inaction. Break the inertia of depression by accepting that these feelings are transitory and taking action even when you don't feel like it. |
| **Behavioral** | Letting slide many activities of daily living , such as changing your clothes | Force yourself to behave as if you were not feeling depressed. Start each day wearing fresh garb. | "I'm too much like a robot to do anything. Wearing fresh clothing means I have to do the wash, and I have no energy for that." | Put yourself on automatic pilot and make yourself go through the paces of washing and wearing one clean outfit a day. |

# YOUR COGNITIVE-EMOTIVE-BEHAVIORAL SOLUTION TO BREAK A PROCRASTINATION-DEPRESSION CONNECTION

Complete your awareness action plan to address a procrastination-depression combination.

| | Depression | | Procrastination | |
|---|---|---|---|---|
| | Awareness | Action | Awareness | Action |
| **Cognitive** | | | | |
| **Emotive** | | | | |
| **Behavioral** | | | | |

# PARADOXICAL REWARDS

What do you hope to gain by procrastinating? Here is a tentative answer. You gain quick relief from momentarily avoiding an activity that you associate with tension. For example, if you tell yourself that you'll do something later, you may feel relief in believing that you have made a decision that you'll soon execute.

Relief from stress is a powerful natural reward. You are likely to repeat what brings relief or pleasure. However, the relief you feel can have a paradoxical effect when it reinforces procrastination. Say you promise yourself you'll stop procrastinating, you feel relief, and then continue procrastinating. Or say you want to stop feeling depressed. Instead of coping, you slug down a stiff drink and temporarily feel numb to depressive sensations. When you dance with procrastination in these and other ways, you may not expect things to turn out worse, yet the same sorry results reoccur. Therefore, the relief you feel in delaying your decision is a paradoxical reward, for it reinforces the opposite of what's in your enlightened interest to do.

Procrastinating is never a good idea in the long run. Instead of taking steps to reestablish relationships with meaningful others, you withdraw. You may feel relief from avoiding contact with others, but keeping positively connected with others during your time of depression would help to address your depression. Another example would be telling yourself that you need to feel inspired before you take steps to curb your depression. You may feel satisfied with delaying for this reason, but all you've done is put off taking steps to quell your depression.

When one reason for delay follows another, you have a clear procrastination problem to face, as you continue to feel relief after telling yourself that it doesn't matter what you do since you'll stay depressed forever. Oddly, this pessimism can feel relieving when you exonerate yourself from your responsibility to act, to do, and to get better.

Paradoxical rewards reinforce problem avoidance. You tell yourself that you are too tired to try. You tell yourself that whatever you do will turn out poorly. You feel relieved that you don't have to do anything to help yourself get up from depression. These excuses can both coexist with and reward discomfort avoidance. As you entangle yourself in procrastination distractions, you fail to get to the heart of what is troubling you. You fail to develop quality solutions for defeating depression.

## Secondary Rewards

You can get a second reward from procrastinating if you engage in a pleasurable diversion instead of doing something more important.

How do you distinguish between diversions and activities as remedies for depression? For rewards to be effective, they follow constructive action. For example, exercise is a remedy for depression. When you play a computer game after getting exercise, you are rewarding yourself for making the effort to exercise. However, the game is a distraction when you do it in place of exercising.

## Reversing Paradoxical Rewards

Here are some things you can do right away to reverse paradoxical rewards:

In the next hour, write a short essay about paradoxical rewards versus other rewards that you think may be productive because they reinforce personal effectiveness in overcoming depression.

Alternatively, speak with a thoughtful and helpful friend about paradoxical rewards. Talk about rewards you receive from taking action instead of procrastinating.

The following rewards-reversal technique will help you defeat procrastination tendencies that sidetrack you from coping with depression.

## REWARDS-REVERSAL TECHNIQUE

Experiment with a procrastination-reversal technique where you reward yourself for putting off an impulse to procrastinate. Say you have shopping to do but you keep putting it off. You agree with yourself that you'll shop for an hour. At the end of that time, reward yourself by doing something pleasurable.

Plan your rewards ahead of time. Follow this pattern for the next two weeks. Then fade some of the short-term rewards as you enjoy more of the longer-term benefits of a job well done.

You will receive several positive psychological rewards for executing this proactive process. You will demonstrate that you can impose reason between impulse and reaction, and this sense of mastery comes from being productive. You also will show yourself that you can assert control over your actions even when you feel depressed. This feels good too.

You will also demonstrate that you can engage in constructive actions instead of impulsive actions, which helps to build confidence. Confidence feels better than helplessness.

By stretching your ability to self-improve, you can rise above a paradoxical procrastination-reward pattern. You show yourself that you can organize and regulate your actions to achieve a positive result. This rewards your growing ability to avoid distractions and to stay on track.

The sense of relief you receive from taking action is always better than the immediate, but only temporary, relief you receive from procrastinating around addressing depression.

## SOLVING THE DOUBLE-AGENDA DILEMMA

Sigmund Freud's horse-and-rider metaphor (1950) illustrates the struggle between delaying and doing. When you procrastinate, it's like being on a horse that is taking you somewhere other than where you are wise to go. The horse is like the powerful primitive brain that goes for pleasure and avoids pain. The horse's normal inclination is to follow the path of least resistance. When the horse is in control, it goes where it wants. The rider is the rational side of your personality. This is where rationality overrides impulse. Instead of automatically collapsing in dispair, your rider guides the corrective actions that you take.

What happens when you take the reins and direct the horse toward antidepression actions? You are likely to experience conflict. At first, you may experience strong resistance. The horse won't budge. But you grip the reins. You channel the horse's energy and strength into a new direction. This takes mental effort, but by using your higher mental powers productively, you are less likely to be diverted.

Another way of understanding the conflict that you feel between taking action and dodging discomfort is to see it as a *double-agenda dilemma;* that is, you want the benefits of relief from depression. That's your stated agenda. But you also don't want to face uncertainties, doubt, and discomfort. That's your second

Believe you are helpless to overcome a depressed mood, and you've given yourself an excuse to procrastinate.

agenda. This is a core procrastination conflict. If you cave in to your second agenda, you are likely to continue to experience depression until it lifts on its own. Unfortunately, without having coping skills in place, depression is also more likely to return on its own. From past experience, you know that taking a walk gives you temporary relief from depression. Yet you also feel sluggish about starting, and that feeling of sluggishness can quickly turn into a source of resistance. You may tell yourself that when you feel sluggish, walking is impossible to do. But if your goal is to walk in order to feel less sluggish, then sluggishness is a weak excuse for not walking.

## Use the "Just Do It" Technique

Florida psychologist Robert Heller (pers. comm.) suggests a way to block the downward spiral of depression. He points out that when depressed, people tend to withdraw from others and from many activities of daily living, and they spiral downward with an increasing sense of isolation and loneliness. As an alternative, he suggests a "just do it" technique where you initially act without inspiration. The key is to interrupt the pattern.

Heller is less concerned about recognizing depressive thinking and connecting the dots between events, thoughts, and depressive feelings. He takes the position that by changing your behavior, you can shift your focus from depressive thoughts and premonitions to antidepression actions.

Heller suggests keeping an activity log as a motivational tool. The purpose of the log is to keep track of what you do each day and to gradually and consistently add activities, regardless of how you feel. This record also provides a way to measure your progress over time.

Through reviewing your ongoing record, you can also recognize gaps in your activities, say, where you avoid personal contacts that might help curb loneliness. You might then add activities where you spend time with others. This can include such simple gestures as greeting your neighbors or asking a store clerk where a product may be found. Instead of shopping once a week, you might choose to shop for a different basic item each day.

To benefit from this method, you would continue doing this exercise even if you experience no initial pleasure. After all, a prime feature of depression is a loss of pleasure. This exercise paves a path to feeling better.

## Increase Your Activity

Dr. Judith S. Beck, president of the Beck Institute for Cognitive Behavior Therapy and author of *Cognitive Behavior Therapy: Basics and Beyond*, is a strong proponent of helping people with depression become more active. Beck (pers. comm.) offers the following: "Many people who suffer from depression believe, 'Once I feel better, I will start calling friends again, going to the movies, playing tennis, making plans for a vacation.' They need psychoeducation. Research shows that they have put the cart before the horse. In order to feel better, people need to start getting actively reinvolved with life right away."

Beck says that even though her clients may understand this point, thoughts of procrastination will often interfere: "I help clients grasp the idea that their thoughts may be 100 percent true, 0 percent true, or some place in the middle. I tell them that I don't have a crystal ball, so I can't predict the validity of their predictions—but I also gently ask them whether they themselves have a crystal ball."

Beck asks her clients to do a little experimentation: "It is highly likely that they have already done the experiment of not calling friends, not going to movies, not playing tennis, or not planning a vacation. I ask them what has been the outcome of those experiments on their mood. Then I see what they're willing to try this week. I give them a low benchmark to aim for: 'It's worth doing an activity if it reduces your suffering by even 10 percent.' Then we predict, and respond to, likely thoughts they may have that will decrease the likelihood of following through with the activity and also thoughts that may spoil the enjoyment or sense of achievement they could receive during and after the activity."

She concludes, "Helping clients develop robust answers to their depressed thinking greatly increases the likelihood that they will follow through."

# APPLYING PROCRASTINATION TECHNOLOGY TO DEPRESSION

Procrastination technology is the application of methods and techniques to improve your performances by staying on track with doing what is relevant and timely. This technology brings a new dimension to combating depression. Here are a few basic counterprocrastination tactics that apply to depression.

**If a challenge is complex, break the activity down into subsets.** Even the most complex of tasks has a simple beginning.

**Take a bits-and-pieces approach.** As an example, here are some sample steps for targeting depressive thinking:

1. Log the content of your depressive thoughts.

2. Look for the flaws in the thoughts.

3. Seek plausible, positive, or neutral alternative views.

4. Play with perspective. Make up a jingle, such as "Mood moves mind." This says that a depressed mood begs for negative interpretations, such as "Life sucks." Remind yourself that you can have this type of overly general thought, but you don't have to take it seriously.

**Use your bits and pieces analysis to create a check-off list.** List the steps in their logical order (what you'll do first, second, and so forth). Check off the activities as you finish them. A sample check-off list follows:

| Step | Done |
|---|---|
| Look for flaws. | ✓ |
| Make up a jingle. | ✓ |
| Log depressive thoughts. | ✓ |
| Identify plausible alternatives. | ✓ |
|  |  |

**To break inertia, attack the items on your list using the five-minute method.** You agree with yourself to work on your self-development project for five minutes. At the end of that time, you decide whether to continue for another five minutes. You continue until your list is completed or you have gone far enough. Then, take a few extra minutes to prepare for the next step at a designated later time. It's easier to start later when you have the next step laid out for yourself.

There will come a time when depression diminishes and your energy returns. A new challenge may surface. You might think that you have too much catching up to do. If this frustrating thought arises, thinking that "it's useless to try to catch up" can follow it. Perhaps there's some truth to this statement. So, what's the other part of the story? The past is kaput. The present is now. Times change, and so do priorities. It's time to realign them and build toward your future.

At this point, you can make a new list of to-do activities representing their current value. This selection process includes dropping what may once have been important to do but is no longer viable. This is not exactly like starting with a clean slate, but it is a reasonable thing to do.

# WOULD BUDDHA MAKE A TO-DO LIST?

In an effort to curb their procrastination, practically everyone will try using a to-do list at one time or another. Is this a necessity or just another distraction? It depends.

To-do lists can be short: one to five items. Short lists are useful when it is important to keep focused on a few important items. On the other hand, throwing everything you can think of to do onto the list may be unrealistic. You might be biting off more than you can chew. Long daily lists are prescriptions for procrastination.

## A Path to Progress

If you asked Buddha how to obtain freedom from procrastination, he might say that you cannot desire freedom from procrastination because the desire would become the wall. You are the problem. Your ego takes up space. Don't desire. Be desireless. Given this view, would Buddha make a to-do list? Would Buddha put "exercising" on that list?

Different people have different goals, values, philosophies, and spiritual interests. So, if you want to follow the path of Siddhartha to a higher spiritual state, then the ordinary world of commerce and achievement is not your cup of tea. You have a different calling and a different concept of achievement. Thus, you probably won't gain from making a to-do list. You already know what you want to accomplish, and awareness and experience are your guide.

Although Buddha would be unlikely to follow a formal to-do list, you still can find value in constructing one to overcome depression. Use it as a tool to shift from diversionary actions to productive actions. Focus on self-improvement.

## Creating a Self-Improvement To-Do List

Self-improvement ranges from growing your musical talents to kicking an addiction to overcoming xenophobia to building confidence. Any of these goals is usually ongoing.

To start work on a self-improvement goal, ground your actions to meaningful, measurable, and attainable goals. Say you choose to work on your efficiency. You would then take three steps a day that are consistent with this goal. For example, to improve your efficiency, you might spend the first half hour of your day organizing and scheduling your activities for the remainder of the day. You then might spend one-half hour at an appointed time each day working on the novel you previously put off writing. You might spend fifteen minutes, from 10:00 to 10:15 a.m., clearing your mind of mental clutter. See chapter 17 for how to turn a schedule from your to-do list into one that gives you rewards for your efforts.

# YOUR SELF-IMPROVEMENT TO-DO LIST

Use the following chart to create a self-improvement to-do list, using the first item on the list as an example. In the left column, list self-improvement activities that you plan to do. If you think you might procrastinate or be sidetracked by another activity, also list the diversion that you will need to avoid. Check off completed activities, and check off the behavioral diversions that you have successfully avoided. This gives you a record of both accomplishments.

| Activity to Do | Done | Sidetracking Diversion to Avoid | Done |
|---|---|---|---|
| Example: *Getting up early to read the newspaper before going to work* | | *Hiding under the blankets* | |

Checking off completed items can feel rewarding.

# SEVEN PRINCIPLES FOR WAGING WAR AGAINST PROCRASTINATION

The nineteenth-century military strategist General Carl von Clausewitz (1968) wrote a classic book titled *Principles of War*. I've adapted his principles so that you can use them in overcoming procrastination.

## Principle of Preparation

You won't break a procrastination-depression barrier by retreating. But by understanding what you do when you needlessly delay, you can direct your efforts toward combating procrastination urges and actions as you address the correctable features in your depression.

A reasonable understanding and preparation for addressing procrastination, and the conditions where it appears, is important knowledge to have. To start your campaign against procrastination, put enough time into preparation to ensure that you know your motivations and mechanisms for procrastination. For example, you may have discomfort-dodging urges and then bicker with your mate instead of addressing depression hot spots that you identified through your procrastination inventory. With that awareness, you open options for changing direction.

> Von Clausewitz found that generals who hesitated and delayed were generals who faced certain defeat.

But avoid overpreparing, such as trying to learn all that you can about depression and procrastination before taking on this joint challenge. This can lead to analysis paralysis, indecisiveness, and more procrastination.

## Principle of Adaptability

Your rules of preparation will not apply in every case; sometimes you have to adapt to the circumstances. But while procrastination has varied causes and different styles, it also has common elements, such as side-tracking yourself at the first sign of a negative feeling. You can adapt this knowledge of diversion to changing circumstances and choose to act to stop procrastination at its inception.

Procrastination may also have unique features. In reactance procrastination, you may see the freedom to drink to the point of inebriation as a defensible right. Using the principle of adaptability, you would reframe this thought to recognize that an addiction like this represents a loss of freedom. You would then adjust your action accordingly.

## Principle of Concentration

It takes a deliberate effort to stay on a direct route to achieve reasonable goals, so concentrate your efforts for maximum impact. Focus your attention in the direction of importance; avoid dispersing your time and energy in frivolous activities. You know where that form of delay will get you.

Procrastination involves a series of distracting actions, such as reading a novel rather than preparing for an upcoming job interview. This form of delay puts you into a holding pattern as you wait for courage or inspiration. Instead, challenge yourself to identify an area where you'd ordinarily delay and concentrate your resources on starting your campaign against procrastination. Resist all distractions. Intentionally assert force to achieve the most productive outcomes.

## Principle of Balance and Momentum

Use only as much time and as many resources as you need to bring about the desired result. Unless hesitation is a tactic, don't waste your time delaying.

You may view actions to address pressing situations as onerous, laborious, and worthy of avoidance. Alternatively, think about where you can expend the least effort to produce the best outcome in changing the controllable aspects of depression, such as shifting negative thinking to at least neutral thinking. Time and pace yourself to follow through decisively.

## Principle of Boldness

Go on the offensive and vigorously pursue each opportunity to advance. Although there is no guarantee of success, advancing is positive. Unless they produce the best outcome, defense and retreat are negative.

Procrastination is a practice of retreat. Use proactive language to motivate your advance, such as "I will" and "I can." Proactive thinking opposes generalized pessimistic thinking, such as "Life is too tough for me to change."

## Principle of Efficiency

It's better to act soon to avoid a problem than to have to experience the stresses and penalties that often result from needless delays.

Delays from indecision can put you in a pickle. If one of your goals is to avoid putting yourself in a position where you have to extricate yourself from the consequences of delays, don't even consider retreat as an option. Instead, take a necessary step in the direction of victory, starting now.

## Principle of Persistence

Keep on the move. Envelop the procrastination enemy. Make each battle a decisive event. Focus on committing resources to decisive action. Disrupt enemy communications, such as the classic "I'll do it later" thinking that interferes with a timely execution of your plan. Expose this thinking for what it is: feeble excuse making. Go after procrastination's defensive positions, such as your urges to diverge. Vigorously pursue a do-it-now process to overpower your procrastination urges.

# YOUR WAR-ROOM CHART AGAINST PROCRASTINATION

Think of an activity that you believe would help alleviate the pain of depression but that you have put off doing. Make it your goal to do this activity. Then, working toward this goal, assemble the seven principles for waging war against procrastination. Write down how you will use each of these principles to forward your goal. Then apply your strategy and record the results.

Your goal:

| Principle | Application |
|---|---|
| **Preparation:** | |
| **Adaptability:** | |
| **Concentration:** | |
| **Balance and Momentum:** | |
| **Boldness:** | |
| **Efficiency:** | |
| **Persistence:** | |

# A POSITIVE CYCLE OF CHANGE

Procrastination can lead to a pileup where you put off so much that you feel overwhelmed. This *primary procrastination* may lead to depression. Even if you escape depression, this is an unhappy state. Depression has many causes. Regardless of the cause, when you feel depressed you are more likely to put things off that you can still do, such as taking corrective steps to stop feeling depressed. This is *secondary procrastination*. Let's look at what happens when primary and secondary procrastination co-occur.

Procrastination is an impediment to overcoming itself. It's also an impediment to overcoming depression when depression is a coexisting condition. Here's a closer look at how to get into a positive cycle of change.

In both procrastination and depression, you may delay or avoid taking corrective action. For example, if you believe you can't succeed in overcoming depression, you are likely to make a half-hearted effort or not try at all. Thus, you are more likely to continue feeling depressed until depression loses strength in time. This is a vicious circle:

1. You feel bound by depression.

2. You believe you can do nothing.

3. Your depression lingers.

If you believe you can do nothing, you are likely to put off trying. But you can break a procrastination-depression connection with a three-step positive cycle-of-change coping process:

1. You choose to cope with depression.

2. You attack procrastination that impedes coping by engaging a counterdepression activity that you believe can help but that you've put off.

3. You persist in coping with depression by sticking with the coping method, thus clearing procrastination from your path. This cycle-of-change activity applies to curbing both depression and procrastination.

As you procrastinate less in coping with depression, you help yourself break a vicious depressive pattern. As you start to feel better after taking coping actions, you have more energy and less reason to procrastinate. Here's a look at how this cycle-of-change technique works when exercise is a coping technique for changing from a depressed mood to a feel-good mood.

1. You put off exercising.

2. You take action to stop procrastinating around exercising.

3. As you engage in exercise, you feel better.

4. You procrastinate less around exercising.

Using this cycle-of-change technique, you can break the depression-procrastination connection and feel better.

# PACE YOURSELF

If you had a seasonal flu, you wouldn't expect yourself to perform normally. When you are mildly to seriously depressed, you'll normally scale back on what you do. But just as you would take care of yourself to get well from a flu, you can take prudent steps to curb your depression.

By addressing procrastination when you feel depressed, you evoke an activity remedy to help disrupt depression. However, when depressed, you may have to prioritize and pace yourself differently around doing things you would ordinarily do more easily.

Some activities are complex. Say you have a competitive analysis to do. If so, you may have to settle for working for shorter time intervals over a longer period of time. By accepting depression as a limitation, you don't expect yourself to be a superstar. You will probably also get more done and have less reason to feel down.

# YOUR "DO IT NOW" EXIT PLAN

"Do it now" is a prescription for addressing both procrastination and depression. The idea is that you do reasonable things in a reasonable way within a reasonable time for the sake of your personal efficiency, effectiveness, health, and happiness. Your pace, however, depends upon your energy and circumstance.

Plodding along, when you are depressed, is perfectly consistent with the do-it-now view. This pacing can actually reduce your risk of feeling overwhelmed. With less to feel overwhelmed about, you'll have less to feel depressed about.

When you are ready, here is the *procrastination endgame*. This involves doing the following to defeat procrastination and end depression:

- Strengthen your capability to execute efficiently and effectively.

- Experience competency.

- Buffer yourself against depression.

- Add to a growing sense of confidence that you can do better to get better.

Resign yourself to the fact that defeating depression requires time and purposeful effort, and you are less likely to walk into a wall constructed from a combination of procrastination and depressive thinking.

# END DEPRESSION PLAN

**Key ideas** (What three ideas did you find most helpful in this chapter?):

1.

2.

3.

**Action steps** (What three steps can you take to move closer to your goal of overcoming depression?):

1.

2.

3.

**Execution** (How did you execute the steps?):

1.

2.

3.

**Results** (What did you learn that you can use?):

1.

2.

3.

By making a small string of efforts—even when you feel lethargic—you may soon enough feel a growing confidence in your ability to take bigger steps.

## PART 2

# Recognizing and Defeating Depressive Thinking

Learn how to recognize and defuse depressive thinking.

Discover the freewill methods that helped the founder of psychology defeat his depression.

Apply Socratic methods to depressive thinking.

Use critical thinking to build a healthy perspective.

Address depression with Albert Ellis's famous ABCDE method.

Build a pluralistic self-view to broaden your perspective.

Use the circle-of-worth technique to build a healthy self-concept.

Boost your problem-solving abilities and get over feeling helpless.

Develop realistic optimism to do and get better.

Escape and stay out of the blame trap.

# CHAPTER 6

# Recognizing Depressive Thinking

Focus on unpleasant experiences, describe yourself as a failure, view your future as hopeless, and you are thinking depressively. These depressive thoughts are a form of double trouble. You experience the misery of the mood of depression. Negative, depressive thoughts make a bad situation even worse.

A depressed cat is free from this extra discord. It may mope, move slowly, and eat less. It may be irritable. Its usual purring and affections temporarily vanish. Thinking that the cat feels ill, you may feel concerned. Meanwhile, the cat just does its thing. The cat doesn't think of itself as a bad mouser, a worthless animal, unable to meet minimal cat standards; it doesn't think that its misery is unendurable or that it should throw itself off a bridge. This negative thinking is a peculiarly human affliction. The affected cat is spared this double trouble. It lives from moment to moment and day to day until its depression lifts.

Depression is nothing to take personally or to view as an indictment against your character. It is something to take seriously, as is double-trouble thinking. If you hear yourself thinking depressive thoughts, you're wise to take steps to neutralize them. Fortunately, these thoughts are far more changeable than the color of your eyes and your height. They are more like the clothing you wear. You can shed them and replace them with something more suitable.

## RECOGNIZING DEPRESSIVE THOUGHTS

Eighteenth-century physician Thomas Fuller said, "A disease known is half cured." When you identify, define, and articulate a problem, you have taken a big step in the direction of understanding and controlling the process.

Your thoughts and beliefs may blend with the physical sensations of depression. They have their own context (your perceptions and emotions) and content (what you tell yourself or believe). Shedding depressive thinking starts with recognizing the context and the content of these thoughts.

## Clues for Detecting Depressive Thinking

How can you tell if a thought is depressive? You can tell by its results. You feel worse. For example, you believe you can't change. That's a downer thought. Here are some other indications of depressive thinking, along with some antidotes:

- If a thought sounds depressive, it probably is depressive. For example, thoughts like "I'll never get over my loss" sound depressive. This extremist thought is likely to wane. Here, the antidote is to allow yourself time to heal.

- Overgeneralizations can deepen depression. Depressive thoughts like "Life is meaningless" can be misery makers. As a positive option, you can demystify what is happening by labeling this thinking as overgeneralization. You can then affirm that your life has meaning through the positive values that you follow.

- Depressive thinking is often circular. You tell yourself that you are going to continue to feel worse, then feel worse because of the thought, and then use the feeling as proof that you have no choice but to feel worse. You can break the cycle by seeing that this self-fulfilling thinking is discretionary.

- Depression may include *should*, *ought*, or *must* demand thinking. You lost a valued job. You tell yourself, "This should not be." You feel stressed. Balance this thinking with acceptance.

- *Awfulizing* is taking a bad situation and making it worse. Awfulizing beliefs, such as "It's awful that I have diabetes," often detract from problem solving. Corrective actions will get you farther than lamenting.

- Catastrophic expectations can worsen depression. You believe that you are doomed to stay depressed forever. You feel powerless and more depressed. You can counter this thinking with a realistic perspective. For example, define "doomed." Identify the overgeneralization in telling yourself that you will be depressed forever.

## Five Folks with Depressive Thoughts

Here's a look into the personal thoughts of five different people with depression.

### ■ Ken's Story

*Ken lost an important sale. He immediately thought, "This should not have happened to me." This thought triggered a negative stream of thoughts: "I can't do anything right." "I'm a failure." "I'm a complete fool." "I'm no good." "My family would be better off without me." "This is horrible." I can't stand it." For Ken, a lost sale—or anything that went wrong—was catastrophic. When these thoughts dominated, Ken felt miserable. This depressed mood could linger from hours to months.*

*Ken shifted from this self-absorbed, catastrophic view to one of objective self-observation. He reminded himself that sales are a percentage game. Although making a sale is a performance measure, it was not a measure of his self-worth. He concluded that while his sales performance can affect his income and standard of living, one lost sale was not an indictment of his whole life. His wife and family were far more important. What he thought of himself was more significant than his level of income.*

*Within a year, Ken felt significantly less pressured and less depressed. Partially because he wasn't so uptight about succeeding, his sales percentage improved.*

> You can tell depressive thinking by its results. You feel worse.

## ◼ Sandra's Story

*A significant depression can signal that something has gone wrong in your life. Sandra suffered a financial setback on the stock market. The market was depressed, and so was she. She told herself, "I've lost a fortune." "I can't retire." "I ought to have seen this recession coming." "I'm such a fool." "This is awful." This catastrophic thinking morphed into depressive thoughts, such as "It's hopeless." "I'll never recover." "I'll die poor and alone." This escalation in her distressful thinking added an emotional burden to her negative financial situation.*

*Because she felt depressed, Sandra thought her feelings of depression validated her depressive thinking. Sandra is not unique. When people get into distressful self-talk, they typically believe that the distress they experience validates their thoughts and vice versa.*

*Sandra made significant progress when she realized that the value she gave to her financial loss overshadowed another value, which was to act kindly toward others, including herself. That awareness helped break her circular-thinking loop.*

## ◼ Donna's Story

*Donna sobbed that she had married too soon and that must be why she felt so depressed. She wanted a divorce. She said she had been feeling this way for the past year.*

*"Marrying too soon" had nothing to do with Donna's depression. It was a desperate attempt to find a reason to explain her misery.*

*Donna was thirty when she married. She dated her husband for over a year before their engagement. Before that, she believed that she was getting too old to find a suitable mate. She paused when asked, "If you once saw yourself as too old to get married but now see yourself as having married too soon, how does this compute?"*

*Donna quickly saw the incongruity. She understood that these two ideas could not both be true. As she accommodated to this new awareness, she began to accept her depressed mood as unpleasant. As she stretched to think from a more objective perspective, she saw that the causes for her depression were likely more biological than social or psychological. This answer seemed palatable.*

*By accepting that her thinking about her depressed mood was manageable, Donna felt less depressed and finally not depressed. Around that time, she viewed her marriage as solid and her husband as loving. She was happy with her choice of a mate. She later mused, "I can't believe I once thought that my marriage caused my depression."*

*To help prevent depression, Donna acted to defeat passing depressing thoughts when she found herself slipping back. She called this her "mental workout," a mental discipline like jumping rope every day to stay in shape. (She also jumped rope each day to stay in shape and to buffer herself against future depressions.) Since then, she has experienced depressed moods from time to time and stoically lives through them. Compared to her past depression episodes, her depressive episodes are less frequent and intense.*

## ■ *Tim's Story*

*Tim was working at a low-paying, dead-end job where he felt pressured and stressed. He was living alone in a dangerous neighborhood. He drank too much and blamed the world for his problems. These conditions were risk factors for depression. Tim was depressed.*

*It took Tim over a year to stop drinking, work his way out of his depression, go back to school, and establish friendships to replace his loneliness. Once past the fog of depression, he discovered an interest in exploring and writing about the history of Native American tribes.*

*Tim's pivot point was simple and quick. At my suggestion, he did a cost-benefit analysis of continuing to blame the world for his problems versus assuming he was responsible for his depressive thinking and drinking. He recognized that he couldn't change the world but that he could change his thinking and life circumstances. He needed to stop drinking and take proactive steps to do and get better. Tim joined a self-help group to work on his addiction. He worked at changing his depressive thinking. He learned to cope more effectively at his workplace. As his anger and depression diminished, he took a series of career tests.*

*As of this writing, Tim has been sober for eight years, is in a new career that fits with his interests and talents, lives in a safe neighborhood, and is engaged to the "woman of [his] dreams." His life is far from perfect but great in comparison to his darker period.*

## ■ *Sally's Story*

*For most of her life, Sally described herself as a happy person. In the days before her depression, she looked forward to coming home from work and seeing her children at play. If the children were not doing their homework, she would tell them they could play after they finished it. She would do this in a good humor but with a quiet determination that got her message across.*

*Following an ugly divorce and unusual job pressures, Sally found herself slogging through her day. She felt cranky, irritable, and moody.*

*One day Sally came home from work, walked into her living room, and went wild when she saw "the mess." Her children were running and playing in the living room. She saw toys strewn everywhere. She saw their backpacks by the door. She knew they had not done their homework.*

*As a rush of negative thoughts went off like firecrackers in her head, she experienced a strong wave of tension. She found herself emotionally unraveling, screaming, and finally collapsing into a corner, sobbing uncontrollably.*

*Her outburst frightened her. She decided she needed to get help before her children hated her. In counseling, Sally began working on the connection between her thinking, mood, and behaviors. At first, this seemed like a mishmash to her, but by recognizing and writing down the sequence of her depressive thoughts, Sally turned a chaotic process into an orderly chain of thoughts:*

1. "I've had a difficult day."

2. "The kids should be quiet."

3. "They should have picked up before I came home."

4. "They should have done their homework."

5. "They're little monsters."

6. "I can't control them."

7. "I'm a bad mother."

8. "I can't control anything in my life."

9. "I'm doomed."

*Sally was struck by the negativity of her thoughts. She could admit to having a difficult day, but the rest of her thinking wildly misrepresented reality. Her kids' behavior was not the main issue. It wasn't even a major trigger. Her problem was her depressed mood and negative thoughts that were too general to be credible.*

*Sally gradually experienced peaceful acceptance of her depressed condition. She still felt depressed. Her job remained stressful. She felt sad over the loss of her marriage. However, as she felt more in command of herself, her depression lifted.*

*Ten years later, Sally was in a new and solid marriage. Her children were all doing well in their young adult lives. She reported no more than a few scattered days of feeling depressed.*

# A COLLECTION OF CRIPPLING COGNITIONS

Negative cognitions strongly contribute to the development of depression. To free yourself from the extra burden of these cognitions, it's important to recognize them, learn self-corrective actions, and then work toward executing these actions. The following overlapping cognitive distortions coexist with depression and reflect and spur negativity (Burns 1999).

## *Overgeneralizing*

When you overgeneralize, you draw conclusions on the basis of one or a few factors, even invented ones. For example, after making an error, you think you can't do anything right. When you feel depressed, such overgeneralizing can take on a life of its own. Your lover ditches you. Your mood turns dark and worsens when you think, "I'll never be able to find anybody to love me." But can you prove that you'll never find anyone to love you? Ask yourself this question, and you are likely to discover that you're overgeneralizing.

The key is to look for exceptions. First, you can expect yourself to feel little satisfaction when you feel depressed. That goes with the territory. Now, using your objective self-observation abilities, explore the positive parts of your life. What do you value that you can still achieve? What conditions are improving or can improve?

> "There is nothing either good or bad, but thinking makes it so."
>
> —William Shakespeare

If you have difficulty recognizing overgeneralizations, a clue resides in the verb "to be." The statement "I am helpless," for example, is a generalization because of the verb. Can you be only one way? What if you were to label yourself "wonderful"? When you are depressed, the word has little credibility. Nevertheless, while labeling yourself "wonderful" is far better than labeling yourself "helpless" or "worthless," it's an overgeneralization too. Who can be only one way?

There is a quick technique for addressing generalized "to be" thinking in depression. Substitute the phrase "I act" for the phrase "I am." By saying that you "act helpless," instead of saying that you "are helpless," you can examine whether you can act in only one way or not.

## Magnifying and Minimizing

Have you ever met anyone who does not, from time to time, make a mountain out of a molehill and dwell on a situation long after its moment has passed? It's human nature to fall into this magnification trap. However, when you exaggerate the negative, you are likely to suffer longer than if you were to take most matters in stride.

Some people are masters of understatement. They downplay their positive attributes and accomplishments and take negative incidents and make them unimportant. Although this may be a form of humbleness, depression minimizing is different. If you have a stressful job, you minimize the role stress plays in your depression. You do nothing about the situation because "it is not that important." A cost-benefit analysis can yield a different perspective. What are the short- and long-term advantages and disadvantages of dealing with the situation? What is a reasonable first step to take?

## Catastrophizing

*Catastrophizing* describes how people exaggerate negatives: a small event explodes into an end-of-the-world situation. The observation that people catastrophize goes back at least as far as Buddha. The concept of *catastrophic howling* (Williams 1923) is a later ancestor of this idea, but Albert Ellis is best known for applying it therapeutically.

Here is an example of catastrophizing. A friend sounds short with you. You tell yourself, "My friend hates me. I can't maintain my relationships. I'll die old and alone." However, what would it then mean if you discovered that your friend had been coming down with the flu and later acted as friendly as usual?

When depressed, you may have medically unexplained symptoms, such as headaches, fatigue, and lower-back pain. You may jump to conclusions and imagine having a serious but unknown disease. You may catastrophize by telling yourself that your physicians are incompetent because they can't find a medical cause, and you'll surely die because of this omission. However, if you successfully question your catastrophic thinking, you add to your chances of gaining longer-term relief from depression (Steinbrecher and Hiller 2011).

To help yourself break the links in a catastrophic chain, seek alternative explanations that suggest different results. Separate facts from exaggerations. Label exaggerations as "exaggerations." Focus on what you can do. Make a plan. Take the steps.

## Dichotomous Thinking

In the world of depressive thinking, variability is ruled out and replaced with dichotomous thinking. This is a black-and-white form of thinking. You are either a good person or you are a bad person. There is no variability, no middle ground. If you declare yourself a bad person, you combine overgeneralizations with magnifications.

The dichotomous thinking fallacy lies in its lack of variability. To combat this line of thinking, look for exceptions. Look for shades of gray.

## Mental Filtering

In mental filtering, you exclude what doesn't fit with what you want to hear. It's typical in mental filtering to look for the one negative within a general picture and to exclude the rest of the image. For example, Ben is depressed and loathes himself. Kathy tells Ben, "You work so well with your hands. You do exquisite carpentry work." Ben replies, "But I have calluses," which is a response that shows his negative bias and allergy toward compliments.

If you don't expect to have pleasant experiences, as a rule of thumb, you are probably going to discount and filter out such experiences. You can use a balancing exercise to restore some perspective, however. This means intentionally adding a contrasting view when you're inclined to only see the negative. For example, cite in writing as many factors as you can—good, bad, and neutral—that relate to a situation where you show a filtering bias. This balancing approach interferes with the automatic part of mental filtering. You may still give disproportionate weight to the negative. But you have set your mental wheels in motion to balance your view.

## Jumping to Conclusions

Jumping to conclusions means that you are guessing before you have justified the facts. When depressed, you are likely to judge situations based upon your depression-related expectations. For example, your depression lingers, so you jump to the conclusion that you are helpless to break free from the web of depression.

You can practice suspending judgment until you have the facts or a reasonable basis for a conclusion. Putting reason between an impression and a conclusion can give you a sense of increased mental flexibility. You'll increase your chances of drawing wiser conclusions.

## Fortune-Telling

In a pessimistic state of mind, you see only gloom and doom in your future. But you can no more predict your future than a fortune-teller could read it using a deck of tarot cards. Avoid fortune-telling of all sorts. Rather than foreclosing on your future, stay open to your experiences.

## Mind Reading

Some people make a studied habit of trying to read other people's motives, temperaments, intentions, and even thoughts. But mind reading requires a telepathy that humans don't have. True, you can anticipate what some people believe because you know them well enough, or you can pick up cues from what they say. Mind reading, however, involves reading into an interpersonal situation more than is actually there.

When faced with a situation where you speculate on what someone is thinking about you, consider suspending judgment until you get credible verification or learn something different.

## Emotional Reasoning

In emotional reasoning, you trust your feelings too much. You act as if your emotions were evidence for your thoughts, beliefs, and perceptions. This is a classic circular form of reasoning. You think of yourself as being inadequate and believe that the feeling validates that you are as you think. The emotions you experience are real enough. But the thoughts behind the emotions can be gross distortions of reason.

To break through emotional reasoning, examine the thoughts you associate with the emotions. Weed out the thoughts that feed the emotional part of the circle. Separate facts that you can objectively verify from subjective impressions. Imposing reason between emotion and reaction is a classical way to break the circle.

## Labeling

Put a belittling label on yourself, and you strip away positive aspects of your humanity. You may call yourself a "failure," an "idiot," a "jerk," a "knucklehead," a "loser," "worthless," or "useless." To confront this cognitive distortion, define what you mean by the label you use. Ask yourself how this label, and only this label, applies 100 percent to you 100 percent of the time. If you think you are a failure, consider that a failing action is not the same as being a total failure as a person. Next, think of ten ordinary things you do that do not fit the definition. Can you see why labeling yourself is an overgeneralization?

## Personalizing

In personalizing, you take credit for the blame in situations that you neither control nor influence, and you may feel guilty about what are often fictions.

You may feel self-conscious about another's behavior. For example, your mate gets drunk and acts like a jerk. You think all eyes are on you. However, if you saw a similar circumstance played out by another couple, you'd probably focus your attention on the person who was drunk and not blame his companion. You might even feel sorry for the companion.

If you find yourself in a personalizing trap, ask and answer these questions: "Do I think it is a bit excessive to think that what goes wrong is always my fault? Do I have the kind of power to cause others to think largely about my foibles? If I feel insecure because I think I lack worth, then why would people pay attention to me?"

# RECOGNIZING COGNITIVE DISTORTIONS

Hopefully, you now have a better understanding of the cognitive distortions that commonly coexist with depression. It's also important to know that cognitive distortions are usually some blend of magnifying, over-generalizing, and catastrophizing. Instead of many forms of depressive thoughts, you may have many examples of a few distortions.

## *Turning Feelings into Thoughts*

You say, "I feel hopeless." Is hopelessness a thought that evokes a feeling or a thought that reflects a feeling? Either way, hopelessness is a bridge from mind to mood.

When you tell yourself that you feel "hopeless," "helpless," or "worthless," you have identified the thoughts behind some negative feelings. To expand your understanding of the meaning behind these emotive expressions, you can translate your thinking into a framework for recognizing depressive thoughts. As in the chart, you preface each statement with "I tell myself…"

| Depressive Feelings | Translation into Depressive Thoughts |
|---|---|
| "I feel hopeless." | "I tell myself that my situation is hopeless when I experience depression." |
| "I feel helpless." | "I tell myself that there is nothing I can do to make positive changes." |
| "I feel worthless." | "I tell myself that I have no value, and therefore, there is nothing to do to change this outlook." |

Notice how in doing this, you take ownership of your depressive thinking. Thoughts like "I feel worthless" can seem permanent. Preface this thinking with "I tell myself," and you've logically removed this sense of permanence. For example, you can tell yourself something different.

## TRANSLATE YOUR FEELINGS INTO THOUGHTS

Use the following chart to translate your depressive feelings into correctable depressive thoughts. In the left column, write down how you feel, starting with "I feel…." In the right column, translate this expression into a depressive thought, starting with the phrase "I tell myself…."

| Depressive Feelings | Translation into Depressive Thoughts |
|---|---|
|  |  |
|  |  |
|  |  |

## Detecting Depressive Deceptions

People normally don't consciously go out of their way to fool themselves. Rather, they have some self-deceiving habits of mind.

When you are depressed, how do you know when you are deceiving yourself? Use the following five-point plausibility checklist:

1. State the suspected depressive idea.

2. Ask yourself five plausibility questions.

3. Answer each question with a simple yes or no.

4. Give your reason for your conclusion.

Here is an example: Your friend Bart borrowed money from you under the false pretense that he needed a temporary loan to keep his business going. Instead, he gambled the money away in an ill-fated hope that he could make enough money to pay his business expenses and pay you back. Now he can't and won't repay you. Here is a plausibility check on a depressive idea.

# PLAUSIBILITY CHECK

Depressive idea: "I'll never get over Bart's betrayal and will suffer forever."

| Plausibility Questions | Yes | No | Basis for Conclusion |
|---|---|---|---|
| 1. Does this idea seem plausible? | | ✓ | There is a partial truth here. Betrayals will negatively affect most reasonable people. Suffering a dollar loss from deception can be emotionally rattling. However, saying you will suffer forever is jumping to a conclusion. |
| 2. Does the idea fit with expected life experiences? | | ✓ | Betrayals are inevitable. |
| 3. Is this idea consistent with known facts or probabilities? | | ✓ | Loaning money to a gambler is risky. It's also risky making a prediction that you stay burdened with the results of a betrayal forever. It's like making a magical leap from what is remotely possible to what is certain. |
| 4. Is there an advantage to believing this idea? | | ✓ | There is no healthy advantage in believing that you will suffer forever. |
| 5. Would knowledgeable and rational people agree with this idea? | | ✓ | Most would agree that Bart's deception was costly. Feeling bad about the betrayal and loss is reasonable. Distrusting Bart now makes sense. There is no requirement to overgeneralize and expect to suffer forever. |

All in all, the idea of suffering forever doesn't fit with experience. Depression lifts. Dollars lost can sometimes be recovered.

The plausibility test helps you to get a perspective on your own thinking and to eliminate self-deceptions. Try it and see.

# YOUR PLAUSIBILITY TEST

First state your depressive idea. Then answer yes or no to the following five questions and give a basis for your conclusion.

Depressive idea: _____

| Plausibility Questions | Yes | No | Basis for Conclusion |
|---|---|---|---|
| 1. Does this idea seem plausible? | | | |
| 2. Does the idea fit with expected life experiences? | | | |
| 3. Is this idea consistent with known facts or probabilities? | | | |
| 4. Is there an advantage to believing this idea? | | | |
| 5. Would knowledgeable and rational people agree with this idea? | | | |

## *Statements in Disguise*

Some questions that depressed people ask themselves are statements in disguise. They are rhetorical questions with a known answer. The question "Why can't I do anything right?" is a statement in disguise. Rather than indict yourself, indict the idea.

You may ask the question, "Why is this happening to me?" Let's assume your default answer is that you deserve punishment. You've now identified a statement in disguise.

By translating this question into a statement, you have taken a step forward in identifying a punitive depressive belief. Once you catch yourself expressing this belief, you can flip it. If you believe you deserve punishment, in what ways and for what reasons do you deserve to give yourself self-acceptance?

When you think depressively, you look through a distorted lens. The lens stays distorted until you dial it into focus.

As an alternative to closed-ended, statement-in-disguise questions, switch to open-ended questions, such as "How might I uproot depressive thinking in order to increase my chances for getting relief from depression?" Open-ended questions promote inquiry and discovery.

Recognizing depressive thoughts, categorizing them, and questioning their validity is an activity remedy for depression with a big side benefit. You may find yourself increasingly alert to the overgeneralizations, biases, and distorted thinking of others, including well-known news commentators and political pundits who routinely skirt issues and distort reality through overgeneralizations and other forms of cognitive distortions. However, the most important change is that you may recognize that there are many ways to view and categorize negative thinking, and you can choose how you go about doing this. A crucial issue, however, is what you do about the thoughts that you categorize. That is the subject of the next chapter.

# END DEPRESSION PLAN

**Key ideas** (What three ideas did you find most helpful in this chapter?):

1.

2.

3.

**Action steps** (What three steps can you take to move closer to your goal of overcoming depression?):

1.

2.

3.

**Execution** (How did you execute the steps?):

1.

2.

3.

**Results** (What did you learn that you can use?):

1.

2.   .

3.

# CHAPTER 7

# Confronting Depressive Thinking

In his old TV sitcom in which he played a psychologist, Bob Newhart came up with a two-word solution for any problem: "Stop it."

I wish it were that simple and easy to correct complex mental health problems. But making important personal changes ordinarily takes more than a slogan. The process of defeating depression normally takes learning, understanding, and following guided problem-solving actions directed toward exposing the flaws in depressive thinking and dismantling depressive thoughts and themes.

You can't automatically erase a tendency to feel depressed. You can't just stop it. But you can take corrective actions. You can choose how to change depressive thinking. This chapter will show you how to make positive changes in three ways, by exercising free will and choice, applying Socratic reasoning, and using critical thinking.

## CHOOSING TO CHANGE

When your future is shrouded by depressive pessimism, you may treat pessimism as the truth. But what if you were to decide to act as if you could free yourself from this thought affliction? That choice could be transformational.

The French philosopher Charles Renouvier (1842) saw that people often act as if they are blind to the power of their negative habits, yet they don't intentionally bring bad things upon themselves. Freedom from these negative habits comes from freely and willfully choosing a different path.

William James, the nineteenth-century founder of American psychology who suffered from repeated bouts of a debilitating depression, found relief using Renouvier's philosophy of free will. James decided to believe that by changing his thinking, he could turn his life around. He then did what he thought he could do.

Is freedom from depressive thinking a choice? Although free will may be a trick of the mind, people do change their depressive thinking by adopting a more pluralistic perspective. For example, hopelessness is a thought. You can exercise free will by considering ideas that contradict hopelessness thinking. That action can give you a broader perspective and help you be less negative in your thinking.

"Why has the will an influence over the tongue and fingers, not over the heart and liver?" asked the eighteenth-century philosopher David Hume (2008, 48). Hume rightly points out that you'll face limitations in asserting control over aspects of yourself. Nevertheless, you can act to gain freedom from depressive thinking when you do the following:

- Monitor mood-related thinking.

- Extract depressive thoughts.

- Formally apply depressive-thought recognition criteria to separate reasonable thoughts from depressing exaggerations.

- Put depressive thoughts into categories.

- Determine which categories of thought represent a choice. (Blaming yourself for being depressed is a choice.)

- Look for exceptions to depressive thoughts. (Helplessness represents a general idea that can be true in specific situations but not at all times.)

## Freedom and Restriction

Feeling an itch is not a choice. Automatically scratching the itch is an impulse. Choice comes into play when you exercise restraint, such as stopping yourself from scratching when it could cause or worsen an infection.

Choice and change are pivotal to most forms of psychotherapy, including therapies for addressing depression. In general, this process involves developing realistic awareness, engaging in problem-solving actions, restricting negative activities, and building on positive thoughts and actions. Change is earned and comes from an effort to do and get better by reducing the negatives and increasing the positives in your life.

You can approach change from different but related angles. You can sometimes change the context for events by making environmental changes. You can change the concepts (values, beliefs) you apply to events. You can change the content of your thoughts. These choices involve restrictions of old habits and assertions of new actions.

If you choose to correct your negative thinking, you are likely to do yourself considerable good. You can quell your current depressive thoughts, build confident composure (active acceptance of self, others, and life), and create barriers against future depressions. Even when you have a biologically based bipolar depression, by lifting the extra burden of depressive thinking, you may feel considerably better if you cycle into a depressive episode.

## Can't, Won't, and Will

You feel immobilized by depression. It's not that you absolutely can't, say, sharpen a pencil. You just think you can't. You'll get beyond depression sooner by accepting that you often need to push yourself to do some of the smallest activities of daily living, even when you tell yourself it's impossible.

You can hold two contradictory thoughts: "I'm too depressed and immobilized to move, so I can't" and "I feel depressed, but I can still blink my eyes and sharpen a pencil." The second belief is true. Accepting it as the truth means you can assert measured control over your actions.

You can't go back to an earlier time, but you can reset a clock that gives the wrong time.

How do you sharpen a pencil when you hear yourself say *I can't*? Change course by transitioning from *I can't* to *I won't* to *I will*. In fact, "I can't" means that something is impossible to do. You can't pick up a giant Sequoia tree by its roots and single-handedly toss it into space. When it comes to sharpening a pencil, "I can't" really means "I won't."

If you tell yourself something like, "I don't feel like sharpening the pencil, so I won't," you are being honest about how you feel. However, if your goal is to use activity as a remedy for depression, and sharpening the pencil is one of those remedies, you'll need to push yourself further.

Saying "I will" sets a different tone. You can *will* yourself to sharpen that pencil, provided that you give yourself the mental instruction and stretch to do so. Although depression may weaken your force of will, this inner resource doesn't go on vacation. Rather, it awaits your call to action. You can activate it by asserting the phrase "I will" and then mechanically acting on the assertion.

## Powerlessness and Procrastination

"I can't" may signal a form of powerlessness thinking and resignation. When you feel depressed, telling yourself that you are powerless to sharpen a pencil is a belief and not a fact. In fact, this is a form of procrastination thinking, where you identify a solution to a problem but believe that you can do nothing to execute the first step. With this kind of thinking as your guide, you'll keep delaying.

What if, instead of saying "I can't" to describe how you feel, you were to substitute the words "it's impossible for me"? For example, "It's impossible for me to sharpen a pencil. It's impossible for me to stop feeling anxious or depressed. It's impossible for me to stop drinking." Really? Is this true? Are these actions as impossible as throwing a giant Sequoia into space? If they are less impossible, then they are possible. However, they still may be difficult actions to undertake.

# THE SOCRATIC METHOD

The ancient Greek philosopher and teacher Socrates was renowned for his ability to ask pointed questions to get to the "truth." Socrates invited his students to examine their premises and opinions in order to gain knowledge about themselves and their surroundings.

Socrates used a three-pronged method to distinguish truth from falsity, and you can apply this method to defeat needlessly depressing thoughts. You will need to do the following:

1. Define a specific depressive thought.

2. Give examples that support the definition.

3. Give exceptions.

If you said you were helpless to escape depression, Socrates might ask, "Can you tell me what you mean by 'helpless'?" You might respond, "I can't change." Socrates might then ask you for examples of how you can't change. You might respond, "Whatever I do, I stay depressed." Socrates might then ask you to give examples of when depression has lifted. You might respond, "When I take a fast walk." Socrates might then point to the truth with the following question: "If you can't change, then why do you feel better when you walk?"

Here's another example of the Socratic method applied to the depressive thought, "I can't do anything right."

1.  Define the thought: "Whatever I do, I will do wrong."

2.  Give examples that support the thought: an error on a tax return; a missed opportunity by applying for a job too late.

3.  Give exceptions: obtaining an education and advanced degree; finding a wonderful mate; taking charge of a crisis when a neighbor was injured.

When you tell yourself that you "can't do anything right," it may help to look more closely at the context in which this thought occurred. Does this "can't do" view refer to acting less effectively than you'd prefer in a specific situation? If so, you may have caught yourself in an overgeneralization. By shedding this distortion, you may get closer to a core issue: you may be hard on yourself because you are intolerant of your imperfections.

If you define yourself as helpless, you may be in a circular-thinking loop: "I can't do anything right because I'm helpless, and because I'm helpless I can't do anything right." Recognizing this circular thinking opens opportunities to start to break free of it. If you have defined "helpless" as an inability to do anything right, what is "anything"? What is "right"? Defining your terms, you may cast light on how to exit from the loop. You may indeed be helpless to change a past loss, if this is how you define being "helpless," but even so, you have a choice. You can lament the unchangeable. You can accept that you can't go back, but you can apply what you learned as you move forward.

# YOUR SOCRATIC THINKING EXERCISE

Use the following chart to examine a depressive thought, using the Socratic method. First identify the thought. Then define it and give examples that support the thought and any exceptions that come to mind.

| | |
|---|---|
| Depressive thought | |
| Definition | |
| Examples | |
| Exceptions | |

Use this variation on the Socratic method as a tool to help break the links between a depressed mood and its associated thoughts. Through this exercise for gaining clarity, you may find that you have fewer depressive thoughts to address. You will get the added benefit of practicing a thinking tool that you can use in other situations where it's important to separate truth from fallacy.

# USING CRITICAL THINKING

Critical thinking researcher Richard Paul (1990) developed another Socratic questioning process that you can adapt to defeat depressive thinking. In this six-point process, you ask yourself a series of questions to help you define and examine the truth of any depressive thought.

You can apply this technique to practically any form of depressive thinking. The following chart gives hopelessness thinking as an example, with sample questions, responses, and conclusions.

# CRITICAL THINKING EXPERIMENT

Example of a depressive thought: "I have no hope for the future."

| Clarifying Questions | Questions about Assumptions | Questions about Facts and Evidence | Questions about Viewpoints | Questions about Consequences | Questions about Questions |
|---|---|---|---|---|---|
| Question 1: "What do I mean when I tell myself that I have no hope?" | Question 2: "What am I assuming about the future?" | Question 3: "Does hopelessness thinking reflect a factual reality?" | Question 4: "What could disprove a hopelessness outcome?" | Question 5: "What are the consequences of pessimistic thinking?" | Question 6: "Do the previous five questions refocus my thinking?" |
| Response 1: "Nothing changes." | Response 2: "I have a crystal ball that tells all." | Response 3: "There is no compelling evidence that hopelessness is factual." | Response 4: "Finding exceptions to hopelessness thinking." | Response 5: "Doom thinking layers depression onto depression." | Response 6: "The questions can help me restructure my thinking from depressive thoughts to suspending judgments." |
| Conclusion 1: "That's implausible." | Conclusion 2: "That's implausible." | Conclusion 3: "Hopelessness depressive thinking reflects a subjective impression, not a factual reality." | Conclusion 4: "Defeating hopelessness thinking is doable." | Conclusion 5: "Beyond creating its own self-fulfilling prophecy, pessimistic thinking does not necessarily accurately predict the future." | Conclusion 6: "It is possible to shift thoughts from narrow pessimism to a realistic perspective?" |

# YOUR CRITICAL THINKING EXPERIMENT

Following the previous example, test this critical thinking system against one of your depressive thinking themes. First state your depressive thought. Then define what you mean with a clarifying question, question your assumptions, question the facts and evidence, look for other viewpoints, question the consequences of this kind of thinking, and finally ask yourself if this exercise of asking questions has changed how you think.

Your depressive thought: _____

| Clarifying Questions | Questions about Assumptions | Questions about Facts and Evidence | Questions about Viewpoints | Questions about Consequences | Questions about Questions |
|---|---|---|---|---|---|
| Question 1: | Question 2: | Question 3: | Question 4: | Question 5: | Question 6: |
| Response 1: | Response 2: | Response 3: | Response 4: | Response 5: | Response 6: |
| Conclusion 1: | Conclusion 2: | Conclusion 3: | Conclusion 4: | Conclusion 5: | Conclusion 6: |

Well-articulated questions can point to gaps in knowledge and possibly to wisdom in an area where once there were gaps. By using this method, you can recognize gaps in your knowledge, and you can take steps to fill them.

# END DEPRESSION PLAN

**Key ideas** (What three ideas did you find most helpful in this chapter?):

1.

2.

3.

**Action steps** (What three steps can you take to move closer to your goal of overcoming depression?):

1.

2.

3.

**Execution** (How did you execute the steps?):

1.

2.

3.

**Results** (What did you learn that you can use?):

1.

2.

3.

# CHAPTER 8

# Albert Ellis's ABCDE Method

When you feel depressed, you will often have multiple distressing thoughts that go through your mind. You may think about events that you associate with your depression and then think about a specific event. Then your mind may jump to pessimistic ideas and then on to something else that is negative.

In fact, depressive thinking is rarely linear. It's more like a cacophony of clashing sounds. These thoughts can go from pessimism to feelings of worthlessness to self-blame to blaming others, and so on. As you monitor, recognize, and give these depressive thoughts a linear order, you will find it easier to examine and correct them. Albert Ellis's (2003) ABCDE method for doing this is easy to learn and use.

## LEARNING YOUR ABCDE'S

The letters ABCDE stand for activating events, beliefs, consequences, disputation, and new effects. Here's how the system works.

### Activating Events

A neighbor's cat enters through an open window and shreds the fabric of your expensive couch. You get a flat tire. As you're standing in line, a person in front of you gabs with a clerk while you're in a hurry. Your best friend comes for a visit. You get a pay raise and a letter of commendation for your work. What do these situations have in common? They are activating events: how you evaluate and judge them can evoke emotional and behavioral reactions. For example, you might become angry upon seeing the cat scratch your couch if you were to think, "The owner of this damned cat should have kept it locked up. I can't stand this." You'd likely feel differently if you disliked the couch and now had an excuse to buy another—perhaps at your neighbor's expense.

## *Beliefs about Events*

We are a believing species. We all believe in something, whether it's believing in god or believing in freedom or believing that it's bad luck to walk under ladders. Some beliefs are fact based, such as believing that weather patterns vary in New England. Others may exist without substance, such as believing that angels dance on the heads of pins.

The power of belief was recognized and used by the ancient Babylonian king Hammurabi to control his population. When Hammurabi introduced his legal codes, he faced the problem of enforcement. He knew his agents could not be everywhere to apprehend people violating any of his 281 laws, so he told his people that the laws came directly from the sun god, Shamash. He said that if his agents did not discover those who violated the god's laws, the god would surely see the violation and sooner or later punish the offender.

If anyone doubts the power of beliefs, consider what motivated the kamikaze pilots of World War II. Some—perhaps the majority—of these suicidal pilots believed that by crashing their planes into US ships, they would go directly to heaven.

It is impossible to have human intelligence and not have beliefs. These beliefs weave through our lives and give a certain sense of constancy and stability to what we do and to how we feel. Some, however, cause more harm than good.

> It isn't so much what people tell themselves to get themselves depressed. Most will pick up on that right away. Rather, it is the mental structures that lurk beneath negative thought patterns that are the troublemakers and normally take time to change.

Depressive beliefs sprinkle melancholia with dispiriting ideas. An extreme idea is that you can never escape the grip of depression. If you take this proposition as truth, it feels real. However, while the emotions that can extend from this thought are real, the underlying idea is seriously flawed.

When you feel depressed and are guided by harmful beliefs, a basic challenge is to cull out the false from reasonable beliefs about yourself, your abilities to make changes, what you can do to shape your future, and how to escape the grip of these and other harmful beliefs.

Examining what you believe is the centerpiece of Ellis's system. If you believe that you can't escape depression, you are likely to deny that you have any exceptions to this belief. However, using and strengthening reasoned thinking is a prescription for combating depressive beliefs. Finding exceptions creates an incongruity to resolve between not being able to escape depression and recognizing exit points that you have already found and used.

Ellis divides beliefs into rational and irrational categories. He links rational beliefs to functional motivations and actions and connects irrational beliefs to dysfunctional emotions and behavior.

## RATIONAL BELIEFS

Rational beliefs are propositions of truth that are functional and based in reality. Healthy rational beliefs are ordinarily objective and lead to constructive actions. They support personal development and the pursuit of happiness, including the reduction and prevention of depression.

How can you tell if a belief is rational? Such beliefs represent reasonable, objective, flexible, and constructive conclusions or inferences about reality that support survival, happiness, and healthy results. The questions that follow can help you determine if your belief is healthy and rational.

- Does your belief promote productivity and creativity?

- Does your belief support positive relationships?

- Does your belief prompt accountability without unnecessary blame and condemnation?

- Does your belief encourage acceptance and tolerance?

- Does your belief strengthen persistence and self-discipline?

- Does your belief serve as a platform for conditions that propel personal growth?

- Does your belief correlate with healthy risk-taking initiatives?

- Does your belief link to a sense of emotional well-being and positive mental health?

- Does your belief lead to a realistic sense of perspective?

- Does your belief improve your career performances and opportunities?

- Does your belief stimulate openness to experience and an experimental outlook?

- Does your belief direct your efforts along ethical pathways?

If your belief fits several of these positive criteria, it is likely to be rational and lead to positive results. For example, believing that it is important to meet your responsibilities is a rational belief that normally yields advantages.

Rational beliefs can be tested by their results. If you believe that you can help yourself overcome depression by successfully disputing depressive thinking, and you act according to this belief, the chances are you'll gain relief from depression.

## IRRATIONAL BELIEFS

We all have flaws in our thinking (see the discussion of cognitive distortions in chapter 6). Like blind spots, some are hard to see. But by accepting that you will have blind spots, you are more likely to think about your thinking and act to change harmful beliefs once you can see what they are.

Irrational beliefs refer to any thoughts that are inconsistent with reality, though not all are harmful. For example, you may believe that grasshoppers can communicate with crickets because they both make sounds with their legs. This belief is irrational because, as far as we know, there is no interspecific communication between grasshoppers and crickets. However, this belief is unlikely to have any meaningful effect on your mood, behavior, or life. It may be irrational, but it is probably harmless.

Harmful irrational beliefs are arbitrary, subjective, unscientific, and lead to negative results. By definition, harmful irrational beliefs are unhealthy. They cloud your consciousness with distortions, misconceptions, overgeneralizations, and oversimplifications. They limit and narrow your outlook. They lead to pernicious feelings and dysfunctional activities.

Here are some questions you can use to help yourself identify harmful depressive beliefs:

- Does the belief link with a mood of depression and exaggerate that mood?

- Does the belief promote a sense of pessimism, fatalism, or defeatism?

- Does the belief evoke a sense of helplessness?

- Does the belief generate feelings of worthlessness and self-blame?

- Does the belief interfere with your relationships?

- Does the belief impede your ability to manage basic activities of daily living?

- Does the belief detract you from pursuing meaningful personal goals?

If your belief meets any of these seven criteria, it is likely to be irrational. When irrational depressive beliefs actively dominate your consciousness, your rational thoughts can sound like a faint murmur in the background. But you can bring your rational thoughts out of hiding so that they become active, dominant thoughts. When rational thoughts are the active thoughts, the depressive beliefs tend to fade.

## Consequences

In Ellis's framework, *consequences* refers to both emotional and behavioral results that stem from your beliefs. Mapping the connection between depressive thoughts, emotions, and behaviors opens opportunities to cut those connections and thus change the consequences.

Rational beliefs usually have beneficial consequences, or outcomes. Self-efficacy is a belief in your abilities to organize, regulate, and direct your actions to accomplish positive results. Possible emotional and behavioral consequences of self-efficacy are confident composure and motivated actions. Increasing positive activity levels can help counteract depression. All things being equal, act on a self-efficacy belief, and you are likely to overcome depression quicker than someone who believes that he has no hope.

Harmful irrational beliefs have both emotional and behavioral consequences. When you believe that you are helpless to change and you have no hope, and then you blame yourself for what you claim you can't control, you have an irrational thought with the power to evoke negative emotional consequences. When you believe you can't do anything to defeat depression, you are likely to languish with a downtrodden emotional sense of helplessness.

A behavioral consequence can be withdrawing from activities with significant others. Another is procrastinating on following through on self-help measures to curb depression.

## Disputation

It's human nature to be suggestible, to develop false beliefs, and to hang on to those beliefs. It is here where you have an opportunity to shift from a self-absorbing depressive perspective to an objective self-observant perspective. For example, you can observe what you think and do and apply objective methods to the task of escaping the trap of depression thinking.

A person who has never experienced significant depression may feel puzzled about how people with depression can hold on to depressive beliefs. Can they not see that the premises behind the thoughts only serve to perpetuate an already miserable state? But depressive thoughts are well connected to each other and to depressive sensations. When you are depressed, it takes time to recognize and weed out depressive thoughts and develop competitive networks of rational thoughts.

Knowing the difference between depressive beliefs and their rational counterparts is no assurance that the rational perspective will prevail. But by actively questioning the negative, plus seeking positive alternatives, you can create a new response pattern within your brain in the form of a powerful new set of antidepression beliefs. For example, disputing depressive thoughts can lead to a more reality-based way of thinking and doing. By recognizing and disputing depressive thinking, you can show yourself that you are not helpless. Thus, you have hope. By developing an antidepression belief system, you build a coping frame of reference.

Disputation is where you apply scientific ways of knowing and doing, along with common sense, to counteract your depressive thinking. By disputing depressive thinking, you will do two positive things. You will deflate the effects of negative thinking, which can have a calming effect. You will also free your thoughts and time for pursuing experiences that you are more likely to value. The following disputation methods show how to strengthen your rational connections while weakening harmful depressive beliefs.

## PIT REASON AGAINST UNREASON

Believing that you will stay depressed forever is an example of depressive hopelessness thinking. Here is a way to dispute, or question, hopelessness thinking and build your clear-thinking skills.

Start with these observations: Hopelessness is an overly generalized prediction that people who feel depressed often make. It is also a conjecture. Since you can't know the future (and thinking that you do know the future is a false belief), you can't predict what will happen with any certainty. So how can the future be hopeless?

When you rationally articulate your observations and questions with the goal of countering depressive thinking, you increase your chances of gaining relief from such thinking. For example, if you have tools to defeat depression, then how does it follow that you cannot put some to use to test the hypothesis that you can't change anything about yourself?

## TAKE ACTION

Challenging helplessness thinking can be accomplished in part through practical actions. You tidy your abode even though you'd rather withdraw into darkness. At a fixed time each day, you jog in place for five minutes, or you do some other form of exercise. You do something altruistic, such as anonymously sending toys to an orphanage.

You may find that by taking practical actions, you don't feel quite so emotionally drawn into yourself. You may find that you dwell less on events that displease you and that you have fewer negative thoughts about yourself. But you may also begin to experience a growing sense of confidence in yourself as a doer rather than a stewer. Such a perspective shift can initiate positive motion forward, which leads to a disengagement from a downward spiral of depression.

By teaching yourself to think about your thinking, by separating sensible from depressive thoughts, and by engaging in problem-solving behaviors, you position yourself to disengage from automatic depressive thinking, feelings, and behavioral habits. The skills you develop to counter this thinking will grow in strength through practice.

## *Effects*

When you engage in activities to counteract depression, you identify and challenge depressive thinking and engage in problem-solving activities. Through this objective self-observation approach, you act to do and to get better. The effects of your efforts will show you if your cognitive behavioral strategy is working. If you find that by acting against depressive thinking, feelings, and actions, you feel a growing sense of relief and control, you've produced a positive effect. As this effect increases, depression decreases.

# PSYCHOLOGICAL HOMEWORK ASSIGNMENTS

Ellis is famous for his psychological homework assignments. Following the preceding ABCDE analysis, he might ask what you would do over the next week to practice what you've learned. That would be your psychological assignment.

Any of the following exercises can serve as a weeklong homework assignment, where you practice Socratic reasoning skills to sharpen your intellect and to buttress yourself against depression.

**Question truth in advertising.** Most advertisements contain logical flaws and omissions. Some provide great opportunities to practice logical thinking. Weight-loss advertisements can prove especially interesting. When you see an advertisement for a weight-loss product, you'll likely hear multiple testimonials attesting to the value of the program. You'll see before-and-after photographs. You can use these advertisements to practice your reasoning skills. First, look for the omissions (exceptions) in the ad. Does the advertiser show people who gained weight following the use of the diet? Does the advertiser show people who started the diet and then stopped using it? Does the advertiser cite relapse-rate statistics?

**Watch the news.** News channels that favor extreme political positions are a wonderful opportunity for practicing your reasoning skills. Whenever an ideologically driven group presents a slanted point of view, you can properly ask questions about definitions, omissions, and exceptions.

**Critique negative labeling.** The human tendency to label other people provides a rich avenue for sharpening your critical thinking skills. People apply labels to other people with frequency, such as "Jack's a wimp." Such negative labeling is an obvious target for practicing critical thinking skills. What is meant by the word "wimp"? What examples apply to Jack? What are the exceptions? This simple three-phase exercise is likely to show that Jack isn't totally one way or another.

**Critique positive labeling.** Positive labels provide yet other opportunities for developing your critical thinking skills. Suppose a friend tells you, "Jane is a wonderful person." But Jane is no more likely to be 100 percent wonderful than Jack is likely to be a 100 percent wimp. Here are some sample questions to ask: What is the definition of "wonderful"? What examples apply to Jane? What other views about Jane are possible?

Psychological homework assignments are skill-building experiences for separating sense from nonsense. You'll find examples throughout this book. Challenge yourself with those that seem to have the best fit with what you'd like to accomplish in your work to overcome your depression.

# THE ABCDE PROGRAM: A CASE STUDY

Following a bitter divorce, Amy had been mildly to moderately depressed for approximately three years. This conscientious and sensitive person's depression was complicated by a highly self-critical attitude, brooding, self-doubts, and a decline in her ability to tolerate frustration and anxiety. She saw herself as a "wet mop" that was pushed around by others. Amy believed that she got no respect from members of her family and her employer. She felt trapped.

In her second session Amy appeared weepy and upset over unkind comments about her appearance made by her older sister, Molly. She saw Molly as the "perfect person" who never admitted to any faults but was quick to find fault with others. Amy saw herself as vulnerable and unable to defend herself against her sister. During this session, she showed elevated depression and anxiety. She flitted from one thought to another, creating a kaleidoscopic picture of different distresses. She found it difficult to focus.

Following an upsetting event, Amy, like many who feel both anxious and depressed, had a difficult time organizing her thoughts. She found it especially challenging to separate her depressive and anxious thinking from her legitimate gripes. She and I took extra time that day on problem organizing so that she could move toward her goals of reducing her distress over her sister's comments, standing up for herself, and getting better control of her thoughts and life.

As Amy progressed with a problem-solving analysis, she used the ABCDE model to get a fix on her problem and figure out what to do. The following is Amy's ABCDE exercise.

## Amy's Activating Event

First, Amy looked closely at what had triggered the kaleidoscope of distressing thoughts. Molly had paid a visit and said, "You didn't answer my e-mail quickly enough." She then added, "What's wrong with your hair? You need to get your act together. You need to lose weight."

Amy, at first, focused on what had happened and on how bad she felt. This is common. Thinking about your thinking is usually far down on the list when you feel distressed.

Amy noted the conditions she associated with feeling upset and then described her emotional and behavioral experiences under the heading, "consequences." She described what she thought at the time. (Note that if you, at first, find it natural to jump over the beliefs category and then come back, that is an acceptable practice.)

## Amy's Beliefs

We broke out Amy's beliefs into a dichotomy of irrational and rational thoughts about the event. As the former were clearly the more dominant, we started with the irrational thoughts first. Then we worked on teasing out the rational thoughts. This proved somewhat challenging. Her rational ideas about the event were present but obscured by her stressful and somewhat catastrophic depressive thinking. (Sometimes you will find yourself inferring your rational thoughts. That is a positive step on the path to teaching yourself to develop a rational perspective.) Here's a table outlining Amy's irrational and rational thoughts.

| Irrational Thoughts | Rational Thoughts |
|---|---|
| "I'm not attractive enough." | "I don't like being put down." |
| "I'm not smart enough." | "Molly's negativity annoys me." |
| "I can't do anything right." | "I'd prefer not to deal with Molly's putdowns." |
| "I'm overwhelmed." | "It's better to stand up for myself than quit." |

After seeing her irrational-rational dichotomy of beliefs in writing, Amy's first comment was, "Wow. I sure did a number on myself. Molly was a pain, but I was a bigger one." Amy felt encouraged that her awareness of her depressing thoughts and their rational counterparts suggested that she was not locked into negativity. She had an alternative. In making this irrational-rational belief comparison, she felt freer.

## Amy's Consequences

On hearing Molly's comments, Amy's stomach dropped. She reported feeling a variety of negative emotions followed by discernible behaviors. Her emotional consequences included anxiety, anger, and depression. Her behavioral consequences were that she became sick to her stomach, vomited, and withdrew.

Later, after she'd thought about her thinking at the time, she saw how she had been dramatizing. She felt less tense and depressed knowing that she could develop a rational perspective.

## Amy's Disputation

Both Amy and I thought that the process of recognizing the irrational and rational elements in her thoughts was a useful exercise. This connecting of the dots between event, thought, emotions, and behavior gave her an organized way to map what was going on in her mind when her emotions felt muddled.

As she was doing this exercise, Amy significantly calmed down. She reported that she could clearly see how her thinking ballooned to catastrophic proportions. This awareness, she believed, could help her to maintain her perspective in the future when she faced her sister's negativity.

However, beyond recognizing the dichotomy of irrational and rational thoughts, Amy took the next step of self-questioning and disputation. Here is an example of how Amy went about disputing her irrational thinking about her sister's comments.

| Questions | Answers |
|---|---|
| "What if I'm not as attractive as my sister wants me to be?" | "My attractiveness is partially controllable, but I am more than my looks." |
| "Where is the law that says I need to be as thin as my sister insists?" | "Maintaining a reasonable weight is a reasonable goal. It's my choice, however, whether to change my weight." |
| "How does my worth depend on my sister's opinion about my appearance and intelligence?" | "My worth is contingent on my appearance only if I let it be." |
| "If I'm not the person my sister wants me to be, what's wrong with being the person I am?" | "I can always give myself unconditional self-acceptance." |
| "What do I mean when I tell myself that I'm overwhelmed?" | "I'm accepting hogwash. I can rethink my situation by looking at what I can control and what I would best work toward improving." |

## Amy's Effects

By learning to organize her thinking, Amy felt hopeful. She also figured out how to express herself constructively with her sister.

Molly continued to harp about Amy's weight and appearance. Amy was able to put her sister's statements into perspective. She also asserted herself more with her sister.

With trepidation, Amy told Molly that she appreciated her concerns; however, she liked her own hairstyle, her weight was on the low side of the average range, and she was satisfied with her choice of clothing. Molly defended her comments. Amy could see that she wasn't going to change Molly's views, but she did get Molly to agree to keep her comments to herself.

Amy saw that she could stand up for her rights. She stopped seeing herself as a wet mop.

Here's a list of effects that Amy produced for herself:

- "Stopped vomiting."

- "Have a sense of optimism that I can learn to recognize and question negative thinking."

- "Stick up for my rights by telling my sister that her criticisms are both unhelpful and alienating. If she wants to get along with me in the future, she had better stop the negativity."

- "Improved positive sense of self-worth."

- "Reduced helplessness and hopelessness depressive thinking."

- "Gained personal control of thinking, emotions."

# YOUR ABCDE EXERCISE

When you find yourself in a depressive rut, use the following ABCDE self-help form to address your depressive thinking. Fill in the blanks.

**A** (the activating event): _____

**B** (your beliefs about depressive sensations, events, or thoughts)

Irrational beliefs (depressive self-handicapping beliefs, misconceptions, distortions, and so forth):

_____

Rational beliefs (functional, factual, plausible, reasonable, predictable):

_____

**C** (consequences)

Emotional consequences of irrational beliefs: _____

_____

Emotional consequences of rational beliefs: _____

_____

Behavioral consequences of irrational beliefs: _____

_____

Behavioral consequences of rational beliefs: _____

_____

**D** (disputing depressive belief systems)

Prime questions to ask and answer: _____

_____

Prime actions to take: _____

_____

**E** (new cognitive, emotive, behavioral effects)

Results of prime questions: _____

Results of prime actions: _____

The ABCDE method is appropriate when you can identify an activating event that triggers a series of depressive thoughts. However, when you have a variety of depressive thoughts that do not seem to stem from any single event (or where you can't locate the triggering event), what I like to call a "stepping-stone" approach can be useful. Using this method, you organize your depressive ideas and beliefs under certain themes, such as worthlessness, helplessness, and hopelessness. You then rank the importance of each theme according to the distress or discomfort you associate with it. This ordering is like laying down stepping-stones to cross the stream of depression. To get to the second step, you take the first. To get to the third, you take the second. But here's the rub. You may start with the toughest step first and break it down into simple parts. When the most depressing theme is evaluated, challenged, and derailed, the weaker themes will sometimes collapse.

## THE STEPPING-STONE APPROACH: BETTY'S STORY

Betty became depressed after her company went bankrupt and she lost her job. She had the symptoms of moderately severe depression. She woke early and couldn't fall back asleep. She complained of a depressed mood, difficulty concentrating, and forgetfulness. She isolated herself in her apartment, often refusing to answer the telephone. She viewed herself as a worthless person with no future. She believed that she could do nothing to help herself.

After Betty entered counseling, she began educating herself about depression and getting regular physical exercise, and she started to show signs of improvement. Her depressive thinking was still especially burdensome, however, so she agreed to take a stepping-stone approach to counter her depressive thinking. Here are the steps that she took.

1. First Betty organized her depressive ideas and beliefs under specific themes. Betty identified four major depressive themes: worthlessness, helplessness, hopelessness, and self-blame.

2. Then she ranked these themes in importance according to her distress or discomfort level when the theme was on her mind or the ideas were active. Her feelings of worthlessness were stronger than either her sense of helplessness or hopelessness, and her sense of hopelessness was more distressful than her sense of helplessness. Self-blame, though painful, was the least powerful theme.

3. Betty's next step was to come up with examples of beliefs that supported each theme. She ranked each of these beliefs according to the level of stress that they produced for her, from least to greatest degree of stress. For example, the worthlessness theme included this order of ideas: "I'm stupid. I'm not living up to my potential. I can't do anything right."

4. Betty made a chart for each theme. Within each chart, she wrote down the depressive beliefs that supported the theme, listing them from least to most severe.

5.  She rationally challenged, or disputed, each of her depressive thoughts and recorded the results. Each time she detected new depressive messages, she added them to her chart and came up with ways to challenge them. She now had a coping tool that she had fashioned for herself.

6.  Through persistence and practice, Betty began to build her skills in disputing negative depressive thoughts and constructed a frame of reference to use against her depressive thinking.

While your depressive thinking may follow different themes, or patterns, you can use the stepping-stone approach in the same way. Here's a further breakdown of how Betty used it, including the charts she made for each of her depressive thinking themes.

## The Worthlessness Theme

Betty's most troublesome theme was worthlessness. She believed that her self-worth depended on her performances and upon what others thought about what she did. For example, she took her company's bankruptcy personally. She thought that if she had done more, the bankruptcy would not have happened. Beyond falling into this *demandingness* trap, Betty worried about interviewing for a new job. She feared that she would not present herself well and no one would hire her.

Self-blame and worry thinking had predated her depression by years. Indeed, she recalled thinking as a child that she could only be good if she did perfectly well. Her parents recalled that she was too hard on herself. They wanted her to do well, but they were also remarkably accepting and tolerant of her mistakes. They would have been happy for her if she were happy flipping hamburgers at a fast-food restaurant.

In her worthlessness theme chart, Betty wrote down three ideas that supported her feeling of worthlessness: "I'm not smart enough," "My performances are inadequate, and that's awful," and "I am inadequate." The following chart describes Betty's disputations and results:

# BETTY'S WORTHLESSNESS THEME

| Beliefs | Questions for Disputations | Results |
|---------|---------------------------|---------|
| "I'm not smart enough." | "If I were more intelligent, how would my life be any different?" | "More intelligence can speed my ability to solve problems. Still, I can make good use of my current abilities rather than lament about not having more of what I already have." |
| "My performances are inadequate, and that's awful." | "What is wrong with doing reasonable things reasonably well instead of having to do perfectly well?" | "I can still do well without having to do perfectly well, and that's not awful!" |

| "I am inadequate." | "How does my global worth depend on each performance I make?" | "My 'self' can't be defined as totally one way or another. Much of what I do and think changes according to my mood and situation. I act fairly toward others, meet my responsibilities, and routinely seek ways to improve. That observation dismantles my global inadequacy belief." |
|---|---|---|

By recognizing, evaluating, and challenging demanding, perfectionist thinking, Betty gained ground in defeating an irrational process of negative beliefs that had promoted considerable anxiety, inhibition, and grief since her childhood.

Next, Betty looked at the circularity in her worthlessness depressive thinking. She thought that she was inadequate because she was not smart enough. Yet she thought she needed to be smart enough to feel worthy. Not being smart enough meant that she could never be worthy. With this line of thought, she was in an impossible bind.

Betty took a logical approach to the idea that to be worthy she had to be smarter. Her primary premise was that she was not smart enough. Her second premise was that she needed to be perfectly smart to be worthy. Her conclusion was that she was inadequate because she wasn't perfect. Now her job was to break the circle by questioning the premises and conclusion. She found all three points logically flawed.

As Betty evaluated her belief that she was not smart enough, her first question was, "Smart enough for what? To invent time travel? To rule the world? To live a fulfilling life?"

She did not want to invent time travel, which was impossible. She did not want to rule the world; that was too big a responsibility. But she could do things to increase her odds of living a fulfilling life. She was clearly smart enough to do that.

Next, she looked at the idea that to be worthy, she had to be perfect. She had already partially dealt with that issue. The following question sapped more power from her perfectionist belief: "If I can't be what I can't be, what's wrong with enjoying and developing the self that I am?" She had only one reasonable answer. She had a right to enjoy her life. One problem was to find ways to improve her life experiences without judging her global self.

In an innovative way, Betty applied a perfectionist standard to her perfectionist thinking. If her thinking was flawed, it was her thinking that was worthless! She graded her perfectionist thoughts on a worthlessness scale. She quickly saw that the basic premises, upon which her sense of inadequacy was based, were flawed beyond belief, and therefore, so was her worthlessness conclusion.

In doing this, she discovered that she'd been assuming that something was wrong with her because she was not living up to her potential. She questioned this distressing conditional-worth idea in the following way:

| Belief | Question for Disputation | Result |
|---|---|---|
| "I'm not living up to my potential, and that makes me worthless." | "Even if I'm not living up to my potential, how does it follow that failing to achieve my full potential renders me totally worthless?" | "Reaching full potential is a vague and probably unrealistic ideal." |

Betty hadn't originally connected the idea of not living up to her potential with her sense of worthlessness. It is common for people to add to their thought logs as they go. They often discover dysfunctional core beliefs that they can then beneficially address. Once Betty recognized the negative implications of this core belief, she went to work to challenge and purge it.

Betty periodically had a revival of contingent-worth ideas. (They are practiced, habitual, and thus retrievable.) But now she had powerful tools to recognize and contradict them.

## The Hopelessness Theme

You can be in a hopeless position when you have twenty minutes to get to the airport and you are stuck in rush-hour traffic. Hopelessness in depression is another matter. Here you have options, yet you believe you can't change. In this mind-set, you have no possibility of succeeding, improving, getting help, or finding a solution.

But this idea of hopelessness is a myth. Like the Sirens who captivated the minds of sailors and lured them to shipwreck and disaster, you can transfix yourself with such fatalistic thoughts.

Hopelessness is a myth because the human mind is made for adaptability. We can generate different ideas, make predictions, and move toward positive future opportunities. We can avoid excessive risks and visible dangers. We can solve problems. Yet, we sometimes forget that these capabilities are within reach if we reach for them. Here is the adaptive approach Betty took to deal with her sense of hopelessness.

# BETTY'S HOPELESSNESS THEME

| Beliefs | Questions for Disputations | Results |
|---|---|---|
| "I don't have what it takes to change." | "What can I work at changing that is both worthwhile and within my control to do? " | "I started exercising to work against depressive sensations and mood. I've made progress. I can make positive changes, for I'm doing that already." |
| "I'm going to suffer forever." | "Where is the proof that my mood will remain constantly negative?" | "The answer is that there is no proof that my depressed mood will continue forever. Education about depression gives me a different prediction. The odds favor that I will free myself from symptoms of depression. Unrealistic ideas are subject to evaluation and revision. Physical exercise helps boost endorphins, or feel-good brain chemicals. In short, I have many ways to change that I have the power to initiate." |

Hopelessness can be among the more painful of the depressive themes. But like the worthlessness theme, this belief is so general that it is not provable.

## The Helplessness Theme

Helplessness is ordinarily high on a depressed person's theme list, but on Betty's list, helplessness ranked third. Here is how she examined and dealt with her thoughts of helplessness.

# BETTY'S HELPLESSNESS THEME

| Beliefs | Questions for Disputations | Results |
|---|---|---|
| "I am helpless to change the discomfort I feel or the events around me." | "How does that view compare with what I actually do? What other perspective is likely to prove productive?" | "Complete control is a myth. New understandings are a softer, progressive approach toward meeting challenges and solving problems." |
| "I can't do anything right." | "Where is the proof that I can do nothing right? What is 'nothing'? What do I mean by 'right'?" | "I can challenge the idea that I can do nothing right by making a list of ten things I do okay every day. This can range from brushing my teeth to getting a refund for a greeting card to writing a poem. This action provides a set of contradictory data to compare to a blanket 'can't do anything right' statement. The statement is false when the facts contradict it." |
| | | "'Nothing' is an overgeneralization. Such blanket statements as 'I can do nothing right' don't take specific situations into account." |
| | | "'Right' is a matter of definition. The effectiveness of actions occurs in degree. It's impossible that all of my actions are not right." |

## Dealing with Blame

Blame was subtly woven through Betty's worthlessness, hopelessness, and helplessness depressive themes. Betty blamed herself for the way she thought. She told herself it was her fault for putting herself into a situation that she saw as hopeless. She also thought it was her fault that she felt so helpless.

# BETTY'S SELF-BLAME THEME

| Belief | Question for Disputation | Result |
|--------|--------------------------|--------|
| "Everything bad that happens is my fault." | "How can any human being legitimately take credit for all that does or can go wrong?" | "Taking credit for matters outside of my control makes no sense. Even in those instances where I am clearly to blame, fixing a problem is better than blamefully dwelling upon it." |

Betty's depressive themes thinned in frequency and intensity as she moved from worthlessness to hopelessness to helplessness thinking. By the time she got to her self-blame belief, she was in a position to quickly brush it off as an illegitimate conclusion about herself.

Betty got a big boost up from depression by learning how to think about her thinking. By defusing her depressive thoughts, she gained relief from depressive thinking and the physical symptoms of depression that she experienced. She felt calmer.

## Betty's Relapse-Prevention Program

After she drafted her thought charts, Betty made revisions. As she learned more, she added questions and challenges to her four negative themes. For example, she had a strong interest in the history of the ancient world. Several weeks after drafting the helplessness chart, she looked up the Roman orator Cicero's "Six Mistakes of Man" and copied down "the tendency to worry about things that cannot be changed or corrected." She saw that helplessness could be legitimately understood as things that cannot be changed or corrected. She also mused that her tendency to worry about possible disasters was something that she could change.

By forcing herself to follow through, even when she felt inhibited by depression, Betty gained an experiential understanding that she was not helpless. If she could act to change, she realized that her life was not hopeless. By meeting tough challenges, she could see that worthlessness was an illusion and self-blame was normally without merit.

As Betty learned more ways to negate negative thinking, she found a growing sense of tranquility. Here are some of the positions she adopted to promote that tranquility:

- Accept that negative depressive thoughts may be automatic, but you don't have to take them personally.

- Recognize that automatic depressive thinking will arise from time to time, especially following a twinge of mild depression, a negative mood swing, or an unpleasant experience.

- Disengage from believing the depressive-thinking message. Thinking habits are habits because they attach to activating events, such as depressive sensations, down moods, and losses. Put them into perspective by matching them against the criteria for rational and irrational thought, separating the rational from the irrational components, and challenging the erroneous emotive content, which is vulnerable to questions about proof and evidence.

- Refuse to engage in any form of global self-blame. This theme often distracts from problem solving.

As a reminder against perfectionist and self-blame thinking, Betty put on her refrigerator an observation from Plutarch, a first-century Greek biographer and essayist: "To make no mistakes is not in the power of man; but from their errors and mistakes, the wise and good learn wisdom for the future."

In time, Betty conquered her depression. To prevent a recurrence, she continued to refer back to her thought charts. Twenty-seven years after her depressive episode, she reports having experienced no more than a few days of mild depression. She is genuinely pleased with what she has accomplished in her life so far. She looks forward to the next decade.

# END DEPRESSION PLAN

**Key ideas** (What three ideas did you find most helpful in this chapter?):

1.

2.

3.

**Action steps** (What three steps can you take to move closer to your goal of overcoming depression?):

1.

2.

3.

**Execution** (How did you execute the steps?):

1.

2.

3.

**Results** (What did you learn that you can use?):

1.

2.

3.

# CHAPTER 9

# Ending Worthlessness Thinking

At one time or another, most people wonder who they are and what makes them tick. There is no single answer to the question, "Who am I?"

At one moment, you impress yourself with your wisdom and the next you disappoint yourself by uttering a foolish statement. With a sharp focus, you sink a hoop. At the next shot, you get distracted and miss the mark. You are charming with a stranger and then sullen with your brother. If nothing else, you are marked by countless attributes, motivations, and actions that are influenced by the situations you're in and your perceptions of them, but you also create unique conditions for yourself and can orchestrate your own reality by the choices you make about what you think, feel, and do.

Your sense of worth definitely influences your perceptions of yourself and the realities that you experience. Depression can change this view and reflect and influence what you think of yourself.

This chapter will explore the self in depression and look at how to separate your sense of worth from this condition. It will begin with a look at what we mean by "the self," then probe a self-worth dichotomy, and finally show how to break away from worthlessness thinking that may cloud your vision and bring on more depression.

## THE SELF ON THE HORIZON

In an allegorical sense, the self is constantly scanning the horizon. When you stand in different places, you can see the horizon in different ways. You can have different perspectives about the horizon, as you can have different perspectives on your "self." Yet, as scenes change, the horizon remains. Likewise, your self remains constant, even as perceptual changes take place within the self, based on changing scenes and shifting perspectives.

Looking at the horizon, you may think that you see the earth meeting the sky. This perception is real, but it is also an illusion. Although you can see the horizon, you can never touch it. The same

> We can't grasp the full essence of the self any more than we can see all possible horizons. Does that invalidate the existence of a self or of other horizons?

paradox is true for the self. There is both a real and illusionary experience of self. Your experience of what you know and feel is you. You know you have recognizable qualities that distinguish you from others. These qualities also occur to degrees in others, but the configurations vary, making each of us unique.

Some human characteristics are dominant, and those cardinal traits influence your views and what you do. With strong leadership skills, you'll tend to initiate, organize, and coordinate the efforts of others. With creative talents, you may shift from new insights to innovative productions. Kindness extends into compassionate activities. Your sense of self can change with shifting circumstances. You may tend to be introverted and yet feel and appear lively and extroverted when you speak before a group.

Like changes on the horizon, changes in our lives are inevitable. The horizon sometimes appears bright (when we feel optimistic, successful). Dark clouds cloak the sky (we feel sadness, gloom, depression). Coming storms appear foreboding (we have anxiety). Your inner perceptions invariably affect your perspectives on what you see and what you do. A pessimistic perspective that clouds the horizon is different from a realistically optimistic perspective that draws you toward taking actions to get past pangs of depression. To the extent that you can orchestrate your experiences in different ways, you can change your perceptions and perspectives when you are ill served by them.

In the seasons of our lives, the horizon can appear different. The horizons that you see as a kindergartner at play will vary from what you see as a middle-aged adult engaged in working on a job. Yet you may exhibit conscientiousness as a child and conscientiousness in the various roles that you play as an adult.

An inner consistency lends predictability and stability to your life, but this consistency often gets messed up when you're depressed, which can affect your sense of self and identity. An inner consistency lends predictability and stability to your life, but this consistency often gets messed up when you're depressed, which can affect your sense of self and identity. A negative sense of self and identity may also presage depression. With effort, you can clear up your distortions about the self during periods of depression. You may also clean up a distorted self-concept that is like a slippery slope to depression. You can find positive new ways to look at your horizon and see beyond these distortions to better times.

> The mind is everything. What you think, you become.
>
> —Buddha

# A THEORY OF WORTH

In a practical sense, people who display special skills gain certain advantages. Highly skilled performers in the arts, business, sports, and the professions gain financial advantages, as does the mechanic who quickly diagnoses and fixes an automotive problem. There are big advantages to performing effectively and disadvantages to performing weakly. But are either top or lower levels of performance a measure of human worth?

It is possible to define human performance and worth as one and the same. The seventeenth-century British philosopher Thomas Hobbes described human worth as a measure of what people contribute to society. Personal contributions can provide us with a way to feel esteemed by others and to esteem ourselves.

## Self-Esteem and Contingent Worth

Equating your worth with what you contribute or with your performance can lead to trouble. You may come to esteem yourself for your accomplishments and degrade yourself for less-than-adequate performances.

The word "esteem" comes from the sixteenth-century French word *estimare,* meaning to set a value on. Esteem basically means to value or judge someone or something as favorable. Self-esteem ordinarily is a prelude for judging self-worth. But seeking self-esteem can have a boomerang effect. What starts out as positive can turn into something negative, such as when what you base your self-esteem on ceases to be available or doesn't occur in the degree you desire. You earn money as an athlete. As you age, you lose your edge. If you base your worth on athletic prowess at professional levels, does your worth disappear when your abilities decline?

A contingent-worth process boils down to labeling yourself based upon how you rate what you do and what you think others think of you. So if you see yourself doing good things or getting praised, you can feel good about yourself. But what happens if you get criticized for what you do, or if you believe that others think badly of you? What happens to your self-esteem then?

Throughout life, there are disappointments, reversals, losses, and frustrations. Does that mean that the horizon changes and your worth is diminished when such events occur? When fortune smiles on you and you hit a home run on the stock market, or a rival leaves a field open to you, do such conditions elevate your worth as a person? Only if you think they do.

People who ordinarily operate on a contingent-worth theory are likely to feel good about themselves when they do well and feel frustrated when their performances fall below their standards. When depressed, you are likely to operate at a slower place, do less well, or may not care about yourself or anything or anyone else. However, if you accept depression as a temporary state, and not a global measure of you, you are less likely to fall into this version of the contingent-worth trap.

## Failure vs. Failings

When depressed, you are more likely to view yourself as a failure compared to when you feel upbeat. If you fall into this failure-thinking trap and are looking for an exit, you can look at the failure issue from another angle on your horizon.

All human beings have failings. One failing is succumbing to failure thinking. You can work to change this form of thinking. For example, failure can characterize an action, but telling yourself that you are a failure is an overgeneralization, a statement that's too sweeping to characterize you.

Failings are part of a changeable human process that also includes successes, accomplishments, and capabilities. You are normally better off working to rectify failings than to engage in the rash act of branding yourself a failure. You have the option of stretching to improve.

While it is true that you can fail at some of the things that you undertake, these failures do not make you a failure. A realistic perspective can mute this thinking. For example, the inventor Thomas Edison made many thousands of attempts to find a filament for the lightbulb he was trying to develop. When asked how he was able to tolerate such failures, he quipped that he saw them not as a series of failures but as a process of discovering what didn't work.

Unlike Edison's approach to discovery, some failures can be hard to accept. You may have lost the love of your life to a rival. Such experiences are dramatic and memorable, and if you didn't feel bad, something would be odd. Nevertheless, significant losses do not make a complex person a failure.

# HOW YOU DEFINE YOURSELF

Most of us think about ourselves a lot. But what is this self that we think about? Is it a theory or a fact? A theory reduces complex data to a short, simple formula. Here's an example: "Global features of personality and an individual's objective life circumstances influence the ways in which the person interprets the circumstances of his or her life, and these interpretations, in turn, directly influence subjective well-being" (Brief et al. 1993, 647).

You may believe that your self is what you think about yourself. Or you may go to the opposite extreme and argue that the idea of self is an illusion; it's something you feel, but this essence isn't real.

The self paradoxically consists of realities and illusions. It's a collection of familiar characteristics that makes your persona recognizable. It is your sense of identity. If you were to look at films of yourself as a child, you'd recognize features in yourself that you see today. Some traits, such as introversion and extroversion, were present shortly after birth. Comparing them to now, you'd also see that the self evolves with those basic traits bearing influence over the choices that you make. The values you acquire from your family and culture have a similar influence. Value responsibility and integrity, and be guided by these values, and you are likely to lead a life that is different from someone whose values are subjective and changing based on what is most expedient at the moment.

## *What Goes into an Identity?*

The English language has thousands of words to describe the complexities that go into a picture of the self. In their search for what makes up the self, psychologists Gordon Allport and Henry Odbert (1936) found 18,000 human qualities listed throughout a standard English dictionary. These words included emotions, talents, and traits. They found about 4,500 trait words, including "warm," "dominant," "sanguine," "inventive," "friendly," "quick-witted," "motivated," "bold," "shy," and "stubborn."

There may be over 150 factors that go into what we call "intelligence" (Guilford 1967). Our intuitive abilities, insights, imagination, and creativity add to this intellectual complexity and come about in different configurations. Albert Einstein's son was as intellectually bright as his father, but have you ever heard of him? Albert Einstein showed a special creative ability.

You can project your identity using externals, such as the type of clothing you wear, the automobile you drive, your job status, or how much money you have invested. These factors reflect and blend into the composite picture we call "self." Some of these qualities, such as a sense of humor, hibernate when you are depressed. You can find them again.

Your unique combination of psychological factors and the life circumstances that shape them may boil down to your sense of identity, or who you think you are. However, when you feel depressed, you are unlikely to feel like your normal self. You may feel like an alienated self.

## *Broadening Your Self-Definition*

When depressed, you may find it challenging to escape a worthy-worthless dichotomous thinking trap, in which you see yourself as either worthy or worthless. If you define yourself as "worthless," you've fallen into this trap. Here are four probable consequences of narrowly defining yourself:

1. By looking through a warped dichotomous lens, you have a distorted view of the horizon, and this can affect your judgments.

2. You layer misery onto an already bad depression by defining your worth negatively.

3. Believe you're not worth the effort to improve, and you may act according to this self-fulfilling prophecy.

4. With a hangdog self-view, you may distance yourself from your important relationships and then complain that no one likes you.

But if your theory of self were comprehensive, including facts about human variability and changeability, then you could take steps to avoid the trap. The solution is simple. Think pluralistically about yourself. This gives you a broader perspective.

Here is a pluralistic solution. As a person with countless attributes and experiences, there are too many permutations and combinations of characteristics that can surface in different situations. You can't be only one way or another. Thus, logically and legitimately, you can dump "I'm worthless" as a self-description. When combined with self-acceptance, this view may be highly useful as a platform for advancing self-improvement efforts, even when you feel depressed.

If you are not used to thinking pluralistically about yourself but want to explore this option, you can do so by immediately entering the accommodation phase of change (see chapter 4). When you first try to think pluralistically, you can evoke a conflict of concepts: dichotomous thinking versus a pluralistic perspective. To resolve the conflict, you'll need ammunition—perhaps a lot of it. Old thought habits rarely retreat without a struggle. Depressive thinking habits, when they reflect and propel a depressed mood, seem credible even when they are mistaken.

Doing a personal features experiment can give you an opportunity to explore attributes that flow into a pluralistic self-concept. You can start broadening this perspective by writing down your major personal features, including your values, faculties, emotions, attributes, and roles. These features are defined as follows.

**Values.** What you value you view as important. Your values may include higher order values of integrity, responsibility, honesty, tolerance, and freedom. Values with utility may include following the rules, reciprocity, politeness, and assertiveness. Values can involve preferences, such as a warm meal. We are all touched, in one way or another, by cultural values and national values. What do you value?

**Faculties.** Our faculties, inborn abilities and learned skills, come into play practically every day. You may have artistic talents, leadership capabilities, and organizing strengths. You may have faculties for doing such things as sensing whom you can rely upon, structuring plans of action, inventing, learning, teaching, protecting, and changing. Your faculties include reading, writing, calculating, cooking, negotiating, and repairing. Each faculty will have related skills. For example, you restore furniture as a hobby. That process can break down to acquiring what you need, repairing, sanding, staining, varnishing, and so forth. You may take your faculties for granted, but they are extraordinary. You may operate with some diminished capacity when you are depressed. That is normal. Having diminished energy is a symptom of depression, not a negation of your capabilities.

**Emotions.** In their simplest form, emotions divide into pleasant and unpleasant states. But as practically everyone knows, we think of emotions in diverse ways. Human beings have primary emotions, such as happiness, fear, surprise, disgust, awe, sadness, love, anger, delight, and anxiety. We have several hundred cognitively toned variations on these basic themes, such as angst and lassitude. Emotions can be mixed, such as feelings of disgust and anger, or anxiety and depression.

**Attributes.** You may be outgoing, quiet, bold, friendly, quick-witted, passive, active, caring, compassionate, sensitive, or hard-nosed. These distinctive attributes can stand out to other people. They may change when you feel depressed. But dormant attributes can come alive again as the leaves of deciduous trees do in springtime.

**Roles.** Your roles are the various parts you play throughout the day and throughout your life, such as student, teacher, protector, or organizer. Your complexity grows when you consider what goes into the many roles you play, such as parent, prophet, pal, or patriot.

The following personal features experiment can help you defuse worthlessness thinking. List what you know about yourself and then see whether the results add up to a pluralistic perspective or myopic perspective on the self.

## YOUR PERSONAL FEATURES EXPERIMENT

What are your personal features? Record your values, faculties, emotions, attributes, and roles.

| Values | Faculties | Emotions | Attributes | Roles |
|--------|-----------|----------|------------|-------|
|        |           |          |            |       |
|        |           |          |            |       |
|        |           |          |            |       |
|        |           |          |            |       |

| | | | | |
|---|---|---|---|---|
| | | | | |
| | | | | |

If you think of yourself only as worthless, ask yourself, how can you be only one thing, worthless, and at the same time, operate with changing perspectives and judgments that are influenced by your mood, values, faculties, emotions, and other attributes?

If you work to adopt a pluralistic theory of self, would taking this view decrease your degree of depression and improve the quality of your life? There is no guarantee, but you probably won't sink yourself with one-way dichotomous thinking. This can feel emotionally freeing. You may also find that you have an easier time separating this pluralistic self from a temporary state of depression. If you are not just a depressed person but are a multifaceted person with depression, you are less likely to identify with your disorder. Instead of thinking of yourself as a depressed person, you may think of yourself as a person who happens to feel depressed at this time.

# HOW TO DEFUSE WORTHLESSNESS THINKING

When I ask people about their theory of worth, I commonly hear that your worth is based on your performances and what others think of what you do. However, when I ask them to compare a pluralistic theory of self with a dichotomous theory of worth, some seem stunned.

## *Pluralism-Worth Comparisons*

The act of pitting a pluralistic theory of self against a contingent theory of worth creates an opportunity to resolve a paradox when you define your worth in a narrow sense yet also can see your "self" as extensive.

If you are more than what you do, then how can what you do be all there is to you? If you are, for example, a person with multiple characteristics, multiple roles, multiple abilities, multiple dimensions of intelligence, and multiple experiences, then how could you be worthless, even if you made a colossal mistake, if an acquaintance despised you, or if you suffer from depression?

Contingency-worth theories are radically different from pluralistic theories of self. From a self-development point of view, it's important to separate the two. If you have a choice—and as a pluralistic thinking person, you absolutely do—why not rate your performance rather than yourself? You can grade performances, but defining your global worth based upon ever-changing performances is arbitrary and absurd.

You have a choice between thinking pluralistically about the self and accepting a simplified depressive label like "worthless." Adopting a pluralistic self-view helps negate a narrow negative self-view.

## Getting Past Mental Entanglements

Both the individual therapist, Alfred Adler, and the rational emotive therapist, Albert Ellis, have wisely asserted that you would best work against negative habits of thought, as this process has entanglements and traps that need to be discovered and defeated. Defaulting to worthlessness thinking when you feel depressed is such an entanglement.

> You are what you think. But what you think you are when you are depressed may represent how you feel and not your human complexity.

Most people follow the same patterns, beliefs, and interests. Once an idea is fixed in the mind, it tends to persist. That's one reason why self-change normally proves to be challenging. For example, as a habit of mind, worthlessness gets etched in memory. As an antidote, you can add new coping memories that you can call upon later. You can do this by practicing thinking pluralistically. This effort can eventually create coping memories that you can use to compete with worthless-thinking memories.

If you daily find a few novel ways to use some of the abilities you've listed, and you note to yourself three good things that happen each day, you are likely to experience a reduction in depressive symptoms within a six-month period (Seligman et al. 2005).

# ABCDE METHOD FOR DEFUSING WORTHLESSNESS THINKING

A small egg rested on the top of a haystack beneath an oak tree. Upon seeing the egg, a farmer picked it up and put it into the henhouse. A chicken sat on the egg. It hatched. The baby bird grew into a chicken hawk. Growing up among the chickens, the hawk pecked kernels of corn from the ground. Believing it was like any other member of the flock, it lived its days thinking it was a chicken.

Fables like the hawk among the chickens suggest that you are what you believe yourself to be. There is certain validity to that view. What you generally think about yourself will normally influence how you feel about yourself. However, your traits don't disappear.

Depression typically includes worthlessness thinking such as, "I'm no good. I'm worthless. I'm a failure." When active, these pronouncements can influence how you feel and what you do. But, there is a big difference between self-labeling and *being*.

The following example shows how to use ABCDE method to defuse worthlessness thinking.

| |
|---|
| **Activating event (experience):** "A series of errors due to difficulties paying attention and concentrating." |
| **Rational beliefs about the event:** "Lapses in attention and concentration happen when I'm depressed. This is unfortunate but it is as it is. "I would prefer to concentrate better." |
| **Emotional and behavioral consequences for the rational beliefs:** "A sense of regret for lapses in concentration. Acceptance of a temporary disability." |
| **Irrational worthlessness beliefs:** "I make too many careless mistakes. I'm a failure. I've always been a failure. I'm worthless." |
| **Emotional and behavioral consequences for the irrational worthlessness beliefs:** "Shame. Disparagement. Anxiety. Depression. Withdrawal. Avoidance of challenging activities." |
| **Disputes for irrational worthlessness beliefs:** (1) "Although lapses in concentration are unfortunate, how does having such lapses make me a total failure?" Sample answer: "Lapses in attention and concentration are expected when I am depressed. There is no reason to expect anything different." (2) "How does a temporary lapse in concentration result in a permanent sense of failure?" Sample answer: "It doesn't. An extreme overgeneralization about the self does not prove that the self is the same as the overgeneralization. This is as illogical as saying that I am a completely noble person for throwing a piece of trash into a wastebasket." (3) "How does a lack of concentration mean I am worthless?" Sample answer: "This conclusion is the result of a faulty major premise, that there should be no lapses in concentration when I am depressed. This premise is unreasonable: lapses in attention and concentration are part of the depressive process. The secondary premise is that I am a failure because of errors resulting from lapses in concentration. This premise reflects an overgeneralization and is disputable. The worthlessness conclusion that follows is assumptive. It is based upon primary and secondary premises, and both lack validity. When matched against a pluralistic theory of self, this conditional-worth theory collapses under the weight of its own absurdity." |
| **Effects of the disputes:** "Despite depression and disappointment about operating less efficiently than normal, a calmer outlook." |

If worthlessness thinking surfaces before or during the course of your depression, use the following ABCDE chart as a guide for challenging this self-negating habit of mind:

**Activating event (experience):**

**Rational beliefs about the event:**

**Emotional and behavioral consequences for the rational beliefs:**

**Irrational worthlessness beliefs:**

**Emotional and behavioral consequences for the irrational worthlessness beliefs:**

**Disputes for irrational worthlessness beliefs:**

**Effects of the disputes:**

# THE CIRCLE-OF-WORTH TECHNIQUE

Based on his more than thirty years of clinical experience, REBT therapist Dr. Russell Grieger finds that helping people totally and unconditionally accept themselves, no matter how badly they perform, how lousy some of their traits may be, or how poorly they feel, is probably the most significant thing he can do to help them relinquish depression. Grieger (pers. comm.) suggests that you "use the visual image of a circle filled with thousands upon thousands of dots. The circle represents yourself or being, while the dots represent all the actions or performances you have ever done, all the characteristics or traits you possess, and all the acquisitions (for example, family, career, house) you have acquired."

As you look at this circle, you can see that because "you are made up of thousands, even millions of dots… it is an illogical overgeneralization to rate or judge your whole circle (self) based on any one [dot] or combination of dots." The white space in the circle shows you that "there is room for millions of more dots to be added…you are a work in process, always changing, not a snapshot, never to be frozen in time as always anything (for example, a good or bad person)." Grieger adds that while it may be "wise to rate or judge the dots—performances, traits, and acquisitions—as that provides an opportunity to improve…it is never desirable or necessary to jump from judging the dots to judging the circle."

He concludes, "To get past depression, you repeatedly recognize these self-damning beliefs in operation, depthfully question them, and energetically replace them with a pluralistic sense of self-acceptance."

# END DEPRESSION PLAN

**Key ideas** (What three ideas did you find most helpful in this chapter?):

1.

2.

3.

**Action steps** (What three steps can you take to move closer to your goal of overcoming depression?):

1.

2.

3.

**Execution** (How did you execute the steps?):

1.

2.

3.

**Results** (What did you learn that you can use?):

1.

2.

3.

# CHAPTER 10

# Defeating Helplessness Thinking

When you are depressed, do you feel overwhelmed and too helpless to act? If you believe that you can do nothing to exit from your depression, chances are that you view yourself as powerless and defenseless, and that is a bleak way to experience life.

Helplessness in depression is the belief that you have no ability to assert control over life's events or your depression. This belief frequently accompanies a depressed mood.

But such thinking is changeable! You have the power to think about your thinking. You can learn to develop competing systems of thought and actions to counteract depressive helplessness thinking. You can change your views when you experience yourself looking at this horizon. Read on and start now.

## WHEN YOU FEEL HELPLESS

What is helplessness? Simply defined, it is an inability to act or succeed or a feeling of being depleted of strength. When depressed, you may feel helpless or believe that you are generally unable to act, but this is a mental myth. You have the power to act against depression. True, you may experience difficulty paying attention and concentrating. Your mood is down. You can feel as if you are trudging through the day. You may feel fatigued and disinterested in acting. Every bone in your body can resist action. Nevertheless, most of the capabilities you had before depression did not vaporize. They may be available in lesser degrees, but they remain accessible.

You probably do experience a depletion of strength when you're depressed. A persistently depressed mood, lower energy levels, and higher levels of fatigue are to be expected.

On the other hand, if you view depletion as part of a temporary state of depression, this is radically different from defining it as permanent. When you interpret the thoughts and sensations of depression as temporary, you are less likely to encounter the double trouble of feeling depressed over feeling depressed. However, using helplessness as an excuse to

> Helplessness is like a bird that thinks it has wounded wings, yet the wings are strong enough for flight.

delay actions to overcome depression is just another form of procrastination. It is usually better to do less to break free than to do nothing at all.

# WHEN HELPLESSNESS IS REAL

There are many things in life that you can't control but that don't evoke depression. You probably can't prevent earthquakes. Unexpected events can disrupt your interests and goals: you train for months for a marathon race and then accidentally break your leg on the morning of the race. Most people can unhappily accept these occurrences without faulting themselves or thinking helplessness thoughts.

When you feel a sense of helplessness over understanding or controlling what is happening around you, consider Helen Keller, who was born both deaf and blind. She found a way to gain meaning in a dark and silent world and to make meaningful contact with others. This didn't happen overnight, but it did happen.

Depressive ideas can fall.

# BOOSTING YOUR PROBLEM-SOLVING EFFECTIVENESS

In Aesop's fable of the crow and the pitcher, a crow is thirsty and wants water. It sees a pitcher nearby, but the water inside the pitcher is just out of reach of the crow's beak. What does the crow do? Keep pecking its beak inside the pitcher with no success? Instead, the clever crow drops pebbles into the pitcher until the water rises to where it can be reached.

As the story of the crow and the pitcher illustrates, a problem exists when we have a gap between what we want and what we have, and the process of finding a solution is still to be found or applied. The story also shows the value of problem solving. But can problem solving be employed in the service of defeating helplessness in depression? Yes! By focusing your efforts on solving problems related to your depression, you can help yourself defeat depression (Nezu 1985). Actively engaging in cognitive-behavioral problem solving is a scientifically supported method for addressing depression and improving your quality of life. Developing a problem-solving attitude has a long-term benefit, especially when you do this in the early stages of depression (Nezu and Nezu 2010). One problem is that of resolving the helplessness dilemma.

There are many reasons for the observed increase in the prevalence of depression. Since the 1960s, a shift has taken place from relying on your own efforts toward assuming that external forces have a greater controlling influence over your life (Twenge, Zhang, and Im 2004). By addressing problems in everyday living, you can add to your sense of self-reliance. By shifting from an external locus of control (others are at fault) to an internal locus, where you believe you can act to help yourself, you'll feel more inclined to see helplessness thinking as a problem to resolve.

If you have an issue with feeling stigmatized because you feel depressed, a disease model of depression may seem appealing. If you suffer from a chemical imbalance, you're not at fault. You are likely to feel less to blame. That is generally a positive conclusion (see chapter 12 on blame). However, there is a downside. By putting the cause outside of your control, you may set the stage for a worse outcome. This includes rejecting evidence-based psychological corrections for depression (Deacon and Baird 2009). In short, you may be inclined to see your locus of control as being out of your hands.

This is not an either-or situation, where you are either going to take corrective psychological actions or you are stuck with a disease called depression. Indeed, this is a false dichotomy. You can realistically accept that your biology is affected when you feel depressed, but that doesn't preclude you from taking corrective actions. You may not be responsible for your tendency toward depression, but it is your responsibility to take reasonable actions if you intend to both do and get better.

## Questioning Helplessness

Helplessness beliefs commonly morph into hopelessness beliefs, and vice versa. This combination forms a vicious circle of depressive thought. However, the fact that you think helplessness thoughts is cause for some optimism. It means your mind is active. With an active mind, many things are possible, including using your mind to reverse depressive helplessness thinking. To resolve the paradox between helplessness thinking and mental activity, identify the helplessness message, question the message, and see if you can come to a nonhelplessness resolution. The following chart shows how you can do this.

| Helplessness Message | Self-Questioning | Resolution |
|---|---|---|
| "I'm helpless to change." | "Is helplessness a depressive thinking example? Is it a fact-based belief that predicts for all time that I am utterly unable to take any step whatsoever to break from a depressive rut?" | "Helplessness thinking represents an example of depressive thinking. Since people cannot guess the future with certainty, helplessness is a hypothesis. There is practically always something to do to step out of a depressive rut." |
| "I feel overwhelmed with too many responsibilities without the energy to act." | "What does 'overwhelmed' mean? What constitutes 'too many'? What does 'without energy' mean?" | "These key words and phrases in helplessness thinking point to exaggerations. Instead of accepting the key words in a helplessness-thinking monologue, clarify the meaning. This exposes the myths in the words. An exposed erroneous myth soon loses credibility." |

# YOUR HELPLESSNESS QUESTIONING EXERCISE

List your own helplessness messages, question them, and see what results.

| Helplessness Message | Self-Questioning | Resolution |
|---|---|---|
|  |  |  |
|  |  |  |
|  |  |  |

By disproving negative helplessness beliefs, you can see for yourself that you are not helpless.

## The Puzzle Technique

It's common in depression to abandon your otherwise good problem-solving skills and to feel indecisive and unable to choose between various options. Barry Lubetkin, cofounder of the Behavior Therapy Institute in New York City and an internationally known cognitive behavioral therapist, has come up with a puzzle exercise to help defeat this helplessness thinking. Lubetkin (pers. comm.) suggests doing the following:

Have a friend with a watch draw a design on a sheet of paper and then tear it up into several pieces. Then you put the puzzle back together while paying very close attention to your thoughts and out-loud verbalizations. You may hear yourself say, "I can't do this…It's too difficult…I'm not good at puzzles… Turn the timer off, I can't work under pressure." If you hear yourself saying or thinking these unhelpful thoughts, switch to these positive strategy thoughts and then follow them: "Let me figure out a plan, perhaps placing the straight edges along the outside… I've done this before, just take a breath and proceed… The hell with the timer, just relax and proceed at my own pace." The point is to begin to practice developing a "problem-solving mind-set" and eliminate useless helpless mind meanderings that will always interfere with being successful at any project.

## The HelpFULL-HelpLESS Paradox

New York City psychologist Diana Richman (pers. comm.) points out the paradox that people create for themselves when they purchase self-help books and yet describe themselves as helpless. People can still believe they are helpless, even as they take steps to achieve their desired outcomes. Since individuals so often negate actions that reflect the reality that they can, and do, help themselves, Richman suggests a "helpFULL-helpLESS" exercise to resolve this paradox and break from a cycle of depression.

To define these terms, *helpFULL* thinking is more conducive to combating depression and attaining your goals than maintaining a helpless style of thinking. This thinking involves three primary beliefs:

- "I can organize and direct my efforts toward achieving my goals."

- "I can explore areas of uncertainty and unknown outcomes."

- "I can withstand the discomfort of hard work."

*HelpLESS* thinking involves these three primary beliefs:

- "I am not able to take actions toward achieving my goals because of external life conditions."

- "I could not stand not knowing if I will attain my desired outcome."

- "I cannot bear the discomfort of hard work."

Richman's exercise challenges the perception that you have been helpless to achieve your goals throughout your life.

## YOUR HELPFULL-HELPLESS EXERCISE

List some goals in the left column that you achieved when you believed that you could (and you did) take actions toward achieving those goals. Next, list goals in the right column that you failed to achieve (and/or outcomes that might have resulted) as you avoided the discomfort of taking action. You can use the given examples as a guide.

| Goals Achieved with HelpFULL Thinking | Goals Failed with HelpLESS Thinking |
|---|---|
| Example: "Obtained job in desired field." | Example: "Avoided job interviews from fear of rejection; no job." |
| Example: "Negotiated price on new car." | Example: "Avoided salesperson thinking I'm a cheap person; paid a higher price." |
| | |
| | |
| | |
| | |

Compare the lists and review the choices that you have made throughout your life. Revisit how you perceived and experienced the process of executing short- and long-term goals that included a healthy helpFULL thinking outcome. Then, revisit what you perceived and experienced during the process when you were thinking in a helpLESS style. Through this comparison, you may discover that in those situations in which you thought helpfully, your actions did create the desired difference. You truly do have a choice in how you shape your perspective. You can take action now to defeat your helplessness thinking.

List your current goals and the helpFULL thoughts that you will maintain during the process:

| Current Goal | HelpFULL Thoughts |
|---|---|
|  |  |
|  |  |
|  |  |
|  |  |

The choice between thinking in a helpful or a helpless manner can exist in a phase of mind that is independent from the sensations of depression. That is, you can feel depressed and still think helpful thoughts and take helpful actions. Apply this approach, and you might soon discover that helpful thoughts can result in self-help actions for getting out of a depression abyss.

# ABCDE METHOD FOR DEFUSING HELPLESSNESS THINKING

Helplessness thinking can be so much a part of daily life that you take it for granted as you partially build your identity around this belief. In a helplessness mind-set, there is a hidden message: "Techniques to curb depression may work for others, but I can't do them." Thus, helplessness thinking can impede initiative.

Believe that you can't manage or cope, and you can experience anxiety that can extend to resignation and hopelessness. Acting against helplessness thoughts has several bonuses. You will gain a sense of pleasure from a calmer state of mind and body. You will be able to think more flexibly. You will see better through the lenses of realistic optimism.

The following example shows how to use the ABCDE method to defuse helplessness thinking and to advance competency thinking.

| |
|---|
| **Activating event (experience):** "A strong sense of inertia that seems like a wall preventing acting against depressive helplessness thinking." |
| **Rational beliefs about the event:** "This dull, resistant feeling is a natural impediment to positive relief from depression. However sluggish I feel, I will take the initial step of applying the ABCDE approach, and see what results." |
| **Emotional and behavioral consequences for the rational beliefs:** "A feeling of sluggish resistance is likely to continue, for a while, even following focused actions. Eventually, acting on the rational belief can promote a valid reason to experience a sense of control over the helplessness-thinking process." |
| **Irrational helplessness beliefs:** "I'm helpless to change. The feeling of depression is too heavy, too weighty." |
| **Emotional and behavioral consequences for the irrational helplessness beliefs:** "Helplessness thoughts amplify the feeling of inertia and that gives credibility to the thinking." |
| **Disputes for irrational helplessness beliefs:** (1) "Where is the proof that there is 'nothing' that I can do to change?" Sample answer: "This judgment makes no sense. Making an effort may not guarantee a desired result, but making an effort can represent a change." (2) "In what way is depression too weighty?" Sample answer: "The key words are 'too' and 'weighty.' It is a reality that depression can feel weighty. Adding the word 'too' suggests being overwhelmed with depression. Sticking with 'weighty' to describe the experience of depression sounds valid. 'Too' sounds like an exaggeration." |
| **Effects of the disputes:** "An acceptance that depression may continue, but a growing sense of mastery over depressive thinking demonstrates an ability to organize and regulate my efforts to deactivate this form of thinking." |

When helplessness thinking flows with your depressed mood, use the following ABCDE chart as a guide to map, question, and counteract helplessness thoughts that mingle with your depressed mood.

| |
|---|
| **Activating event (experience):** |
| **Rational beliefs about the event:** |
| **Emotional and behavioral consequences for the rational beliefs:** |
| **Irrational helplessness beliefs:** |
| **Emotional and behavioral consequences for the irrational helplessness beliefs:** |
| **Disputes for irrational helplessness beliefs:** |
| **Effects of the disputes:** |

# END DEPRESSION PLAN

**Key ideas** (What three ideas did you find most helpful in this chapter?):

1.

2.

3.

**Action steps** (What three steps can you take to move closer to your goal of overcoming depression?):

1.

2.

3.

**Execution** (How did you execute the steps?):

1.

2.

3.

**Results** (What did you learn that you can use?):

1.

2.

3.

# CHAPTER 11

# Overcoming Hopelessness Thinking

Hopelessness is a powerful generator for depression (Joiner et al. 2005; Liu and Alloy 2010). If you believe that you have no hope, you are likely to use this as an excuse to procrastinate and to create a self-fulfilling prophecy. Self-fulfilling prophesies were known at least as far back as ancient Greece. Harvard professor Robert Merton (1936) noted that making self-fulfilling prophecies may have unanticipated consequences. For example, believe that you have no hope, and you are likely to affirm this prophecy. An antidote is to create a productive self-fulfilling prophecy where you act as if you had hope.

## ACCEPTING REALITY VS. HOPELESSNESS

In some situations there is no hope for change. There is no fountain of youth, so aging is inevitable. But you don't have to feel miserable about this reality. Even when one situation is hopeless, you can find other opportunities. For example, by living healthily and reducing the stresses in your life, you may age more slowly.

In some situations, reality works against you. You are a four-foot-eight adult with dreams of being a National Basketball League center. You can't fulfill that dream, but you are free to go about making the most of your life in areas where you can assert control.

When you compare the reality of hopeless situations with hopelessness thinking, the difference can be dramatic. Hopelessness thinking includes overly generalized beliefs such as these:

- "My future looks dismal."

- "Nothing will ever work out."

- "Whatever I do will be futile."

- "I will never get better."

- "This is the way I am. I always feel miserable."

Hopelessness thinking is double-trouble thinking, where you layer despair on top of the unpleasant aspects of unfortunate situations. It's a mental trap. You have the key to unlock the trap and can use it if you see it.

Of course, unfortunate events happen, but the fatalistic resignation of hopelessness thinking is optional. Here are three examples of factually unpleasant situations with double-trouble thinking added (in the parentheses):

- "I lost my job (and will be out of work forever)."

- "I botched this sale (and may as well quit because I can't do any better)."

- "My pet, Puffy, died (and I can't go on)."

Some situations are generally bad or sad, even unforeseeable and catastrophic; your home could be torn from the ground by a tornado. It is the situation plus what you make of it that makes the difference. If you orchestrate your experiences from a depressive perspective, the expected outcome is more misery.

## The Power of Illusion

Psychological illusions are something you believe to be true but are not that way at all. They are reality distortions about someone, something, or some condition. People who think they drive well after a few drinks are afflicted by an illusion of false competence. Some people believe their intuition is always accurate. But it can't be right all the time, for human intuition is often far from perfect.

The power of a psychological illusion is that even after you see it, the illusion may continue to influence your perceptions, emotions, and actions. When many of my clients first see their own hopelessness thinking, their hopelessness thoughts often continue automatically. That's because hopelessness illusions stealthily flow along the channels of the mind as they merge with mood. Even when you recognize this thinking, you still have the habit to contend with. Yet being able to watch yourself automatically go through a negative thought habit is often a preamble to changing the pattern.

Alternatively, when you first see through the hopelessness illusion, you may feel relief. Often this relief is temporary. It is useful to think of relief as a preview experience. This preview provides a peek into future positive possibilities. You are likely to have a hopelessness thinking habit to break in your future, but now you know the problem, and your challenge is to solve it.

## Questioning Hopelessness Illusions

Seeing a hopelessness illusion is a first step to exiting the trap. But, how do you see what appears veiled from view, especially when you have no feedback except that which comes from you? The answer is simple: you can tell an illusion by its results. If a needlessly pessimistic thought worsens your depressed mood, you bought into an illusion.

Here are some examples of hopelessness illusions: "It's no use going on." "I have no life." "It's all over for me." What can be said about such hopelessness thoughts? They reflect a point of view where you have no way to succeed, can't cope, can't change, or are incapable of improvement. They are ideas. Without them, would or could you do differently?

> Hopelessness is a foreclosure on opportunity.

Hopelessness thoughts convey futility. But is this futility an illusion? Probe a little deeper. What does it mean when you tell yourself, "It's no use going on"? Does this mean that nothing over the next three years could possibly happen to change your thoughts or life situation?

Hopelessness thinking involves fatalistic prognostications that are based upon cognitive distortions, such as jumping to conclusions and overgeneralizaing. Instead of accepting them, you can view them as assumptions or hypotheses. You can't do much about what you view as permanent and negative, such as the loss of a dear friend. But you can do much about a hopelessness assumption.

Asking and answering coping questions is a way to debunk hopelessness thinking. For example, a general sense of hopelessness is a prediction where you assert that the future is fixed. Can you prove that the future is fixed? If it were fixed, then whatever you do would be predestined. You would have no free will. You'd have no cause to blame yourself for anything. That view is seriously flawed. Thoughts do not control chance and probability. The unexpected happens. A rapid and positive change in perspective liberates the mind from depressive torment.

# CHANCE AND CHANGE

"Clickety-clack" went a wheel as it slowly rolled in a fixed circle digging a groove into the soft soil. A small mouse, caught in the rut caused by the rolling wheel, was running in front of the wheel. The mouse couldn't climb out, so the poor creature ran to survive. Then, a sudden rainstorm drenched and shorted the motor that drove the wheel. It stopped. Water filled the rut, and the mouse swam out.

Preoccupied with survival, the mouse had little time for hopeful thoughts. Nevertheless, there was "hope." Chance unexpectedly intervened.

There may be much reason for hope, even when you can't see it. For example, hopelessness thoughts can get short-circuited by reason. The unexpected can happen. Your depression may spontaneously lift.

The story of Kate Adamson (2002) sheds some additional light on how chance and probability can effect a positive outcome. After suffering a stroke, Adamson seemed to be in a coma. She survived on life support. Her physicians thought she was in a vegetative state. At a point in time, they ended her life support. With a blink of an eye, Adamson saved her own life.

Adamson was aware of what was happening around her. She recognized people and heard what they said. Although she was aware, she could not move and respond other than to occasionally blink her eyes, which her husband saw.

Adamson was off her feeding tube for eight days. Her husband threatened to sue the hospital and insurance company that had denied treatment. The tube was put back. Today, Adamson is back to living a full life. Her journey back to a normal life started with an eye blink. She recorded this experience in her book, *Kate's Journey: Triumph over Adversity*.

## *Freewill Opportunities*

Viktor Frankl (1963), an Austrian psychiatrist and founder of logotherapy, was a death camp survivor. Following his death camp experiences, he asserted that social conditions can never fully set the boundaries for the human spirit and cannot deprive people of a freedom of will. Free will remains possible under even dangerous and oppressive circumstances.

During World War II, Frankl was incarcerated in four different Nazi death camps. Rather than dwell on his dismal situation, he looked for meaning in what he saw. Thus, he would find meaning in the smallest events, such as watching an ant move a crumb.

> When you believe you are trapped and have a very remote chance of prevailing, do what gives you the best chance.

His insight, that people can find meaning despite very limited freedom of choice, led to his emotional survival under the most dangerous and disturbing of circumstances. He lived through his reason, not through fear.

Frankl saw that people can live life through their higher mental processes. This provides freedom from unreasonable fears as well as pessimistic expectations. He thought it best to live in the present moment and to prepare for the future. He accepts that life can be hard and that positive change involves work.

## *A Radical Change in Perspective*

Clifford Beers (1908), who spearheaded the mental health movement of the early twentieth century, made a remarkable recovery from a severe bipolar condition. It began when he determined that he need not imprison himself with his past follies, indiscretions, and failures.

Beers described his own exit from depression. Beers turned his world around from a terrifying pessimism to a determination to oppose prejudice toward people with mental illnesses. Thereafter, Beers made great strides.

# BUILDING MENTAL FLEXIBILITY

Pessimistic thinking involves a static view of the future, where nothing good will happen and miseries will remain the same. Shifting from this static thinking to a more optimistic view involves recognizing the fluidity in situations, adapting, and acting to shape parts of the future through what you do in the present moment. A step in this process involves helping yourself build mental flexibility by doing the following:

- exploring novelty, change, and improvisation

- cultivating a willingness to withstand a lack of structure, control, certainty, and predictability

- developing tolerance for ambiguity, complexity, and feeling different

- making independent judgments

- knowing when to suspend judgments

- accommodating to changing information

- inching forward when bold steps cannot be taken

The actions you take to shift from pessimism to intellectual flexibility involve counteracting hopelessness thinking where:

| Acceptance of uncertainty, tension, and suffering |
|---|

converts

| Fear of depressive thinking |
|---|

into

| Acceptance of risk and opportunitites to devise and achieve performance and mastery goals |
|---|

This chart displays a process of maintaining an open perspective.

## The "Prove It" Technique

If you are responsive to the idea that you can improve your depression using cognitive methods, you are more likely to make progress, regardless of whether you feel mildly or severely depressed (Kuyken 2004). However, if you are not so sure, are you likely to feel unresponsive to the idea that you can benefit from learning how to make changes while feeling depressed? If so, the "prove it" technique is a three-phase exercise for challenging your hopelessness thinking and assumptions about the possibility for change. In phase one, you list hopelessness thoughts, such as "My future is dismal." In the second phase, you cite examples to support these thoughts. In the third phase, you explore alternative views and possibilities.

If you think your future looks dismal, give some examples of how it looks dismal. Then look for facts that contradict this view, or look for reasonable alternative ways to view your situation. Next, compare hopelessness with your alternative view. Can you prove that either is absolutely true?

This exercise can help broaden your perspective, and this boost can lead to relief from depressing speculations.

# "PROVE IT" EXERCISE

List your hopelessness thoughts, examples to support the thoughts, and alternative ways of thinking.

| **Hopelessness thoughts:** |
| 1. |
| 2. |
| 3. |
| **Examples of these thoughts:** |
| 1. |
| 2. |
| 3. |
| **Alternatives:** |
| 1. |
| 2. |
| 3. |

## *Punching Holes in Your Hopelessness Theory*

Does hopelessness thinking represent a fact or a theory? It is a fact that people think hopelessness thoughts. But what happens when you treat hopelessness as a theory?

Hopelessness thinking during times of depression often boils down to a short, simple theory, such as "Life is bad and won't get better." When actively believed, this pessimistic theory blocks out hope. Because of the enormous impact that hopelessness thinking has on mood and actions, this belief deserves close scrutiny.

In choosing between a fixed hopelessness theory and the scientific method of discovery, you are normally better off choosing a scientific approach. Granted, applying the scientific method takes extra effort. That effort involves asking probing questions and insisting on factual answers that you can independently confirm. However, through applying the scientific method, you can build cognitive skills to contest hopelessness beliefs.

Is there a role for pessimism in everyday life? Sure! Pessimism is sometimes reasonable. Imagine going to a used-car lot believing that you will get the best price on a great automobile by trusting everything the sales-person says. After all, the lot is called Honest John's. Go into this type of purchase blind, and you probably won't like the outcome.

# ABCDE METHOD FOR DEFUSING HOPELESSNESS THINKING

If you wait for hopelessness thinking to lift, you may be rewarded for your patience. But you also can do something about hopelessness thinking and perhaps shorten the wait.

By acting to recognize and question hopelessness thinking, you need not give up the possibility that an accidental happening can deal a blow to an unrelenting pessimism. You're just increasing your chances to defuse a negative, debilitating form of thinking. The ABCDE method is a proactive way to achieve a growing sense of confidence and optimism, as you can see in the following example:

| |
|---|
| **Activating event (experience):** "A dark, grim, lingering mood." |
| **Rational beliefs about the event:** "A depressed mood is unpleasant, distracting, and inhibiting. I'd strongly prefer to feel different. But the mood is what it is and will continue until it passes." |
| **Emotional and behavioral consequences for the rational beliefs:** "Acceptance of a painfully unpleasant ongoing experience. A realistic optimism that depression will pass when it passes." |
| **Irrational hopelessness beliefs:** "I can't stand this feeling. It will on forever. Things will never change. I will never get better. I'm doomed." |
| **Emotional and behavioral consequences for the irrational hopelessness beliefs:** "The mood remains. The conditions associated with it remain. These dire predictions can lead to desperation without hope. There is a deepening of the depression and immobilization." |
| **Disputes for irrational hopelessness beliefs:** (1) "Although a lingering feeling of depression can feel oppressive, why can I not stand what I don't like?" Sample answer: "I can, but I still don't like the state I'm in." (2) "What do I gain by telling myself that depression will go on forever?" Sample answer: "There is no meaningful benefit for making a fatalistic proclamation. This state has gone on longer than I'd prefer. I'm not in a position to predict all chance and other opportunities to defeat a lingering depression." (3) "What are the 'things' that will never change?" Sample answer: "Forever is a long time. Many things can happen between now and then. Is it possible that my perspective can change with new information and the passage of time?" (4) "Where is the proof and evidence that I am a fortune-teller with certain knowledge that I can't get better?" Sample answer: "Mythologies of the mind fictionalize reality. Their presence may be real, but what they represent can be no more than a figment of reality." (5) "What do I mean by 'doomed'? In what way am I doomed? Can I prove this doom theory beyond a reasonable doubt? Can I show the world that there can be no exceptions to this theory?" Sample answer: "Doom is a form of extremist depressive thinking. As ink can color water, doom can blur clarity. Doom thinking can destroy clarity; however, this pessimistic prophecy is vulnerable to a crystal-clear rationality that comes from a fact-based analysis." |
| **Effects of the disputes:** "Abandon hopelessness thinking." |

When hopelessness thinking is linked with your depression, you can use the following ABCDE chart as a guide to map and counteract this thinking:

**Activating event (experience):**

**Rational beliefs about the event:**

**Emotional and behavioral consequences for the rational beliefs:**

**Irrational hopelessness beliefs:**

**Emotional and behavioral consequences for the irrational hopelessness beliefs:**

**Disputes for irrational hopelessness beliefs:**

**Effects of the disputes:**

# END DEPRESSION PLAN

**Key ideas** (What three ideas did you find most helpful in this chapter?):

1.

2.

3.

**Action steps** (What three steps can you take to move closer to your goal of overcoming depression?):

1.

2.

3.

**Execution** (How did you execute the steps?):

1.

2.

3.

**Results** (What did you learn that you can use?):

1.

2.

3.

# CHAPTER 12

# Restraining Blame

We live in a blame culture where blame is like smog in the air. Although rarely addressed as a mental health issue, blame is probably our greatest social malady. Blame saturates practically every form of human disturbance. It's so much a part of the social fabric that most of us either don't pay attention to it or don't want to deal with it. Yet, sometimes this is necessary to do, especially when blame has a damaging effect on you.

We'd all be better off if we used blame as a means of establishing accountability and steered clear of the coercive and nerve-jolting forms of blame. As a society, we are far from that ideal. Still, you can do much to bring serenity into your life by limiting self-blame, blaming others for normal faults, and blaming events for all your misfortunes.

## HOW BLAME OPERATES

Blame merges seamlessly with everyday experience and takes effort to resist. Blame can be hard to see, yet curbing blame excesses may be the single most important act that you can undertake toward achieving higher levels of positive mental health and avoidance of depression.

Blame is often taken for granted. When something negative happens, people ask, "Who's at fault?" When a nation's economy falters, the leadership is blamed. The grass on your lawn starts to brown, and you blame the hot sun. The clothing you wear could offend someone who prefers a different color, and you get blamed for that. In US culture, political correctness has run amuck. If you use the word "homeless" instead of "residentially challenged," you could get blamed for insensitivity. In a depressive state of mind, you blame yourself for feeling the way that you do. This blame-trap thinking contributes to needless miseries.

You could possibly escape blame if you were in a coma, but someone might blame you for that too! Even if you act with great diligence in your responsibilities, normal errors and lapses can lead to blame. When you are especially self-critical, you can feel pangs of depression for no good reason.

You can't escape blame. The question is, what blame is relevant, what is not, and how do you deal with blame when it is needless, excessive, or coercive?

# BLAME AND DEPRESSION

As practically everyone knows, blame often spreads for no good reason at all. What is not so widely known is that blame is a significant threat to positive mental health and is a factor in depression.

## *When You Blame Yourself*

Self-criticism is a form of internalized blame that is common among people with depression (Beck 1987). If you are highly self-critical, the odds are that you are likely to entangle yourself in thoughts about inadequacies and imperfections. Self-criticism interferes with progress (Bulmash et al. 2009).

Self-blame can come about from damning yourself for imagined deficiencies. You may view yourself as not attractive, smart, or athletic enough. Imagine if your contingency for happiness were a need for something that you thought was impossible to obtain, such as thirty more IQ points? When this deficiency-blame mode of thought is active, happiness, success, and worth are out of reach. However, consider this view: "I am the only me I will ever be, so I might as well act to do the best I can with the resources that I have available." That's an obviously healthier way to think, but it is surprisingly elusive.

A common depression paradox is that of blaming yourself for your problems while declaring yourself helpless to change. If you are truly helpless, which is doubtful, then there is no rational basis for blaming yourself for what you can't control. However, from a social perspective, internalizing blame is healthier than leading the callous life of the sociopath who lacks empathy, views others as suckers, has shallow relationships, and goes through life exploiting others.

## *When You Blame Others*

Another stress from blame can stem from a "Why me?" question. When something negative happens, you play the victim or think that the fates are against you or that you deserve punishment.

There is no universal answer to the "Why me?" question. Things are as they are. The more interesting question remains, "How do I make the most of what I have?"

You can view yourself as the consummate victim of past atrocities. Here is an example: "I suffered a series of losses, including a pet parakeet flying out of an open door, automobile repair problems, a flooded basement, and a reduction of my hours at work that led to financial strains. That's why I feel depressed."

You can typically find others to blame for your depression. The reason you feel depressed is because of government corruption, a sneaky rival, parents who gave you a rotten childhood, discrimination, a lousy education, a narcissistic mate, an unfair boss—the list goes on. By blaming others for your depression, you narrow your choices. Either others must change, or you'll stay depressed. You may be able to influence people, but you can't change them. While aversive actions by others can contribute to depression, how you think about such situations can yield double-trouble distresses and keep depression alive.

Blaming others is a poor solution for overcoming depression. Alternatively, you can explore empathy options where you try to see things from another's perspective without yielding any of your

> It's hard to imagine a best-selling self-help book titled *The Joys of Blame and Self-Deception.*

rights to act in your best self-interest. By preceding a blame statement with a simple "I believe" phrase, you can cause a shift from blame accusations to a discussion.

Whatever the causes of your depression, your present and future depend on your efforts to do and get better now. You have a great ally: yourself and your ability to change perspective and locate exit points from depression.

## The Triple E Factor

The triple E factors of dysfunctional blame include *excesses*, *extensions*, and *exonerations*.

### EXCESSES

Blame excesses are patterns of finger-pointing, denying, and faultfinding. The list goes on. The adage "Who are we going to blame for this one?" characterizes this style. When excesses are pervasive, fear of blame can blend into a depressive outlook. When irritable, you may blame others for your troubles. When insecure, you may be inclined to take the blame. Neither way is healthy.

It is easier to blame parents, education, an indifferent universe, the devil, an unhappy marriage, unfairness, bad breaks, strangers, or genetics for your depression. Blowing off responsibility may be an engaging way to psychologize about depression at a cocktail party, but abdicating responsibilities to others can contribute to a bigger problem: depressive helplessness. At the same time, there is no need to correct faults or make amends as long as you opine that someone else is at fault.

### EXTENSIONS

Blame often has extensions, and they are normally even worse than the excesses. Extensions of blame include demands, intolerance, and condemnation. Thus, when feeling depressed for an unacceptably long period, you might get mad at yourself:

- "I should not have gotten depressed."

- "I can't stand what I did to myself."

- "I did something wrong and should be punished."

When depressive extensions of blame affect your perceptions and judgments, depression can mushroom.

Blame extensions can be verbal, come from outside sources, and take many accusatory forms: "What's wrong with you?" "Can't you get anything right?" or "Were you brought up in a barn?" When subject to such a deluge of blame, some succumb to depression and withdraw.

### EXONERATION

To avoid blame excesses and extensions, it's a normal human tendency to excuse real or imagined blame-worthy behavior. Exoneration ploys are ways to maintain a good public image while cloaking real or imagined faults and actions. These ploys take many forms, including making excuses, telling white lies, identifying loopholes, shifting blame, omitting relevant information, rationalizing, and such defensiveness as, "Nobody told me not to do that." You may exonerate yourself by blaming others or circumstances: "Sam is the problem." "The world is corrupt." "There is too much unfairness."

It is the rare person who seeks and then squarely faces the truth. Why is this ordinarily so hard? If blame were not unpleasant, telling the truth, being open, and leveling with others would be the rule. But the golden rules of honesty are more often the exception when something more important is at stake, such as your personal image.

# ELIMINATING BLAME

Blame and its extensions may make your depression worse. Recognizing the blame factor in depression is the first step toward reducing the stressing and depressing impact of this social affliction.

## An Evolutionary Outlook

*Psychology Today* contributing editor and clinical psychologist Nando Pelusi (2003) notes that most people find that overcoming their depression can prove especially challenging when they blame themselves for being depressed. He suggests a two-step evolutionary perspective to eliminate self-blame and self-downing as a secondary aspect of depression.

As a first step, Pelusi (pers. comm.) suggests that you evoke a *contemporary* explanation for blame thinking. For example, if you catch yourself involved in secondary depressive thinking—where you think you should not be depressed, blame yourself for how you feel, and then down yourself—think again. Telling yourself something like "I'm worthless if I'm depressed" does not change the depression and can deepen this state.

Pelusi's second step involves what he sees as an *ultimate* explanation for taking the burden of blame away from feeling depressed. He theorizes that the depressive tendency may have evolved as a survival function among early humans, when 99 percent of our ancestors lived among small bands of kin. For example, feelings of depression among people in northern climates could routinely occur a few months before the winter solstice. These feelings of depression could trigger an impulse to migrate to a warmer climate. Then, when spring grew near, a biological depressive impulse could trigger a northerly migration. Under this scenario, depression wouldn't have been a flaw but, in some cases, would have served an adaptive function.

With the growth of civilization and language, certain philosophies, such as a need for approval, could attach to this survival mechanism with unfortunate results. This *modern* adaptation is like evolution in reverse.

## Blame and the Brain

There is an observable difference between how the brain looks when you are depressed and when you are not. You can see this difference in the results of computerized neuroimaging methods such as a PET scan (positron emission tomography) or fMRI (functional magnetic resonance imaging). When you are depressed, parts of your brain look cooler. Thus, the depressed brain looks different from the nondepressed brain.

Depression is what it is. It is no more a choice than is vulnerability to the flu. Unfortunately, when they are depressed, many people blame themselves, others, or circumstances for their depression. By refusing to blame yourself for depression, you act kindly toward yourself. You are then in a better position to get tough on the problem of curbing depression.

> Even when some aspects of your life go poorly, other parts are likely to go better.

## Getting Some Perspective

Depression is neither a choice nor a character flaw. It's a psychological, biological, social, and environmentally related condition. Thus, depression is not the fault of the person who suffers from this darkened mood. No one wakes up one morning and says, "I believe I will think depressing thoughts today and cause myself to feel miserable." Choice comes into play in what you decide to do to free yourself from depression.

You can choose to develop a realistic perspective to counter blame excesses. Perspective involves weighing what is going on in your life according to its relevance. This more fact-based perspective insulates you against needless pessimism.

When blameworthy conditions and negative thinking initially dominate your attention, a broader perspective can be a relief. This broader view can involve accepting the right of others to hold views you don't like. It can involve putting up with irritations but also rectifying and correcting problems.

# ABCDE METHOD FOR DEFUSING BLAME THINKING

Blame excesses, extensions, and exonerations are a significant part of our social interactions and are implicated in a broad range of disabling emotional conditions, from road rage to depression. You can cut back on blame excesses by learning to pause before blaming and using that time to substitute confident composure for your blame-trap reactions. The following chart shows how to pause and apply the ABCDE method to blame thinking:

| |
|---|
| **Activating event (experience):** "A lingering depressed mood." |
| **Rational beliefs about the event:** "Down moods are unpleasant." |
| **Emotional and behavioral consequences for the rational beliefs:** "The down mood continues but is not exacerbated by added negativity. Activities continue, but at a pace that reflects the level of depression I experience." |
| **Irrational blame beliefs:** "I brought depression upon myself (and therefore I am to blame)." |
| **Emotional and behavioral consequences for the blame belief:** "A worsened sense of depression. Withdrawal." |

**Disputes for the blame belief:** "How am I totally blameworthy for feeling depressed? Sample answer: "The various causes of depression suggest that this disability occurs because of vulnerability to depression and conditions that evoke it. Unless I can convince myself that I should be singled out for blame, I had better accept that I have this vulnerability and learn to apply my abilities to mute depression's effects."

**Effects of the disputes:** "Relief from the ravages of blame and depression."

When blame thinking is linked to depression, you can use the following ABCDE chart to map and counteract this thinking.

**Activating event (experience):**

**Rational beliefs about the event:**

**Emotional and behavioral consequences for the rational beliefs:**

**Irrational blame beliefs about the event:**

**Emotional and behavioral consequences for the irrational blame beliefs:**

**Disputes for irrational blame beliefs:**

**Effects of the disputes:**

# END DEPRESSION PLAN

**Key ideas** (What three ideas did you find most helpful in this chapter?):

1.

2.

3.

**Action steps** (What three steps can you take to move closer to your goal of overcoming depression?):

1.

2.

3.

**Execution** (How did you execute the steps?):

1.

2.

3.

**Results** (What did you learn that you can use?):

1.

2.

3.

# Building Emotional Resilience

Recognize and overcome agitated depression.

Address the psychology and biology of depression.

Demagnify the biological strains of depression.

Use mindfulness to ease depression tensions.

Stop powerlessness thinking.

Confidently break a mixed anxiety-depression connection.

Stop inhibiting yourself and make progress.

Halt the inertia of depression with the five-minute plan.

Discover fresh ideas from old books on conquering anxiety.

Prevent panic from surging into depression.

Overcome depression from trauma thinking.

Cut the anger-depression connection.

Replace anger thinking with confident composure.

End depressive pain from self-consciousness, guilt, and shame.

Build frustration tolerance for inconvenience.

Defuse a vicious ADD-depression-procrastination cycle.

Exit a depression and substance abuse cycle.

# CHAPTER 13

# Coping with Depressive Sensations

In his Harvard medical school lectures, the French physician Pierre Janet (1913), pointed out that *somaticizing* (the false belief that emotionally related pains have a physical cause) happens outside of conscious awareness. Scattered here and there throughout his lectures, he seamlessly linked melancholia to physical complaints. That observation is largely valid today.

When you feel depressed, your biology is likely to feel off-kilter and you'll experience unpleasant sensations. You may feel lethargic, fatigued, or headachy. You will likely have sleep and appetite problems. If you lose your ambition to communicate with others, you may become reclusive. Alternatively, if you suffer from agitated depression, you may be very irritable.

The focus of this chapter is to help you cope with depressive sensations and improve your mood. It will explore the mind-body connection and give you cognitive behavioral tools to break through a depressive sensation-and-thinking cycle.

## ■ *Marybeth's Story*

*Marybeth slumped in her chair. Aspirin and ibuprofen did nothing to stop her pounding headache. As her melancholic mood ground on from week to week, Marybeth's headaches came, went, and came again. She suffered multiple aches and pains. After extensive medical testing, she found that her vitamin D level was down. So she took vitamin D. She also had a mild hypothyroid condition and took medication to restore balance. Her physician prescribed an antidepressant for her headaches and mood. She found that the side effects were worse than the "cure" and she began to have suicidal thoughts. She said, "I feel like a mess."*

*Marybeth had suffered a series of earlier setbacks. Her husband had run off with her next-door neighbor, whom she'd considered a confidante. A few months later, her mother had died. Initially, she didn't want to think about what had happened, but she gradually came to grips with these losses. At my suggestion, Marybeth listened to "Let It Be" by the Beatles. The music had a temporary saddening but quieting effect.*

*Marybeth was not out of the woods. She suffered from self-doubts, insecurities, and fears of feeling tense that had been with her long before she had met her now-estranged husband. She said she probably would not have addressed and resolved her fears were it not for her desire to defeat her depression.*

*Ironically, the adversities that led to her depression became the occasion for her to feel revitalized. She worked out her core insecurity issues. As she resolved these issues, her depressive sensations disappeared.*

### ■ *Harry's Story*

*People who overfocus on unexplained negative sensations and blow them out of proportion can benefit by refocusing their attention on coping rather than complaining. For example, Harry felt irritable and blamed his boss for holding him back, his wife for her bad temperament, and his parents for undercutting his confidence. As he watched a documentary newscast on the economy, he seized on the idea that "the government" was loaded with corrupt bureaucrats feeding off the public trough. The thought that he was supporting this thievery with his tax dollars brought him closer to the edge of despair and agitation. Harry suffered from agitated depression.*

*As he grasped at straws to explain his feelings, Harry dug himself into a deeper malaise. In therapy, he made modest progress in recognizing his tendency to jump to conclusions about his feelings. At first, he kept slipping back to blaming and complaining when he felt depressed, but then he came to a stoic acceptance of his tendency toward irritability. His complaining was still noteworthy but substantially less so than before. His wife, Laura, was happy that he no longer blamed her for his troubles.*

As Harry's and Marybeth's stories illustrate, depression can have dramatic sensations that beg for explanation. When you concentrate your attention on how bad you feel, and you use your imagination to conjure up reasons why, you are likely to magnify the negative. Separating the psychological from the biological parts of depression gives you the advantage of targeting the right issues with workable solutions.

## THE MIND-BODY CONNECTION

The relationship between your body (*soma*) and your mind (*psyche*) has been known since ancient times. You are a member of a conditional and suggestible species. You can talk yourself into feeling depressed by the negative things that you tell yourself. You can suffer from imaginary crises that exist in your mind and nowhere else. Your thinking also can reflect your depressed mood, and you may magnify conditions that commonly coexist with depression, such as stress-related pain and awakening early and not being able to fall back asleep.

If you are vulnerable to the effects of a combination of negative thinking and depressive sensations, you can feel physically ill. Feel physically ill, and you are more likely to think negatively. Think negatively, and you are more likely to feel stressed and possibly more depressed and physically ill. However, by taking corrective steps to address depressive sensations and depressive thinking, your biological symptoms are likely to ease as your mood lifts.

The mind plays a major role in the interpretation of pain. If you experienced persistent pain prior to your depression, you should know that chronic pain and depression often co-occur. About 60 percent of those who suffer from depression also experience pain (Agüera-Ortiz et al. 2010). Your pain may have an identifiable physical cause that needs to be addressed medically. You also can act against the psychic part of pain. For example, catastrophizing over pain seems to worsen it. Although pain management is beyond the scope of this book, you

> Learning to tolerate—not like—physical signs of depression can lessen their impact.

can apply cognitive behavioral methods—the same techniques you learn here—to end catastrophizing over pain (Turner, Holtzman, and Mancl 2007).

## Depressive Symptoms

Over the ages, hundreds of millions have lived with a prolonged depressed mood and combinations of fatigue, appetite problems, sleep, sluggishness, stomach, or pain problems. Some of these physical conditions coincide with a major depression. If you experience a blend of negative emotions with your depressed mood, you may experience physical symptoms and illnesses without medically identifiable physical causes (Howren and Suls 2011).

Lower-back pain may be easier to report than psychological distress. However, *medicalizing* your psychic distress, or seeking medical treatment for stress-related lower-back pain or other physical symptoms of depression, may keep you going through a revolving door as you seek physical causes for a psychological problem.

Changes in sensations can evoke faulty explanations, and you can increase your risk of experiencing a more severe depression following a misdiagnosis (Perugi et al. 2011). People with depression who believe they are physically ill rather than depressed rarely respond to medical treatment for specific symptoms. If they do, their response is short-lived (Smith 2001). Thus, it's important to start with an accurate diagnosis. This may take a separate review of both psychological and medical areas (McFarlane et al. 2008). Unexplained medical conditions, such as backaches and gastrointestinal distress that are thought to originate in the mind, may effectively be remedied by using cognitive-behavioral manuals (Allen et al. 2006).

# MISREADING THE SIGNALS

If you experience depressive sensations, you can misread and magnify the significance of what you feel, sometimes to your detriment.

### ■ June's Story

*June awoke on the "wrong side of the bed." She explained her distressed sensations by associating them with a harsh comment that her great-aunt had made years earlier about her art. She believed that the comment evoked the negative sensations that she thereafter experienced. She told herself that her great-aunt's comment had deprived her of a career in art, which was why she was depressed. June now had an explanation for her distressed sensations and depression. However, her recurrent depression had started years before the event.*

### ■ Joe's Story

*When Joe's wife cooked his pancakes too long, he felt angry. He thought that his mate's cooking caused his anger and that he would not have been angry were it not for her cooking. Almost instantly, he screamed at her and berated her.*

*The problem did not reside with either the pancakes or Joe's wife. Something else happened in between. Joe demanded that his wife behave infallibly. He thought that she deserved punishment for her imperfection, because it affected him. This demand thinking was automatic; it skipped under his conscious awareness but was associated with his angry feelings and outburst.*

*Eventually, Joe came to understand that he was his own worst pain in the rump and that his outbursts were more of a reflection of agitated depression than his wife's cooking and imperfections.*

## Taking a Closer Look

Joe and June were caught up in depressive sensation-and-thinking cycles, where a sensitivity for unpleasant sensations can lead to negative explanations that then can contribute more stress to an already depressive mood (Knaus 1982). If you follow the arrows in the next diagram, you'll see how these vicious cycles can evolve.

# A DEPRESSIVE SENSATION-AND-THINKING CYCLE

| Depressive Sensations → | Depressive Thinking → | Depressive Sensations → |
|---|---|---|
| 1. fatigue | "I can't stand feeling this way." | 1. agitation |
| 2. depressed mood | | 2. strain |
| 3. dullness | | |
| Depressive Thinking → | Depressive Sensations → | Depressive Thinking → |
| 1. "This will go on forever." | 1. weakness | 1. "I can't do anything to change." |
| 2. "I can't control how I feel." | 2. sluggishness | 2. "I'll never get over this." |
| Depressive Sensations → | Depressive Thinking → | Depressive Sensations → |
| 1. tension | 1. "I'm helpless." | 1. headache |
| 2. upset stomach | 2. "It's hopeless." | 2. fitful sleep |
| | | 3. depressed mood |

## Breaking the Cycle

Fortunately, you can break this cycle of misery. Separating sensations from depressive thinking is a starting point. For example, Atlanta psychotherapist Ed Garcia (pers. comm.) says that when you are depressed, you might wonder, "Why is this happening to me?" This type of question can lead to a "poor me" attitude that takes a negative situation and makes it worse. To separate your psychological interpretation from depressive sensations, Garcia suggests that it is often better to ask yourself simply, "Why is this happening?" This question gives you a greater range of possibilities to choose from. You are now in a position to go from what Garcia calls "soft" to "hard" thinking.

> By tolerating depressive sensations, you can avoid escalating depressive tensions.

Soft thinking is like a floodlight that covers a broad area, giving you a range of possibilities to identify and choose among. By starting with soft thinking, you target a general area to explore and avoid jumping to conclusions.

Selecting among the possibilities is a form of hard thinking. This is like focusing a spotlight on a narrower area. By moving from soft to hard thinking, you are in a better position to examine and evaluate your explanations for depression. By separating depressive thinking from depressive sensations, you can more easily deactivate the depressive thinking, which can be relieving.

# GETTING YOUR INTERPRETATIONS RIGHT

We live in a culture where there is a pill for every purpose. We treat sorrow with antidepressants, ordinary tensions with tranquilizers, and active young boys with Ritalin. Indeed, if you think that procrastination is due to a gene, you might want a pill for stopping procrastination.

When you feel fatigued, you may think it can only have a physical cause. You may come to the same conclusion about headaches, aches and pains, and other noteworthy physical conditions that occur around the time you first feel a downward change in mood. You could look for a magic pill. As an alternative, you can broaden your search (soft thinking) and then focus on fact-based information (hard thinking).

People are prone to make *rogue interpretations* of their somatic sensations (Brown 2004). Say you have an especially painful headache and depressed mood. That combination is understandably straining. When you are depressed, it's easy to escalate the misery by believing that your headache means you have a brain tumor. This rogue interpretation adds a layer of needless misery to your existing strain. You'll need more than speculative thoughts to confirm that dire diagnosis. You'll need evidence.

Faulty explanations for unpleasant sensations will not help you get any better. Here are three thoughts on how to curb a tendency to misinterpret what's going on:

- You can change your mental script from one of blind acceptance of a bogus explanation to one where you look for evidence to support an alternative explanation. Looking for alternative views is a sophisticated way to avoid falling into a common trap of only looking for ways to prove what you already think.

- You can be in a depressed mood with somatic sensations, judge the mood and sensations as unpleasant, and still not exaggerate the negatives.

- You may believe that depressive sensations are unpleasant and stick with this interpretation. This acceptance promises to lessen your level of stress.

It takes work to exit from a vicious cycle of negative sensations and bogus explanations. By keeping a fact-based perspective, you can turn your efforts from magnifying tensions toward easing depressive strains.

## *A Mindfulness Method to Manage Melancholy*

Clinical psychologist John Hudesman (pers. comm.) gives us his top tip on overcoming depression:

One of the most distressing aspects of feeling depressed is the never-ending train of negative thoughts, for example, "I really messed up that job interview." Regardless of the particular thought, a common theme is that we are falling short and are, in turn, diminished in some way. One relatively new approach to dealing with depression is learning to become more mindful of our thoughts and experiences.

Mark Williams and his associates show how mindfulness methods can set the stage for us to look at our thoughts in a new way. For example, it is easy to distinguish between thinking of how it would be great to eat a piece of chocolate cake versus eating a piece of chocolate cake. Clearly, just thinking about a piece of cake is not real. The same distinction holds true for the many negative thoughts we have during the day; that is, these negative thoughts are just that, thoughts.

When you believe that these thoughts are as real as a piece of chocolate cake, you are likely to automatically feel and act in certain ways. An alternative approach would be to recognize that our thoughts could be viewed dispassionately. They do not have to automatically lead to negative feelings and actions. But how can you do this?

Try meditating. Many people use "om" as their sound (mantra) of choice. As you repeat the mantra, it is certain that other thoughts will intrude themselves into your consciousness. They might be neutral thoughts, such as, "Should I go grocery shopping after work?" or they might be more emotionally laden thoughts, such as, "I should have gotten a better grade on the test." As you have these intrusive thoughts, you can recognize them and gently remind yourself to return to repeating your mantra. At first you may only feel comfortable doing this for a few minutes; however, with time you will be able to increase the length of your practice. As you become more comfortable with TM, you will also come to recognize that intrusive thoughts don't have to control you. That realization can be a powerful strategy in helping you to deal with depressive thinking, especially when you see that while you created the thought, the thought is not the same as a piece of cake, nor does it capture the essence of a complex situation or of you.

Mindfulness-based approaches for depression are gaining in popularity, partially because they combine cognitive behavioral methods with a Buddhist philosophy that seems to be helpful in both quelling depression (Chiesa and Serretti 2011; Hofmann et al. 2010) and preventing relapses (Piet and Hougaard 2011).

By following New York City clinical psychologist John Hudesman's prescription, you can reduce the added tensions that come from magnifying the significance of depressive sensations and jumping to conclusions about their significance. Alternatively, you can sing "Let It Be" to yourself and see what will be.

# ABCDE METHOD FOR THINKING ABOUT UNPLEASANT SENSATIONS

Although acceptance may lessen the intensity and duration of depression, you may experience residual physical effects and a lingering down mood. However, this can feel like paradise compared to double-troubling yourself by jumping to rogue conclusions and catastrophizing.

The following chart shows how to apply the ABCDE method to negate needless negative thinking about unpleasant depressive sensations.

| |
|---|
| **Activating event (experience):** "A sensation of general tension." |
| **Rational beliefs about the event:** "I don't like how I feel." |
| **Emotional and behavioral consequences for the rational beliefs:** "Acceptance of unpleasant depressive sensations." |
| **Irrational beliefs about depressive sensations:** "I can't control these feelings. They will go on forever. It's hopeless." |
| **Emotional and behavioral consequences for the irrational beliefs:** "Dullness, sluggishness, frustration, agitation." |
| **Disputes for irrational beliefs:** (1) "Why is it necessary to control depressive sensations?" Sample answer: "This would be preferable but not necessary. Accepting the sensations for what they are eliminates double-trouble thinking that magnifies them." (2) "Where is the proof that the negative sensations of depression will go on forever?" Sample answer: "Forever is a long time. Many things can happen between now and then. We have no absolute proof that depression will persist without abatement." (3) "What is the 'it' that is hopeless?" Sample answer: "Does 'it' refer to your ability to think clearly? There is sound reason to believe that people can develop clear-thinking skills. Does the 'it' mean that tension is terminal? If so, where is the proof?" In short, clarify what "it" is. Next, look at what you mean by "hopeless." Seek alternative views for an acceptance that changes are inevitable. Chances are you'll find loopholes in hopelessness thinking. |
| **Effects of the disputes:** "Reduced frustration. Improved tolerance for tension. Decreased negative thinking about unpleasant depressive sensations. A quieting sense of acceptance. A lessening of depression." |

When negative thinking about depressive sensations is linked with your depression, use the following chart as a guide to map and counteract this thinking.

| |
|---|
| **Activating event (experience):** |
| **Rational beliefs about the event:** |
| **Emotional and behavioral consequences for the rational beliefs:** |
| **Irrational beliefs about depressive sensations:** |
| **Emotional and behavioral consequences for the irrational beliefs:** |
| **Disputes for irrational beliefs:** |
| **Effects of the disputes:** |

# END DEPRESSION PLAN

**Key ideas** (What three ideas did you find most helpful in this chapter?):

1.

2.

3.

**Action steps** (What three steps can you take to move closer to your goal of overcoming depression?):

1.

2.

3.

**Execution** (How did you execute the steps?):

1.

2.

3.

**Results** (What did you learn that you can use?):

1.

2.

3.

# CHAPTER 14

# Attending to Your Anxieties

When anxiety and depression co-occur, your misery index is likely to rise. This combination is common. Anxiety and major depression appear to have a shared vulnerability; one condition is a magnet for the other (Middeldorp et al. 2005; Kessler et al. 2011). If you suffer from generalized anxiety, you are prone to worry about such things as alien abduction or being diagnosed with cancer at any time. With generalized anxiety, you have an 80 percent chance of having significant depression at some point during your life (Judd et al. 1998). If you suffer from a major depression, you have a 58 percent chance of experiencing social anxiety (Stein et al. 1999).

Mixed anxiety and depression contribute to higher levels of work and social problems, a slower recovery, and a higher relapse rate (Sartorius et al. 1996; Das-Munshi et al. 2008). Yet only a small percentage of people take appropriate measures to alleviate their suffering (McQuaid et al. 1999; Young et al. 2008). That's unfortunate.

It's time to improve those numbers. You can apply cognitive, emotive, and behavioral methods, and bring yourself considerable relief from these co-occurring troubles. This chapter will take you on a cook's tour of how to take corrective actions against the family of anxieties that may coexist with depression.

## STOP WORRYING

Worry is a big deal for those who worry. Worry and rumination are core cognitive processes in both anxiety and depression (Papageorgiou 2006). *Depressive worries* reflect a lack of confidence and the feeling that you have no control over the future, your finances, and your relationships. This form of worry intensifies depression (Diefenbach et al. 2001). Stop worry at its inception and you can help yourself sidestep a combination of recurring anxieties and depression.

Depression brings inertia and lethargy. Anxiety begets an electrifying tension and deadening inhibition. When combined, discontent rises.

## *A Top Tip to Stop Worry before It Becomes Worse*

Elliot D. Cohen (2011) is the founder of logic-based therapy and author of *The Dutiful Worrier: How to Stop Compulsive Worry without Feeling Guilty*(Cohen 2011).

Cohen (pers. comm.) offers this tip for defeating worry before this state of mind fuels anxiety and depression:

Recurrent worry is often the result of anxiety stemming from the demand to control future events in your life. This includes a demand to be certain about the future so that control can be guaranteed. However, this demand is unrealistic, as human beings have limited control over their environment and it is not possible to predict the future with certainty. So there are two prongs to overcoming recurrent worry and anxiety. First, stop demanding that you control what is not in your power to control; second, stop demanding certainty about the future.

The ancient Stoic philosopher Epictetus had something very instructive to say about the first demand. He admonished us not to try to control external events, including attaining the approval of others, for such events are outside human control. Instead, you should stick to trying to control your mental attitudes, such as your desires, wishes, hopes, and preferences. These, he said, are indeed under human control.

As for the demand for certainty, I would admonish recurrent worriers to reframe living in terms of probability. This means taking a scientific view about living, where you proportion the degree of your belief to the strength of available evidence. All scientific truth is probabilistic. Were it not for this fact, science would never be revised. Certainty is a stale construct. If you could be certain about things, then there would never be risk. If there were no risk, then life would be boring. Welcome possibilities; they are endless and make life exciting!

# COPING WITH PARASITIC ANXIETIES

Nature has made us vigilant for signs of possible risk and danger. You feel tense at the thought of walking home alone after midnight along a path through a graveyard where members of a satanic cult gather. Your knowledge of this risk has survival value.

Unlike this natural form of anxiety, a parasitic anxiety is where you exaggerate or make up terrors and then shrink into a ball of tension. Your apprehension over imaginary dangers drains your time and resources, offering nothing of meaningful benefit in return.

Parasitic anxieties may coincide with imagined catastrophes involving social situations that have little to do with your physical safety or social responsibilities. You may worry too much about your status, image, performance, and so forth.

### ■ *Mike's Story*

*Mike was worried that he would lose his job. He'd been worried about this possibility for several years. Despite having good performance reviews, he continued to fear the worst. One day, when his supervisor walked past him without appearing to notice him, Mike jumped to the conclusion that he was going to be fired. His stomach became tied in knots. He had trouble sleeping that night as the thought of the possible job loss kept buzzing through his mind. The next day, his supervisor appeared in good spirits. Mike wasn't fired. He felt relief. But it only lasted until he found something else to worry about.*

If you've experienced parasitic anxiety mixed with depression, chances are you've experienced at least some of the following:

- feelings of tension and difficulty relaxing

- moodiness, irritability, and grouchiness

- difficulties falling or staying asleep

- evaluation anxiety (expecting that you will make mistakes and be harshly judged)

- diminished spontaneity

- procrastination

- fear of disapproval

- feeling that you can't cope

- difficulty in paying attention and concentrating

- feeling uptight

- self-consciousness

- experiencing one imaginary crisis after another

- believing you are at the center of attention when you want to fade into the background

Luckily, you can do something about your parasitic anxieties and alleviate your suffering.

## Fresh Ideas from Three Old Books

You may be surprised to find ideas from old books on conquering anxiety that are as fresh as the morning dew. Here are some ideas from three of these treasure chests that I unpacked and reworked with literary license.

> As Mark Twain quipped, "I've had many troubles in my life, most of which didn't happen."

### THE STOP-THINK SOLUTION

Psychologist John Dollard (1942) had this core idea for quelling needless anxiety: "When afraid, stop and think. Examine the feared situation. See if there is any real danger in it. If not, try just that act to which the fear is attached" (22). Dollard uses a basic stop, look, and listen technique for this process.

**Stop.** When you find yourself in an anxious pickle, an essential step is to stop and think about your thinking (the metacognitive way). If you don't figure out what is in your head, you'll run from what you feel in your gut. When in doubt, write out the thoughts. What are you saying to yourself when you have a parasitic form of anxiety? Do you worry about what is wrong with you? Do you hear an inner voice saying, "What's the use? Why bother trying?" Dollard admits that thinking about thinking doesn't come naturally. However, you can develop a nose for sniffing out problem thinking by taking this on as an awareness challenge.

**Look.** When you look, you examine the meaning of your self-statements: "What is going on? What is the problem? Is there a thinking fiction I need to become aware of and correct?" Through this self-examination, you may find that you have a correctable problem to solve.

**Listen.** Dollard struggles with his definition of listening to make the problem-solving mnemonic work. Here is the gist. When you listen, you prepare yourself to separate vexing from useful thoughts and learn to solve the problem of anxiety thinking. For example, if you think you are powerless, what are the exceptions? By asking the question, you've shown yourself that you are not powerless.

Dollard is explicit about what happens next: changes in thinking must include new actions if you are to make the new thoughts useful.

## A BALANCING APPROACH

Anxiety is complex, and the parasitic variety commonly blends with other conditions, such as perfectionism, self-doubting, and worry. These conditions have a common exaggeration factor that distracts and drains your resources, giving nothing of value in return. Swiss psychiatrist Paul Dubois (1909) understood the relationship between exaggeration and anxiety and had much to say about it.

Spinning your wheels by exaggerating what has gone or could go wrong leaves you with little time to examine what's going right. When you get stuck in this defect-detecting cycle, you can feel as if you were living life in a tumbler. You may worry about what will happen tomorrow. If you meet your dream lover, will you lose out because you are not good enough? What will you do if your pet runs away? In this tumbler, worry spins into anxiety, which can eventually extend into depression.

Dubois thought that provocative events happen every day. Some lead to acute symptoms. For example, someone acts aggressively toward you. You react. A friend betrays your trust; you feel devastated. It's easy to lose perspective in this tumbler world. It may seem as if you can't live past these events. However, if you are in this tumbler, you can *will* yourself to try a different way.

If you accentuate the negatives and ignore your positive abilities, Dubois promoted the following psychological homework assignment. In a notebook, make two columns and label the left column "troubles" and the right column "favorable." In the evening, list what troubled you (annoyances from that day) in the left column. In the right column, list favorable things that occurred. Make at least one favorable entry for every trouble. Add as many more favorable occurrences as you can. You may find that that there are more positives in your life than vagrant negative events.

If you conscientiously perform this psychological homework assignment for thirty days, Dubois thought you'd improve your chances of balancing out your life and finding a favorable life direction.

## A COGNITIVE BEHAVIORAL APPROACH

Psychiatrist Tom Williams (1914; 1923) thought that your conscious ideas trigger anxious feelings and that normally you can quickly identify your anxious thoughts. What's more elusive are the underlying conceptual errors, such as filtering reality through a pessimist schema or a distorted self-concept.

Williams offered the following clarifying ideas:

- A persistent destructive anxiety is unnecessary and can be changed.

- A willingness to act with self-discipline counterbalances anxiety.

- An acceptance that it takes time and effort to break an anxiety habit moves you farther on the path to change than expecting illusive immediate relief.

He suggested taking the following cognitive, emotive, and behavioral actions to quell parasitic anxieties:

- Remind yourself that how you view an event determines its fearfulness.

- Obtain clarity of vision through honesty of purpose. (What do you want to accomplish?)

- Examine the idea and reset the mind to accept alternative affirmative ideas.

- Parroting new, positive slogans will get you nowhere. Work at gradually penetrating the mind with reconstructive affirmations (that is, think of yourself as exhibiting your better capabilities, and then exhibit what you think).

- Prioritize fulfilling responsibilities over avoiding anxious tension. (Escape the procrastination trap.)

- The situation, as a whole, rarely triggers anxiety, so try to isolate parts linked to your anxious tension. If you experience performance anxiety, is it about falling short of a standard? Do you fear the feeling? Attend to the feared part.

- Expose yourself to aspects of the feared situation that most trouble you. Gradually make adjustments in how you engage with the situation. Give yourself time to settle in to to a new way of thinking and experiencing.

Cobwebs may surround these three old books. Still, the ideas stay vital and timeless.

# CHALLENGING YOUR ANXIOUS THOUGHTS

As an exercise, list some examples of your anxious thoughts. Next, do some reality checking with techniques you've learned in this chapter and elsewhere in this book. Record some sensible thoughts that you believe add to a realistic perspective on your situation.

| |
|---|
| **Personal examples of parasitic powerlessness thinking:** |
| **Reality checks and challenges for powerlessness thinking:** |
| **Sensible thoughts for a broader perspective:** |

## Defusing Anxiety in Depression

Anyone who thinks that depression is a simple biological mood has Novocain on the brain. Your biology, psychology, and social world are both reflective of and affected by depression. Your depressive thinking is likely to draw you into an emotional wasteland we can call *dysphoria*. As your perspective narrows to a train of negative ideas, your life loses value. In this deadening morass, you feel morose, but you also can feel irritated, apprehensive, and vulnerable to the point where anxiety seems inseparable from depression.

Parasitic anxiety can be emotionally handicapping. But this parasitic anxiety comes from an *emotive cognition*, or a belief that has the power to arouse fear sensations. That is, you may be responding to a misguided signal. For example, if you tense at the thought of giving a talk in front of a friendly group and you start sweating and dodge the opportunity, you are responding to a misguided signal. By finding and defusing these misleading cognitions, you can gain considerable relief from the needless tensions that extend from them.

## REALITY CHECK

When you feel both anxious and depressed, listen for double-trouble parasitic thinking. Do you hear catastrophizing, powerlessness, or self-downing self-talk? These thoughts may be a form of procrastination against taking action. If you catch these thoughts in motion, you are in a position to take corrective action. You can do reality checking with the cycle-of-change technique introduced in chapter 5 and avoid procrastination by engaging the problem. By engaging the problem, you rely less upon procrastination as a defense against facing your parasitic anxieties and fears.

## SELF-APPROVAL

Most people prefer that others think well of them. This is normal. However, if you must have others' approval to feel worthy and not anxious, this belief sets the stage for parasitic thinking and nervous feelings over the possibility that someone will think badly of you. Parasite anxiety typically has its own dysfunctional logic that starts with faulty premises that lead to terrifying conclusions. Say your premise is that someone's disapproval defines you. This primary premise extends into a secondary one that you are helpless to protect yourself from disapproval. You conclude that you will be irreparably harmed if someone disapproves of anything that you do. Look for loopholes in this parasitic logic and you are likely to find fictions galore.

Premises one and two are conjectural and disputable. Conclusions that come from conjecture are dubious. However, parasitic logic can bring about a self-fulfilling prophecy. Therefore, it's important to spotlight faulty logic that can trigger feelings of anxiety.

The second-century Roman physician Galen described melancholia as a state of "fear and depression, discontent with life, and hatred of all people."

If you think you are unworthy and can't protect yourself, think about your thinking. What does "unworthy" mean? You may quickly see that saying you are unworthy is an overgeneralization.

You can protect yourself from the emotional harm that comes from overgeneralizing by probing both the substance and meaning of the overgeneralization. For example, how does it follow that other people's approval or disapproval defines you? Disapproval can sometimes result in a disadvantage, but this does not change the essence of you.

Here's another probing question: Do you believe you can be harmed because of your unworthiness? Expand upon the issue by asking and answering questions, such as, "Harmed in what way?" If your conclusion is that you will be harmed because you can't cope, look for exceptions and you are likely to find instances where you both coped and were not harmed by disapproval.

Questioning overgeneralizations will help you find realistic ways to quell need-for-approval parasitic thinking and avoid depressive conclusions, such as that you are powerless.

## SELF-EMPOWERMENT

Suppose you believe that you are generally powerless to protect yourself against harm to your social status and, thus, are vulnerable to harm. Remember that although you may not control your destiny as fully as you wish, you still have choices. When you have competing choices, you have decisions to make. You decide to pull five weeds from a garden, open a book, or buy a loaf of bread. When you are in a position to make decisions, you are not powerless. Rather, by taking responsibility for assessing choices and making decisions, you empower yourself.

## ■ *John's Story*

*John saw the stock market tank one morning and felt alarmed at a thought that he would lose his retirement money. This catastrophic idea cascaded into another. He saw himself as ill and handicapped with no one to help him.*

*Because he believed that he was going to be poor, he drew into himself and deeply thought about how he was destined to suffer. Since he could do nothing about the market, he viewed himself as powerless to change his destiny. Now mired in misery, he began thinking that he was not smart enough to survive the economic crash. Then the market rebounded. His portfolio increased in value. His depression dissipated. The market turn was welcome news.*

*John was going to be in danger of feeling up or down based on the ups and downs of the stock market, which he could not control. Nevertheless, he could accept the uncontrollability of the market and still maintain a sense of control over his perspective on the market's volatility. He could be powerless against unexpected twists and turns of the market and empower himself to accept market operations.*

If you experience both anxiety and depression, here is some good news. Cognitive and behavioral methods for dealing with depressive thinking also apply to dealing with parasitic anxious thinking and the inhibitions that typically go with that territory.

# DEFEATING INHIBITION

Inhibitions are restraints or suppressions of feelings and actions. Some are healthy. You don't go 120 miles per hour at rush hour. You don't argue with airport security if it might mean prolonging the search through your luggage and possibly missing your flight.

However, some inhibitions are unhealthy. You are excessively self-conscious and hide in the shadows of life. You think your views are worthless, so you stay silent to appear agreeable. You feel so uptight and unexpressive at times that you could cry. You intellectualize everything to avoid feeling anything.

Andrew Salter (1949), an early behavioral therapist, emphasized acting assertively and expressively to loosen up and shed excessive social inhibitions. While his early work has its share of flaws, it also has its fair share of diamonds in the rough. Here are three of Salter's thoughts on inhibition:

- "In a sense, reason and emotion are two nostrils of the same nose…they are one neurological thing…. There is nothing wrong by being guided by our emotions. The only question is, 'What emotions?' Are they the sterile, stultifying, fearful emotions of inhibition, or are they the free, healthy, vigorous, and healthy emotions of excitation? (58)"

- The proverb "Know thyself" is a vacuous statement unless you have the tools to do so. When you have only yourself to refer to in order to acquire new self-knowledge, acquiring this knowledge is not easy. This often takes expressing emotions that differ from your stultifying habits.

- Getting rid of enslaving inhibitions often feels like going against the grain. This action produces friction. Thus, expect discomfort at first. Expect to stay at this stage of work for a while. Eventually you'll do the right thing without thinking.

Here are more tips adapted from Salter (ibid.) for this book:

- Correct and happy words neither correct nor cure depression or anxiety. Instead of parroting positive phrases, dig into the meaning behind negative thinking. Work at undercutting misleading mental habits.

- Inhibition is a form of emotional constipation leading to trapped feelings. Break free. Trust yourself to say what is on your mind.

- Express your likes and dislikes to others using feeling words such as "like" or "detest." You'll sound more real and alive. (Note: watch out for exaggerating emotionally laden terms, lest you fall into the catastrophizing trap.)

- When you differ with someone, avoid acting as if you were in agreement. Disagree with conviction. (Note: You'll be more convincing if your position is fact based and plausible. Otherwise, you may end up in an intellectual fencing match with one vague opinion competing against another.)

- When you are praised, rather than feel unworthy, embrace the compliment. "Thank you for your compliment" is better than saying something like, "Oh, it's nothing."

- Improvise, or react in the moment with what your think and feel.

- Look forward to the next minute without losing sight of the present second. In short, avoid overplanning your life.

These are some handy tips for loosening up and stepping out of your usual patterns. If you view yourself as too inhibited, you can also experiment with stepping-out-of-character exercises.

# STEPPING OUT OF CHARACTER

Stepping out of character may help you shed inhibitions that contribute to depressed feelings. You can confront your inhibitions under controlled conditions to desensitize yourself against false fears. Try one or more of the following exercises:

**Exercise one.** If you find that you excessively inhibit yourself by doing such things as not asking for information or directions, step out of character by going to a convenience store and asking for directions to a nearby location, such as a restaurant. If you already know how to get there, pretend that you don't.

**Exercise two.** Many breakfast spots offer "two eggs, any style" on the menu, and usually this means that you're being offered two fried eggs, two scrambled eggs, or two poached eggs. The next time you're out for breakfast, ask the waiter if you can have one fried egg and one scrambled egg. If the thought of doing this embarrasses you, try doing it anyway as an exercise in stepping out of character.

**Exercise three.** If you are self-conscious about your appearance, try wearing one of the following for a day: a belt that does not match the rest of your outfit, a T-shirt in reverse, or two different-colored socks.

**Exercise four.** Dress neutrally. Take off your watch. Go to a local mall at a busy time of day. Ask twenty adults for the time. See what happens. Here is my general finding for this experiment: Two to five people are likely to ignore you. They won't give you the time of day. Some may be too shy. A few others will see this as an opportunity for making small talk. Most will give you the time as they pass on their way. And in the unlikely event that twenty people refuse to give you the time of day, you can still ask and answer this question: "How does this make me less of a person if a group of twenty refused to give me the time of day?" If you are honest with yourself, you'll conclude that although you didn't get the time, you can still unconditionally accept yourself. Albert Ellis (2003) calls this the elegant self-worth solution.

By stepping out of character, you can shift from self-absorption to objective self-observation.

# CHALLENGING YOUR INHIBITION THINKING

List your unhealthy inhibitory thoughts, feelings, and actions. Then shift perspective. Force yourself to act naturally and expressively. This is one way to create positive new thought, emotive, and behavioral habits.

| Your unhealthy inhibitory thoughts, feelings, and actions: |
| --- |
| Reality checks and challenges for needless inhibitions: |
| Sensible thoughts, feelings, and actions for authentic self-expression: |

# PUSHING PAST INERTIA

If you're having a hard time getting started working on your anxiety-depression connection, you may be facing a natural inertia barrier. Once you are on an anxiety-depression path, it can be challenging to get past this barrier.

Atlanta psychotherapist Ed Garcia (pers. comm.) tells us that depression and inertia are like Siamese twins standing like a boulder before a ten-ton truck. It takes a lot of power to push the boulder aside. This effort first strains a cold engine. All cylinders are not firing. But once you get the truck moving, even just a little bit, you build momentum. The more it moves, the warmer the engine gets. As the momentum builds, it gets easier to push the boulder aside. Now you've started on a new inertia path. This is the pathway where you point the truck where you want it to go and put it in gear. Garcia goes on to say that as you push yourself past the threshold of inertia, you can reclaim a sense of power that was there all along to discover.

## Exposure Overcomes Inertia

Exposure is the gold standard for getting relief from fear (Wolitzky-Taylor et al. 2008). This is where you face what you fear in the present moment until you no longer react with panic. You can also face your fear in degrees through graduated exposure. Either way, it's important that you allow yourself to experience the fear until it becomes less intense. Otherwise, you reinforce escapist behavior.

Here's an example. You're afraid of the dark, so you expose yourself to darkness. You can go into a dark room and sweat it out. Or you can do this in a graduated way by using a dimmer switch to control the intensity of the light, thus putting this process under your control.

The principle of exposure applies to overcoming the inertia found in procrastination. Here is a practical five-minute technique for cutting through procrastination barriers that are rooted in inertia.

## FIVE-MINUTE EXPOSURE TECHNIQUE

Pick a practical activity for overcoming an anxiety-depression connection that you resist doing and that is in your interest to do. It can be anything from vacuuming your bedroom to filling out a college application. To break the inertia for the activity, commit yourself to working on it for five minutes (like starting the truck). At the end of the five minutes, you can commit to another five minutes of doing the activity, or you can quit. Repeat this five-minute exercise until you finish the activity or decide (at the end of a five-minute interval) to stop.

The five-minute technique is a valuable tool for getting your engine started and keeping your truck moving. It is based on the idea that exposure is easier when you are on control. You decide on the activity. You decide on the rate of activity. You control what you do and the pace. Invoke the five-minute technique when you feel bogged down. Practice it until it becomes a habit.

What happens when you come to a point in this process where you decide to stop but you still have more to do? Take a few extra minutes to prepare for the next time you engage in the project. If you've decided to write the great American novel, make a few notes on what you plan to do next. By recording what you'll do next, you may find it easier to start again later at a designated time.

Of course, there is nothing magical about five minutes. Some people do better working in ten-minute segments, others in half-hour segments, and others by committing all their efforts to the first minute. However, small time frames are easier to commit to than longer ones.

## WHY EXPOSURE WORKS

Exposure is a way to train your brain to stop overreacting to nondangerous situations. The *amygdala*, a pear-shaped part of the brain, responds to real or imagined threat by triggering stress hormones (LeDoux 1998). Primitive and learned dangers are etched onto the amygdala. The amygdala will keep firing whenever it perceives a threat. Thus, it needs to be overridden when it triggers stress hormones in nonthreatening situations. By consciously exposing yourself to needless fears, you increase your chances of overriding the adrenaline surge that is a typical sign of anxiety or fear.

Exposure helps activate the *anterior cingulate cortex* (ACC). This is a control center in the brain that resolves conflicts between cognitive and emotional regions. Following exposure, neuroimaging shows an increase in ACC activity and a decrease in amygdala activity (Goossens et al. 2007; Felmingham et al. 2007). This imaging gives strong evidence that the part of your brain that reacts to a perceived threat becomes less reactive through exposure.

Brain regions that control anxiety and fear are complex, and how they are interlaced may partially depend on the type of anxiety you experience, your vulnerability for anxiety, and the conditions that you face (Shin and Liberzon 2010). Your higher mental process may quickly recognize a silly fear. However, the ACC is a slow learner. It takes time for the ACC to resolve the conflict between the amygdala and higher mental processes. It also takes time to train other areas of the brain that are part of your fear-and-anxiety circuitry. Therefore, it is wise to be patient with your slower-learning brain regions. Give yourself time as you practice exposure.

## *Autogenic Training Techniques*

Psychiatrist Jonathan Schultz developed autogenic training (Schultz and Luthe 1969). This form of self-regulated meditation can promote relaxed feelings while bringing the mind into an optimal state for action. The operating principle here is that relaxation counteracts anxiety, and action reduces some of the causes of anxiety and helps break the inertia of depression.

Autogenic training methods appear effective in producing relief from physical symptoms of depression (Van Dyck et al. 1991; Lowenstein 2002; Ota et al. 2007; Shinozaki et al. 2010), overcoming depressive moods and reducing relapse (Krampen 1999; Stetter and Kupper 2002), and stimulating positive changes in brain activity (Schlamann et al. 2010).

By using positive suggestive phrases, you can put yourself into a state of being both relaxed and ready to launch positive actions. Here is how to use the method:

1. Create relaxing phrases.

2. Create mobilization phrases.

3. Practice this combination of relaxation and mobilization until you get into a rhythm where you feel relaxed and readied for action.

4. Put yourself into a relaxed state followed by a mobilization state. Then launch the desired action from that relaxation-mobilization platform.

# AUTOGENICS EXERCISE

In the relaxation phase, get into a comfortable position, such as sitting in an easy chair, lying on a couch, or floating on a rubber raft in a pool. Using a series of brief suggestive phrases, conjure images that stimulate relaxed feelings. For example, if you associate a feeling of heaviness with relaxation, try to stimulate that condition through words. Use the following suggested phrases if they work for you, or come up with your own phrases:

1. "My arms feel heavy." Repeat this phrase four times. Mentally note how heavy your arms feel.

2. "My legs feel heavy." Repeat this phrase four times. Mentally note how heavy your legs feel.

3. "I feel myself relaxing." Repeat this phrase four times. Mentally note sensations that suggest relaxation.

Note that there is nothing magical about these suggestive phrases. Phrases that contain words like *light*, *warm*, or *floating* may do.

In the mobilization phase, pick three brief phrases that will prepare you to launch an antidepression action that you believe is worth taking, such as having a constructive conversation with a friend, visiting a museum, or going for a bike ride. Choose phrases that stir some of the same feelings you had when you were operating optimally, such as a feeling you had when you achieved a certain goal.

Use the following sample phrases, or come up with your own:

1. "My goal is in sight." (Repeat this phrase four times. Mentally note the value in achieving the goal.)

2. "I know what to do." (Repeat this phrase four times. Mentally note shifts in your attention that go in an action direction.)

3. "I feel ready to go." (Repeat this phrase four times. Mentally note feelings of being driven to start moving toward your goal.)

Practice combining relaxation and mobilization three times a day, or until you get into a rhythm where you feel relaxed, mobilized, and ready to execute actions to reach your goal.

---

As you merge your relaxation and mobilization steps, you put yourself on the brink of action. Action is the concrete steps you take to make changes that are consistent with your constructive goals. It is what you do by an exercise of will.

In combination with cognitive, emotive, and behavioral methods, you can use this autogenic approach for multiple purposes, such as gearing up for a job interview or getting past a procrastination barrier.

# ADDRESSING PANIC

Have you ever suffered a sudden and intense fear associated with a pounding heart and choking sensations where you have difficulty breathing? As this wave of electrifying stress crests, you might grasp your chest fearing that the chest tightness you experience is the start of a heart attack. You have shortness of breath and feel shaky, dizzy, or light-headed. You feel nauseated and think you are going to vomit. Your stomach might cramp, and your legs may tighten. You may break into a sweat, experience hot flashes, or have chills. If you've experienced a similar dramatic combination of sensations, you've experienced a panic reaction.

People in panic often fear a loss of control, feel detached from reality, think they are going crazy, or believe they face imminent death. You might think you are never going to get better and that your condition will worsen. You might feel so frightened that you cry.

Some people with panic reactions have visited emergency wards over fifty times with the fear of having a heart attack. The physical evidence wasn't there, but the panic over the possibility was. As a precaution, you may already have had a medical examination to rule out coronary heart disease or another medical condition.

If you feel panicked, label your panic sensations "a temporary nervous system reaction." This relabeling can put panic into perspective.

More than 50 percent of those who suffer from panic reactions eventually experience a major depressive episode (Tsao, Lewin, and Craske 1998). If you count yourself among this group, the good news is that you have an excellent chance of overcoming panic by using cognitive and behavioral methods (Ruhmland 2001). This family of techniques can yield relatively quick results (Penava et al. 1998).

## How Cognitive Methods Help

Panic is normally experienced as a dramatic negative change in normal sensations when there is no real physical danger. You just believe you have out-of-control and life-threatening physical sensations.

If from past experience, you know that alarming sensations are not dangerous and that they will soon pass, you are less likely to panic over experiencing panic. But there can be no doubt that dramatic physical sensations compel attention.

### BE INFORMED

Here is some information about panic that can help put it into perspective and decrease its frequency and impact.

You won't faint from panic even if you feel dizzy. Fear of fainting is common. But though you may feel dizzy during a panic reaction, it is highly unlikely that you will faint. There is a physical basis for this observation. With a rapid heartbeat, more blood rushes to your brain. Fainting occurs with a slow heartbeat and with less blood traveling to the brain. The next time you panic, remember that you won't faint.

A rapidly quickened heartbeat when you feel panicked is dramatic compared to a resting heart rate. You might be afraid that this is dangerous. But if you were to take your pulse and measure your heart rate, you would probably discover that it is about what you'd expect if you were moderately exercising. If you want proof, take your heartbeat when you are in a panicked state. The knowledge that your heart rate is only slightly elevated may help alleviate your panic. (Note: If your heartbeat suddenly jumps to around 190 beats or more per minute, you should get help immediately.)

## OUTSMART PANIC THINKING

Panic thinking includes such ideas as "I'm going to look like a fool in public," "I'll never be right again," "I can't cope with this experience," "I'm going crazy," or "I'm going to die." You can outsmart panic thinking. Try the following strategies the next time you panic:

- Count the number of people who focus their attention on you. The likelihood is that people around you will not notice you panicking. The sensations you find so dramatic are not dramatically visible to a casual observer.

- Ask yourself whether you have a crystal ball that tells you for certain that you will never feel right again. If you really believed this prognostication, would you bet your home, automobile, or all your future earnings on the proposition "I'll never feel right again"?

- If you have strong feelings of anxiety and also fear that you are going crazy, the chances are that you are panicking yourself by giving yourself that double trouble. If you suspect that this is happening, it is important to think about what you are telling yourself and to match thought against fact. For example, if you were going crazy, you would likely feel confused about who and where you are. On the other hand, when feeling highly anxious, you are likely to be excessively self-aware of sensations that feed panic thinking.

- "I'm going to die" is likely to reflect your thoughts about how you are feeling in the present moment as much as the thought feeds panic feelings. Such a thought-feeling connection can last until your adrenal glands fatigue. In short, there is a time limit on how long you can feel anxiously aroused or panicked.

Note that if you are afraid that you will panic in a particular situation, your anxiety can lead to procrastination in coping. Before it happens again, it can help to map out what happens when you panic. If you know what to expect and what to do, this proactive approach can position you to assert greater control over the panic process.

# CHALLENGING YOUR PANIC THINKING

List some of your panic thoughts. Challenge panic thinking with techniques you've learned in this chapter. Record your ideas so that you can get a broader perspective:

| |
|---|
| **Your panic thinking:** |
| **Reality checks and challenges for panic thinking:** |
| **Sensible thoughts for a broader perspective:** |

## Behavioral Methods to Address Panic

Behavioral strategies for addressing panic can be highly effective. Several basic techniques follow.

### GET ADEQUATE EXERCISE

Getting exercise often results in greater cardiac efficiency, increased lung capacity, the buildup of endorphins, physical confidence, improved body image, a boost in serotonin levels, and so forth. Exercise may take several weeks to start to show effects. While getting enough exercise is no guarantee for overcoming panic reactions, it raises the probability of reducing panic related to depression and depression related to panic.

### WATCH YOUR BREATHING

Some people with panic breathe about twice as rapidly as normal. Often they forget to use their diaphragm in breathing. When this happens, psychological and physiological signs of apprehension can appear. To address this process, intentionally use your diaphragm when breathing. See if this helps override hyperventilation. For example, pretend that your stomach is a balloon. When you breathe in, your stomach expands. When you breathe out, it contracts. Experience the sensations of breathing in and out in a rhythmic way. When you breathe in, think the word "relax." As you breathe out, think the phrase "I'm going to be fine."

### EXHALE INTO A SMALL PAPER BAG

The body's carbon dioxide level is thought to sometimes trigger a sensor in the brain that sends out signals starting a panic cycle. A technique for interrupting a panic reaction involves fooling the carbon dioxide detection sensor. Exhaling into a small paper bag for two or three minutes sometimes helps. Some people cup their hands over their faces and breathe into their cupped hands.

### TIME IT

Although the sensations of panic can be dramatic and terrifying, they are relatively short-lived. Panic sensations normally fade within one to ten minutes. In rare cases, they may last a few hours. But even a short-lived panic reaction can seem like an eternity. To help you get through it, the next time you panic, look at your watch when the sensations start. Then, look at your watch again as the sensations subside. The knowledge that panic is time-limited can counteract fearful thinking that the panic will never end. This gives you factual information you can use to remind yourself of the transitory nature of panic.

# DEALING WITH TRAUMA

Just as depression is an equal opportunity condition (people at all levels of society are eligible), people with *post-traumatic stress disorder* (PTSD) come from all walks of life. Following a traumatic event, PTSD involves distressing images, thoughts, perceptions, dreams, flashbacks of the event, irritability, difficulties concentrating, sleep disorders, or a strong physical response to trauma cues. Such reactions can start immediately or months after the tragic incident and can trigger a fear of reexperiencing the trauma through a flashback.

The traumatic event can be a job loss, the sudden death of a loved one, a violent assault, a financial setback, a natural disaster (losing a home due to a fire or storm), witnessing a crime or accident, early life stress, being in a combat war zone, and childhood sexual, verbal, or physical abuse. Robert Moore (pers. comm.), a Florida marriage and family therapist, tells us that depression is sometimes a lingering aftereffect of a traumatic event. He goes on to say that "*trauma* is just the clinical term now used for the memory of a loss that continues to trigger sad feelings more than a reasonable while afterward."

Depression affects between 30 and 50 percent of people diagnosed with PTSD. According to the National Comorbidity Survey, people experiencing a catastrophic or traumatic event are eight times more likely to experience depression (Kessler, Davis, and Kendler 1997).

Cognitive and behavioral therapies are effective for people suffering from the psychological aftermath of trauma (Bradley et al. 2005; Harvey, Bryant, and Tarrier 2003). You can use these methods to build *emotional resilience*. This is your ability to recover from traumatic setbacks and to manage yourself with reasonable effectiveness in the midst of hardship (Davydov et al. 2010; Masten 2009). This emotional competence extends from your ability to understand your own and others' emotions and to express and manage them to bring about a positive effect (Petrides and Furnham 2003).

## *Managing Trauma Cognitions*

Following a traumatic event, a range of responses is possible. Believing that you did all you could under the circumstances is positive. Even if you believe that you could have done more, you can still conclude that imperfection is part of being human. Monday morning quarterbacking can't change what happened. However, if months after the event passed, your mind keeps retracing the horror, and you believe that you have failed in some way, and you retreat into a world of hopelessness, then you need to address these thoughts, especially if they are embedded in a depressed mood.

When the past is gone, all the "should haves" won't put Humpty Dumpty together again. Grief and loss continue on their own volition. But you can decrease the impact of stressful trauma memories, images, beliefs, emotions, and behaviors.

### USE EXPOSURE

PTSD etches the experience onto the amygdala, the part of the brain that controls the fight-or-flight response. Through exposure to trauma-related sensations and accompanying emotive cognitions, you can train other parts of the brain to switch on and override a primitive amygdala reaction. However, I'd advise professional guidance for addressing such traumatic experiences as witnessing the murder of a loved one. Even though your memories of a traumatic event remain, you can alter your perspective and emotional responses to traumatic memories and relieve yourself from their depressive impact.

### MANAGE DOUBLE-TROUBLE THINKING

While the event happened in the past, the upset is in the present moment. It is in this theater of the mind that you can come to grips with the meaning of the event and the feelings of terror or horror that accompanied it. You can simultaneously work on double-trouble dimensions of trauma thinking using the ABCDE method described throughout this book.

If you experience depression from trauma, you can do the following to start managing the double-trouble thinking of trauma.

1. List some examples of irrational trauma thinking (i.e. "I can't cope with this experience." "I can't stand it." "I am a weak person.")

2. Examine what you mean when you tell yourself such things as, "I can't cope with this experience." Start with clarifications. What does "can't cope" mean? How does it apply in this instance? You may discover that you can live with what you can't change, which is an acceptable form of coping.

3. Name some exceptions to this line of thought. For example, is it possible to learn to live with a disaster without feeling consumed by it?

By exploring constructive alternatives, you can take away excess distress while grimly accepting the experience.

## CHALLENGING YOUR TRAUMA THINKING

If you are among the millions suffering from PTSD who also suffer from depression, do the following exercise to see if you can start to move yourself in the direction of freedom from the unpleasant sensations, thoughts, and images that accompany this stressful state. Record your trauma thinking. Challenge it. Then record some rational thoughts that you believe give perspective to your situation.

| |
|---|
| **Your trauma thinking:** |
| **Reality checks and challenges for trauma thinking:** |
| **Sensible thoughts that lead to a broader perspective:** |

# ABCDE METHOD FOR CURBING WORRY THINKING

Repetitive thoughts can be functional when you direct them toward planning, problem solving, and rehearsing ways to improve (Watkins 2008). However, some repetitive thoughts are preambles to anxiety. Repetitive worrying is a breeding ground for general anxieties that can expand into depression.

This exercise ends with where the chapter began: correcting worry thinking. You can use the ABCDE method to address the circularity in this thinking, where worry over depressive symptoms reinforces a down mood, which leads to depressive symptoms.

| |
|---|
| **Activating event (experience):** "An unexplained feeling of malaise." |
| **Rational beliefs about the event:** "This doesn't feel good. I don't like feeling this way." |
| **Emotional and behavioral consequences for the rational beliefs:** "Acceptance with displeasure about the feeling." |
| **Irrational worry beliefs:** "I know there is something wrong with me. Maybe I have cancer." |
| **Emotional and behavioral consequences for the irrational worry beliefs:** "Mixed feelings of anxiety and a deadening sense of resignation." |
| **Disputes for irrational worry beliefs:** (1) "Where is the evidence that something is wrong with me or that I have cancer?" Sample answer: "Through emotional reasoning, I've made a magical leap from feeling down to assuming a catastrophic reason for the feeling." (2) "How does a depressed feeling prove the premise that the feeling is a symptom of cancer?" Sample answer: "It would take a confirmed diagnosis by a medical expert to determine if I have cancer. If depression were a sign of cancer, we would quickly run out of hospital space." |
| **Effects of the disputes:** "By addressing the circularity in the worry, the reward can be a reduction in tension from such thinking, less stress to evoke depressive thoughts, and fewer depression-provoking thoughts." |

Use the following chart as a guide to curb your own worry thinking.

**Activating event (experience):**

**Rational beliefs about the event:**

**Emotional and behavioral consequences for the rational beliefs:**

**Irrational worry beliefs:**

**Emotional and behavioral consequences for the irrational worry beliefs:**

**Disputes for irrational worry beliefs:**

**Effects of the disputes:**

# END DEPRESSION PLAN

**Key ideas** (What three ideas did you find most helpful in this chapter?):

1.

2.

3.

**Action steps** (What three steps can you take to move closer to your goal of overcoming depression?):

1.

2.

3.

**Execution** (How did you execute the steps?):

1.

2.

3.

Results (What did you learn that you can use?):

1.

2.

3.

# CHAPTER 15

# Confronting Negative Emotions

Just as you can have a headache and upset stomach at the same time, you can have depression accompanied by anger, guilt, shame, and other unpleasant emotional states. The good news is that you can gain command over these negative emotions that so commonly merge with dark moods.

## CONTENDING WITH ANGER

> Holding on to anger is like grasping a hot coal with the intent of throwing it at someone else.
>
> —Buddha

The Freudian theory that depression is anger turned inward is no longer a primary explanation for depression (Cox, Stabb, and Hulgus 2000). But Freud was correct in that as anger and depression are often connected. While not everyone with depression experiences lingering anger, an anger-depression connection is common. The literature is varied on the percentage of people who are both depressed and angry. Between 30 and 50 percent of those suffering from depression are likely to simultaneously experience anger. Here are a few other facts about anger:

- The percentage of those experiencing anger is higher among people with bipolar depression (Benazzi 2003; Perlis et al. 2004).

- Anger tends to coexist with anxiety (Hawkins and Cougle 2011).

- Harmful anger finds expression in verbal or physical abuse (Koh, Kim, and Park 2002).

- Anger attacks (impulsive anger that leads to property destruction, such as throwing dishes or punching a hole in a wall) have been underestimated (Kessler et al. 2006).

- Angry outbursts are associated with irritability, depression, and anxiety. The pattern contributes to degrading the quality of life (Painuly et al. 2011).

You can use cognitive behavioral methods to cope with anger and improve your quality of life. This chapter will first look at where anger comes from and then give you some strategies for defeating anger that can coexist with depression.

## Anger and Evolution

Anger is a natural reaction to a threat where going on the offensive is safer than retreat. This reaction may have been adaptive in prehistoric times, but these days, you are much more likely to encounter ego dangers than actual threats to your life. Anger is a common reaction to status threats. For example, a colleague smears your public image. You feel a seething rage. Day after day, you brood and plot revenge. Your mind is so filled with hate that you have trouble sleeping and concentrating.

When feeling depressed, you may conjure false explanations for why you feel the way you do. Your autocratic boss doesn't appreciate your contributions. You angrily cop an attitude and lose out on a promotion. When you don't feel depressed, you may see your employer in a more favorable light.

> Anyone can become angry. That is easy. But to be angry with the right person, to the right degree, at the right time, for the right purpose and in the right way…that is not easy.
>
> —Aristotle

## Defeating Anger with Confident Composure

Irwin F. Altrows, a psychologist in private practice in Kingston, Ontario, and professor at Queen's University, has over thirty years of experience helping people overcome harmful anger problems. Altrows (pers. comm.) offers this tip:

When you feel anger, you have the options of (A) letting anger control you, (B) trying to tame your anger, and (C) trying to understand your anger and what it is "telling" you, and then change what you can.

Option A is especially risky when you are feeling depressed. You could physically or verbally hurt yourself or others. By doing something you'll regret, you lose influence over those you care about. Option A is a self-defeating choice.

Option B sounds like a wiser choice. By taming your anger, you can avoid serious mistakes. But what is it that you're taming? Unless you understand your anger, "taming anger" is a slogan without a corrective process. If you stop with the idea that you'd like to tame anger, you are procrastinating on a big opportunity to understand and channel your anger productively.

Option C is to understand your anger. Sure, your anger may be based on some of the same negative thinking as your depression, such as judging some people as bad instead of judging some actions as bad. But it may also be an itch telling you that something is due for a scratch, such as allowing yourself to feel irritable without rashly jumping to conclusions about the cause.

You may be reluctant to lose specious rewards that you get from feeling anger: (1) an energizer that can buy you a temporary reprieve from living in the depths of depression, (2) a sense of power that cloaks helplessness, (3) superiority because you can blame others or the world, (4) a reason to bury your stressed emotions in alcohol or other drugs. This list of possible specious rewards scratches the surface.

When you evoke option C, you tune in to what your anger is telling you. Are you telling yourself that life should be sweet for you, that you should not feel depressed, and that people should accommodate your wishes? If you are making demands that are beyond reach, you have two options for deepening your understanding of your anger.

The first is to get perspective. Identify the problem that is causing your anger itch, and assertively scratch it while respecting your rights and feelings and the rights and feelings of other people. Here is a basic question to start this scratching process: "Why *must* life go the way I want?" By asking this basic question, you've taken a big step in defusing needless anger. You've put yourself in a position to shift from expectations about how you think things should be to a preferential view where you, more or less, accept things as they are and change what you can.

The second option is to work toward replacing anger with confident composure. You accept that you can control what you think to a point, and what you do to a greater point. You chose to control what is reasonable for you to do.

The anger message is that you are truly alive, you truly care about something (or you wouldn't be angry), and you have energy with which to take action. Although the impulsive forms of anger are not an ideal mental and emotional state, you may transform them into steps on the road toward hope, self-confidence, and healing. Then with confident composure, you channel your emotional energy toward defeating depression, and you keep at it until you make it!

## The Blame-Anger Connection

Some events warrant an angry response, such as if you were to observe a gang of bullies smacking a small child around, or if a friend were to betray a confidence. Managing natural anger can be challenging. However, when an extension of blame thinking drives anger, you have an anger chain with many links that can aggravate coexisting depression.

For example, say you've been depressed for weeks, with trouble getting up and going in the morning. While you are driving to a late-afternoon appointment, a driver cuts in front of you. You expect other drivers to be courteous, and this driver violated that rule. You flip out and temporarily forget about your depression. You start playing bumper tag to punish the offender. You can choose to play a dangerous but stimulating game, or you can change course by rethinking your thinking and restraining yourself.

If you count yourself among those with an irritability that makes you vulnerable to having angry outbursts, you can use cognitive behavioral methods to impose reason between impulse and reaction, decrease the strain you feel, and buffer yourself against needless future pain (Deffenbacher 2011; McCloskey et al. 2008).

# CHALLENGING YOUR ANGER THINKING

List some examples of what you believe or suspect are your harmful anger thoughts. Use the following chart to challenge this thinking and record some helpful thoughts that you believe will realistically broaden your perspective to defuse angry feelings.

| |
|---|
| **Your harmful anger thinking:** |
| **Challenges for harmful anger thinking:** |
| **Sensible thoughts that lead to a broader perspective:** |

# THE PERILS OF SOCIAL EMOTIONS

Social emotions, such as shame, guilt, and embarrassment, are branches on the tree of self-consciousness. Because they are associated with censure, these emotions reinforce social conformity. However, some people get too self-conscious and become social casualties.

Parents, teachers, religious leaders, scoutmasters, and other authority figures can be helpful guides to children. With patience, they model what the culture considers socially adaptive. Others lean more heavily in the direction of using shame and guilt to shape children's beliefs so as to inhibit their impulses and cause them to behave according to "the rules." Because it is expedient, some people control others through criticism:

- "You shouldn't have done that."

- "What in the world were you thinking?"

- "How could you have been so stupid?"

- "Why won't you listen to reason?"

- "Were you brought up in a barn?"

- "You are selfish and inconsiderate."

Often the origins of excessive social inhibitions are found in patterns of this form of hurtful language. In addition, shame and guilt are imposed upon millions through a political correctness movement perpetrated by shadow figures, which attempts to cause people to think badly of themselves for using the wrong words. Instead of "bum," think "homeless." Instead of "homeless," think "residentially challenged." There is a meaning behind the message: if you don't think politically correctly, you should feel guilty. However, that's farcical. A reasonable person might conclude that attempts to control people's thinking, whether you call it political correctness or something else, is a form of brainwashing.

Some people are vulnerable to developing an excessive self-consciousness on their own. You don't need shadow figures to tell you how you must think. You may need to make a special effort to avoid making too much out of what are only normal human foibles and faults.

Independent of source, when external pressures toward conformity become excessively internalized, you may feel strained by self-conscious thoughts of not being good enough, succumb to excessive inhibitions, and track along a path to depression. Both guilt and shame merit a close look. They contribute to depression in about equal degree (Kim et al. 2011). However, it is the type of guilt and the type of shame that make the difference.

## When Guilt Is Irrational

Guilt, when it is an emotional acknowledgment that you intentionally acted badly, is socially functional. Accepting fault and making amends is a culturally prescribed way to rectify harm. The idea is then to do the best you can to take corrective action.

However, this sense of normal guilt, where you regret your actions and are prepared to make amends, is quite different from *i-guilt*, or irrational guilt. Experiencing i-guilt, you believe that you should not have done what you did and are a rotten person. With this attitude in mind, you may have guilt attacks when you try to fall asleep at night.

To feel i-guilt, you need this combination of cognitive factors: ethical or moral values, scruples, and extensions of blame-trap thinking where you are prone to condemn and demean yourself for either intended or unintended acts. You can cognitively address the excess meaning found in i-guilt and still abide by standards that you find ethical and functional.

### ■ Randy's Story

*Each time he tried to fall asleep at night, Randy felt beset by demons of guilt. He recalled a time when he didn't return a call from a deceased friend's distressed son who had called him for help. He imagined his friend waiting angrily for him beyond the grave. Pangs of guilt ravaged his mind.*

*When reminded that his friend's son's drug problem was so severe that it was beyond his ability to help, and that he'd answered those calls before and given advice that was never heeded, the issue shifted to why he was torturing himself over something that he could not control. Randy slept better from then on.*

## CONTENDING WITH I-GUILT

I-guilt is needless self-torture. If you feel that you are in an i-guilt trap, consider that even if you have acted poorly, self-condemnation rarely leads to self-improvement, nor does it rectify a wrong. Under scrutiny, this guilt often reflects an obligatory perfectionism, where you are obliged to be all things to all people and can only accept yourself if you do the right thing all the time.

The following exercise promotes taking responsibility for your actions while disengaging from extensions of blame that are part of i-guilt thinking.

# CHALLENGING YOUR I-GUILT THINKING

List some of your i-guilt thoughts. Challenge this thinking with techniques you've learned in this book. Record healthy and realistic thoughts that you believe will broaden your perspective and decrease needless guilt.

| |
|---|
| **Your i-guilt thinking:** |
| **Challenges for i-guilt thinking:** |
| **Sensible thoughts that lead to a broader perspective:** |

Using this cognitive exercise, you can eliminate irrational self-blame and guilt, which may be contributing factors to your depression.

## When Shame Is Inane

Shame is a complex social emotion that involves self-consciousness and personal humiliation. When you feel shame, your entire self seems tarnished. Shame can be functional. When you can avoid wrongful or foolish acts, you reduce the risk of having that uncomfortable feeling. You may also avoid social censure for stepping outside of the boundaries of what is acceptable for your social group and culture.

As with i-guilt, there is a darker side to shame as well. Shame is inane when it comes from an extreme self-consciousness. For example, you are ashamed of the shape of your nose. When you look into a mirror, you focus on your nose. Then, you think badly of your entire self.

Or you might feel shame because your neighbor has a newer automobile; your children's grades don't match your expectations; you are too short, too tall, too skinny, or too fat; or the person you are dating isn't drop-dead handsome. These are all examples of inane shame.

Inane shame is an offshoot of the blame game. For example, Johnny's mother tells him that he should be ashamed of himself for getting a C in math, which disgraces the family. She adds, "You can do better than that." And because she thinks he can do better, she implies that he should. This combination of *should* and shame can be deadly.

Exaggerated self-consciousness can arise from early social indoctrination. Shame-sensitive people tend to recall negative messages: "You'll never amount to anything." "You are a useless burden." "You're a failure." "You can't do anything right." "You look like a slob."

As the founder of multimodal therapy, Arnold Lazarus (pers. comm.), has said, "To my mind, the shame game is predicated on views that are inculcated by parents and teachers. Nevertheless, it is far better, I think, to have someone who is capable of shame than to deal with psychopaths who have none."

### CONTENDING WITH INANE SHAME

Shame can come before the misery of depression. When you're depressed, inane shame also can aggravate depression.

You can train yourself to recognize and deal with inane shame. If you are caught in an embarrassing moment and hear yourself saying, "I'll never live this down," take a second look. You can shift from this extreme shame perspective by doing any of the following:

- Balancing cultural shame phrases with another common cultural phrase, such as "Life goes on." Then, consider which statement has the greater validity.

- Singing a song in your mind. Some of my clients have made progress using shame-challenging phrases in an upbeat familiar tune, such as by singing, "I can see clearly now…that when dawn next comes, all my needless shame will be gone."

- Questioning the assumption that you are only one way, for example, "totally worthless," because you exposed a weakness or acted foolishly. You may feel uncomfortable about acting foolishly—a natural and normal human response—and still accept yourself as a fallible person.

# CHALLENGING YOUR INANE SHAME

List some of your shame thoughts. Challenge this thinking with techniques you've learned in this book. Record healthy and realistic thoughts that you believe will broaden your perspective and decrease inane shame.

| |
|---|
| **Some of your inane shame thinking:** |
| **Challenges for inane shame thinking:** |
| **Sensible thoughts that lead to a broader perspective:** |

## *Daily Gratitude Technique*

United Kingdom counselor Jim Byrne recommends expressing daily gratitude to shift your perspective away from inward-directed depressive thoughts and toward a more balanced perspective. You can use his daily gratitude technique when guilt and shame attacks dominate your consciousness and when it would be helpful to broaden your perspective. Byrne (pers. comm.) suggests doing the following:

At the end of each day, write down three things that happened for which you can be genuinely grateful. These can be tiny, almost insignificant events. For example, the sunrise, the sunset, the taste of honey, and the smell of baking bread may all be experiences that can evoke a sense of gratitude. Seeking experiences to feel grateful for can help counteract unhealthy doomsday-type depressive thoughts.

Identify people who have been kind to you or who have helped you. Tell them of your gratitude. It could be as simple as saying, "I appreciated…," "Thank you for…," or "I like it when…" Small acts of acknowledgment from you can help shift your focus from what is going wrong in your life to helping others realize that what they do can make a difference.

# ABCDE METHOD FOR DEVELOPING HEALTHY SOCIAL EMOTIONS

When you feel self-accepting, you are less likely to feel conspicuous and self-conscious. You are more likely to do the right thing in any given situation. The following chart shows how to apply the ABCDE method to address excess self-consciousness and build an enlightened self-acceptance.

| |
|---|
| **Activating event (experience):** "A situation where I risk exposing weakness or vulnerability." |
| **Rational beliefs about the event:** "I'd prefer to be in a situation where I can expose my competencies. However, I must accept limitations if I'm to maintain a realistic perspective on myself." |
| **Emotional and behavioral consequences for the rational beliefs:** "Acceptance and a willingness to do my best under trying conditions." |
| **Irrational beliefs about a risky situation:** "I'm going to look stupid. People will think I'm an incompetent fool. They'll all see me blush, and that would be awful." |
| **Emotional and behavioral consequences for the irrational beliefs:** "Anticipatory humiliation, embarrassment, shame." |
| **Disputes for irrational beliefs:** (1) "What is the basis for concluding that others will universally see me as incompetent and stupid?" Sample answer: "This double-trouble thinking is speculative but does reflect what I think of myself in ambiguous circumstances. Rather than anticipate the worst, let's see what I can do to cope." (2) "What is so awful about blushing?" Sample answer: "Blushing is what it is. Tough!" |
| **Effects of the disputes:** "Reduced sense of inhibition. Improved tolerance for tension. Decreased negative thinking about unpleasant depressive sensations. A quieting sense of acceptance. A lessening of depression." |

When social emotions are excessive and accompany your depression, use the following chart as a guide to map and check this process:

Activating event (experience):

Rational beliefs about the event:

Emotional and behavioral consequences for the rational beliefs:

Irrational beliefs about a risky situation:

Emotional and behavioral consequences for the irrational beliefs:

Disputes for irrational beliefs:

Effects of the disputes:

# END DEPRESSION PLAN

**Key ideas** (What three ideas did you find most helpful in this chapter?):

1.

2.

3.

**Action steps** (What three steps can you take to move closer to your goal of overcoming depression?):

1.

2.

3.

**Execution** (How did you execute the steps?):

1.

2.

3.

**Results** (What did you learn that you can use?):

1.

2.

3.

# CHAPTER 16

# Building Tolerance for Frustration

From time to time, practically everybody experiences frustration. Your frustrations erupt when you have a goal blocked, when you face a barrier that you can't immediately overcome, or when there is a gap between what you want and what you get. As long as you have wishes and desires, you can expect to be occasionally frustrated.

Your tolerance for frustration has a bearing on how you face the ordinary and extraordinary challenges and adversities of life. Unfortunately, when you are depressed, frustrating circumstances don't go on vacation. Depression brings fatigue. Fatigue normally frustrates your wishes to feel more energized. When you feel depressed and fatigued, you are likely to experience a lower than usual tolerance for frustration. Managing the ordinary and extraordinary events of the day can seem especially arduous. Thus, a weakened ability to cope with frustration can add to the depressing perspective that your troubles will never end.

> Is there anything in your life that you've accomplished that did not come about from trying to remove a frustration?
>
> —Atlanta psychotherapist Ed Garcia (pers. comm.)

From a depressive perspective, daily frustrations can seem overwhelming. Faced with unwelcome frustrations, you might further frustrate yourself by saying, "Oh my god. This is awful. I'll never be able to manage. I can't take this." You're in a maelstrom of misery.

This chapter will look at the connection between inappropriately low frustration tolerance and depression as well as how to build emotional resilience. It will also discuss what happens when low frustration tolerance, ADD/ADHD, and substance abuse blend with depression and how to disentangle from this web.

## LOW FRUSTRATION TOLERANCE

*Low frustration tolerance* (LFT) refers to impulsively overreacting to situations that impede what you expect or want. With LFT, you are often easily set off and you overreact to inconvenience and hassle. Here are some examples:

- You have a short fuse when things don't go your way.

- You impulsively gobble handfuls of potato chips even when you are on a diet.

- When you are delayed, you tend to tap your fingers, pace, put your hands on your waist, sigh, or express impatience in other ways.

- You ask questions and then don't pay attention to the answers.

- You interrupt people before they finish.

- You buy on impulse.

- You act cranky and irritable when you don't immediately get what you want.

- You dramatize your complaints.

- You have a lot of manufactured frustrations and miseries over situations that roll off most other people's backs.

At the other end of the spectrum, with high frustration tolerance, you understand what you want to accomplish. You are willing to sacrifice and persist even when the going gets tough. You can act—even though sluggishly—if you feel depressed. Your mind feels freer. You experience more spontaneity. With high frustration tolerance, you are likely to have a positive self-concept, accomplish more, and get greater satisfaction with less stress and strain.

Most of us live our lives between high and low frustration extremes. But the emotional advantage goes to those whose tolerance for frustration is normally high. Getting to a higher level of frustration tolerance takes a lot of hard work, but you can do it. From a self-development perspective, doing this typically involves reducing LFT negatives as you stretch to earn greater tolerance.

## Defeating Low-Frustration-Tolerance Stress Thinking

People with a low threshold for frustration tend to think in low-frustration-tolerance language, such as "This is awful." "I can't stand how I feel." Having awareness of the difference between low frustration tolerance language and rational alternatives can be a positive game changer when you use this information to shift from LFT distress thinking to an objective view. Here's a look at some LFT thinking and alternative views.

| LFT Thinking | Alternative Views |
| --- | --- |
| Alarmist phrases: "I am falling apart." "I can't stand it." These catastrophic thoughts can extend to false conclusions, such as "I'm worthless." "I'm a loser." | Thinking something doesn't make it true. Alarmist thinking may be more reflective of your mood than actual events. Asking the question "Does what I think represent mood, reason, or reality?" can help put your thoughts into perspective. |

| | |
|---|---|
| Self-pity phrases: "I always ruin things for myself." "Nothing turns out right for me." "No one appreciates what I do for them." | Self-pity phrases reflect an overly generalized projection of helplessness and hopelessness. It is normally wise to avoid inflammatory language, such as "always ruin" and "nothing turns out right." Instead, use specifics to describe a situation, such as "I got 50 percent of what I wanted." |
| Ineptitude phrases: "I will never be able to manage." "I can't control anything." | These depressive thoughts blend helplessness with hopelessness. Terms like "never" bear special scrutiny. Look for exceptions to the "never" rule. |
| Self-referent phrases: "I'm a jerk." "I'm stupid." | These thoughts are magnifications and overgeneralizations that represent a self-downing view. |

Another way to defeat LFT thinking is to require yourself to elaborate on any of your negative self-statements. In this case, you follow up a blanket statement like "I can't take feeling frustrated" with the word "because." Then you complete the sentence with an explanation of why you can't tolerate that feeling. By digging deeper, you can get to the core beliefs underlying your negative blanket statements. For example, you may believe that you are too fragile to manage frustrations. By homing in on your negative core beliefs, you are in a position to address these issues.

## THE BECAUSE TECHNIQUE

Write a series of negative self-statements. Then add the word "because" after each of your negative self-statements and fill in the blank.

1. _____

2. _____

3. _____

4. _____

Completing these thoughts helps you to gain clarity. Use this clarity to separate exaggerations from reality. For example, you may discover that saying you can't cope is an exaggeration.

### VISUALIZE YOUR FRUSTRATIONS

When you put off addressing frustrating conditions, they accumulate. As frustrating circumstances increase in number, your frustration tolerance is likely to be further strained. You may experience a sinking feeling of hopelessness.

When you progressively manage your frustrations, you are less likely to fall into a hopelessness-thinking trap and the kind of depressed mood that can result from feeling overwhelmed by too many unresolved issues and tasks. By actively coping with frustrating conditions, your frustration tolerance is likely to grow.

Frustration can stimulate problem solving. However, a low tolerance for frustration can trigger expedient actions, such as problem avoidance or quick fixes that rarely turn out well. Use the following exercise to focus your attention on taking reasonable steps to rid yourself of lingering stresses and frustrations.

# VISUAL EVIDENCE EXERCISE

Start with a clear container, such as a jar or eight-ounce glass. Take some paper labels and write down your current frustrations on each one. If some of your frustrations are bigger than others, use larger labels to illustrate them. Now put all the labels into the container.

Next, pull out one of the larger labels representing a high priority. Identify something that you can do to cope with the frustration listed on the label. Test your idea. As you eliminate a given frustration, remove it from the container. As you acquire other frustrations, add them. Then challenge yourself to cope with these new frustrations as soon as possible so that you can remove them.

When you feel depressed and frustrated, you may lose sight of your efforts to cope, so use a separate container to keep track of your accomplishments. For example, when you are frustrated at the thought of waiting in line for an inspection sticker for your car, you might remind yourself that your goal is to get it done—not necessarily to feel good about the process. After accomplishing a task such as this, write the accomplishment on a label and add it to your container representing frustrations that you've resolved.

As you take proactive steps to resolve your frustrations, you'll accumulate visual evidence for the results of your actions. By chipping away at ongoing frustrations, your stress tolerance is likely to rise. By working to keep the number of stresses in your life down, you are more likely to have energy for coping with pressing matters and to head off trouble before it gets to you.

## TAKE AN INVENTORY

Bridgeport University Professor Emeritus Dom DiMattia (pers. comm.) suggests taking an inventory of what's happened recently, to put things into perspective and reduce the sort of distress that comes from awfulizing, or taking a bad situation and making it worse in your mind. For example, when you've had a bad week, and you think, "Nothing went right, and that's awful," take stock. Identify what happened during the week that links to the emotional commotion you are experiencing. Next, inventory what went well during the week. Then, inventory the ordinary occurrences of daily living that went as anticipated. Compare your "nothing went right" self-statement with the positive and neutral experiences that occurred during the same period. Does that change the picture?

Although this inventory approach can lead to a more balanced perspective, it does not take away the significance of recent

In Aesop's fable of a race between a tortoise and a hare, the speedy rabbit was off to a quick start, then napped as the tortoise plodded steadily forward. As the saying goes, slow and steady wins the race.

negative events. Rather, you can use this technique to decrease the impact of awfulizing thoughts. Feel more in control of your thoughts and emotions, and you are likely to respond correctively to frustrating circumstances.

# LOW FRUSTRATION TOLERANCE AND ADD/ADHD

When fatigued, lacking sleep, or suffering a mild cold, most adults find that they are more easily distracted and more susceptible to magnifying frustrating conditions out of proportion. However, for anywhere between 4 percent and 10 percent of the US population, being highly susceptible to distraction is a daily occurrence.

If you normally have difficulties paying attention and concentrating, you are likely to be easily frustrated in situations that require high levels of attention and concentration. A low frustration tolerance for frustration in those conditions is double trouble. You get frustrated over feeling frustrated, and this distraction just adds to what you want to avoid.

> Low frustration tolerance may mimic attention deficit disorder (ADD) or attention deficit hyperactivity disorder (ADHD).

A combination of frustration avoidance and ADD raises your risk for depression. Major depression and bipolar depression commonly co-occur with ADD/ADHD (Klassen, Katzman, and Chokka 2010; Fischer et al. 2007). Additionally, if your executive functioning (ability to plan, organize, initiate, monitor) is somewhat uneven, you are more likely to procrastinate (Rabin, Fogel, and Nutter-Upham 2011).

You are not responsible for how your brain is wired. It is your responsibility to take corrective or compensatory action.

## Contending with ADD, Procrastination, and Depression

When your brain is hardwired more toward shifting attention than focusing it, you have ADD, which evokes an added layer of frustration. Thus, it would seem that ADD and procrastination are magnetic conditions that attract each other and depression.

The psychological literature is paper thin on procrastination co-occurring with ADD. But clearly, a common link between ADD, procrastination, and depressive ruminations is distraction. By taking corrective actions to improve your attention and executive functioning, you may be better prepared to follow through on your goals and priorities.

### PURRRRS FOR ACTION

"Haste makes waste." "Look before you leap." "Count to ten." "Take a walk." "Think before you act." These aphorisms to slow down are easier to say than to do. Still, the guidance is instructive. You can reduce the effects of distraction by slowing down, reflecting, and coming back to your priorities.

Use PURRRRS when it is important for you to change course from being too easily sidetracked and distracted. The acronym stands for *pause* first, *use* your resources to slow down, *reflect* on what's happening, *reason* it out, *respond* effectively, *review* and revise from feedback, and *stabilize* by practicing the previous six phases.

Think of PURRRRS as representing a process for improving your executive functioning, building frustration tolerance, and improving your efficiency and effectiveness now, while you are depressed, and later, when you are not. The following information expands on the meaning of the acronym.

1. **Pause.** This means that you stop to think about your thinking. In taking this self-monitoring step, you can avoid distraction and impulse by substituting a more critical evaluation. But what if you routinely forget to pause? A reminder system can help. You can use a felt-tip pen to put a small green dot on your wristwatch or thumb to symbolize "pause." You can wear a special ring. When you are thinking negatively, seeing the dot or ring can remind you to pause before distractions overtake you.

2. **Use.** The second step involves using your resources to resist letting your thoughts flow unchecked. For example, put your thinking into slow motion by writing out the thoughts and reviewing what you just told yourself. This thought-log method makes your thoughts visual and accessible to examination. In short, draw on your inner strength and make a conscious decision to face the situation head on rather than avoiding it.

3. **Reflect.** Steps 1 and 2 set the stage for reflecting. In this reflection phase, you expand on the issue. You gather information. You reflect on how you feel. You examine what you are telling yourself. In short, you think more deeply about what is happening to you that would lead to distraction, a depressive mood, or procrastination. You map the process.

4. **Reason.** This is your analyzing phase. By pausing, using, and reflecting, you may already have started to think about your thinking. In the reasoning phase, you take this a step further. You evaluate your self-talk: What does your thinking direct you to do? What is the emotional tone to these thoughts? How does this thinking jibe with your priorities? If you are getting offtrack, what changes can you make to stay on task and in focus? What's your plan? Think about the steps that you can take now.

5. **Respond.** After reflecting and reasoning things out, give yourself a list of constructive instructions for taking these steps, and follow the instructions. Follow your instructions by talking and walking yourself through the paces. As an added measure, wrap a piece of athletic tape around your wrist with the instructions—much as a football quarterback might do to remember the planned plays.

6. **Review and revise.** Reflecting, reasoning, and responding are like sighting a target, pulling a bow, and releasing an arrow. However, you might miss the center of your target. In looking at what happened, you can get new ideas. Your experience may cause you to see what you hadn't thought about before and adjustments that you can make. In the review and revising phase, you readjust your aim. If you've overlooked a step, revision involves adding and testing the missing step.

7. **Stabilize.** Practice to the point where you have developed a habit for recognizing, evaluating, and replacing distracting low-frustration-tolerance thinking with focused, problem-solving efforts to follow through on priority activities. As you act to boost your clear-thinking skills, you can better regulate your actions to stick with what is important. In short, keep practicing and keep your eye on the target.

The following is an example of how a client named Joyce used PURRRRS to attack her low frustration tolerance. In this case, Joyce felt burdened by the thought that her life was one big hassle. She felt over-whelmed and got distracted by this thought to the point where she felt stressed out by lingering frustrations, conflicts, and unsatisfied desires and wishes.

## JOYCE'S PURRRRS PLAN:

1. She *paused* and reminded herself that her first goal was to monitor her thinking by putting it in slow motion.

2. She *used* her capability to subdue her automatic depressive thought flow by exercising an act of free will.

3. She *reflected* on the content of what she was telling herself. She heard herself say, "Life is a hassle and will never get better."

4. She *reasoned* it out. Joyce judged what she told herself as an overgeneralization. She realized that whenever she thought "never" in a variable and changing situation, she fooled herself. She reminded herself that avoiding hassles was not her primary goal. Rather, her primary goal was to get something important done, such as defeat her depressive thinking. Following this insight, she found that her thoughts became more fluid and flexible.

5. Joyce *responded* by mapping out the steps to separate her overgeneralized thinking from her depressive feelings. She expanded on the "never" issue by showing herself exceptions to the never rule. She gave herself verbal instructions to recognize and challenge her LFT thinking.

6. By paying attention to doing *revisions*, she learned more about her LFT thinking and got efficient at detecting it and in modifying how she approached potentially frustrating circumstances to resolve them.

7. She *stabilized* what she learned through practice. As she did so, she applied her growing knowledge to emerging situations where she would previously have overreacted and overgeneralized.

# YOUR PERSONAL PURRRRS PLAN

Use the following outline to construct your PURRRRS plan for defeating LFT thinking (depressive thinking, procrastination, and so on).

Target frustration: _____

| |
|---|
| **Pause (Stop):** |
| **Use (resist)** |
| **Reflect (think about what's happening):** |
| **Reason (think it through):** |
| **Respond (put yourself through the paces):** |
| **Revise (make adjustments):** |
| **Stabilize (persist and repeat):** |

# LOW FRUSTRATION TOLERANCE AND SUBSTANCE ABUSE

Between 25 percent (Kessler et al. 2003) and 33 percent (Davis et al. 2008) of people who abuse addictive substances also suffer from depression. Some are unaware that they have depression; others have difficulty accepting that they are depressed and self-medicate to alleviate the pain. Whatever your situation, if you couple alcohol or drug abuse with depression, this is promoting a vicious cycle.

When you are thinking that life is too painful to bear, you may want to numb your sensations and distract yourself from distressful thinking with mind-altering substances, such as alcohol, marijuana, or cocaine. Over the long run, these self-medication efforts backfire.

## *Kicking the Habit*

It is challenging to kick a substance abuse habit even when you are not feeling depressed. Nevertheless, breaking an addictive cycle is often a prerequisite to breaking a coexisting depressive cycle.

Breaking this cycle partially involves building a tolerance for urges and cravings and learning not to capitulate to them. The higher you build your tolerance for this form of frustration, the more likely you are to stay away from your substance of choice.

Kicking your habit can give you a sense of control over your life. With this sense of control, you are less likely to have depressed feelings that link to the habit. You are also in a more clear-headed position to deal with depressive thinking and related conditions. However, if you go from alcohol dependency or abuse to sobriety, your depression may seem worse, at least initially. The masking effects of the substance are gone. Issues originally connected with depression may remain. It takes a while to get past this stage.

New challenges can surface from how to handle sobriety to how to find purpose and meaning in your life. You also may have to address the residual effects of the habit (substance-related behaviors that cause personal harm and possibly harm to others) and come to peace with yourself about past drug-related events.

The following story illustrates how LFT and self-doubts weave through both depression and alcohol abuse.

### ■ *Carl's Story*

*To a casual observer, Carl was a success. He had a loving wife and three great kids. It looked as if he had it all. Yet Carl viewed himself as a loser. He saw himself as destined for failure. His tolerance for discomfort was low. Carl suffered from lingering dysthymic depression and would periodically lapse into major depression.*

*Carl masked his depression well. He dressed sharply. He had a mellow, soothing tone of voice. He forced a smile. But that is not how he felt. He kept himself going through the day by thinking that he'd drink at night and relax. He then drank to dampen his tension. The more frequently he drank, the more troubled his sleep was and the worse his life became.*

*Carl made a major breakthrough when he made the connection between his depressive sensations, drinking thinking, drinking patterns, and low frustration tolerance. That awareness gave him an important insight: his intolerance for tension and discomfort invited greater intolerance.*

*When Carl kept a record of his thinking, he found that his mind switched from thinking about how rotten he felt to thinking about drinking. To remind himself of how this combination of depressive sensations, drinking thinking, and alcohol consumption worked, he made up a card for his wallet. He wrote these four lines, drawing arrows to show their relationship:*

*Depressive sensation*

↓

*Depressive thinking*

↓

*Drinking*

↓

*Depressive sensation*

*Carl used a credit-card-sized note that he put in his wallet as a reminder to pause and think through what was happening when he felt an urge to drink. He continued this reflective process until he tolerated his depressive sensations, refused to give in to LFT urges to drink, and stopped using alcohol as a solution for medicating his depression. This change took place over a nine- month period. In this area, quick cures are nice, but what's nice doesn't always happen.*

Combined masked depression and alcohol abuse practically guarantee a life of misery. However, millions have broken this cycle, and mostly on their own. If you find yourself in a situation that is similar to Carl's, you are wise to face up to the fact that both conditions represent frustrating problems to resolve. It is wiser still to take steps to progressively master techniques that apply to shedding both conditions. You can ready yourself for change by avoiding procrastination pitfalls that interfere with corrective actions for both of these problematic conditions.

It's not necessary to deal with substance abuse before addressing depression. Start with whatever is most salient and pressing. This strategy is supported by a recent analysis of thirty-three years of scientific research on people with both substance abuse problems and depression by two Columbia University professors (Nunes and Levin 2004).

## Nicotine and Depression

You feel depressed. You light up. You distract and relax yourself. But smoking is no magic medicine. Take a look at these facts:

- Nicotine is an addictive substance.

- Smoking and depression can occur together and derive from common, as well as separate, mechanisms (Stage, Glassman, and Covey 1996).

- The risk of developing depression increases as the number of nicotine dependence symptoms increases (John et al. 2004).

- Night smoking increases the risk of sleep disturbances (Peters et al. 2011). Sleep disturbances are a risk factor for depression.

- Approximately 60 percent of smokers who had significant difficulty quitting smoking had previous episodes of major depression (Glassman 1997).

- Current and former female smokers are more likely to experience depression and go on antidepressant medication for depression than nonsmokers (Pomerleau, Zucker, and Stewart 2003).

- There is a correlation between increased smoking and depression among the elderly. Smoking can be associated with increased depression or vice versa. Also, the incidence of depression increases with other unhealthy lifestyle changes, such as reduced activity level (van Gool et al. 2003).

- Smoking elevates the risk of developing chronic diseases, such as coronary heart disease and emphysema. Chronic diseases increase the risk of depression.

When people smoke to dull depressive sensations, nicotine appears to have some antidepressant effects (Balfour 1991). Nicotine affects brain regions that influence mood and feelings of well-being (Gilbert and Spielberger 1987). Nevertheless, depression will not normally lift if nicotine is used as an antidepressant. Once you're addicted, smoking creates repeated cravings for nicotine and does not appear to effectively address depression.

When anxious and depressed, you may believe that you can use nicotine to regulate your mood and reduce stress. However, this is a questionable assumption; smoking may increase your level of negative affect should you relapse (Kassel, Stroud, and Paronis 2003).

You may believe that quitting is risky when you are depressed. Quitting a smoking habit involves withdrawal, and withdrawal can have a depressing effect on your mood. There is evidence that quitting smoking can negatively affect your mood (Edwards and Kendler 2011). Thus, you may put off quitting until your depression is under control. After having defeated depression, however, I have found that many people later procrastinate on quitting, for they fear a relapse.

Smoking has documented negative consequences, including premature death. Procrastination on quitting can have serious consequences. I advise finding the best way for you to quit and then doing it. If you experience depressed sensations and withdrawal sensations at the same time, so be it. That might be an advantage. You can act to rid yourself of both conditions at the same time.

Decide to quit, and you have an opportunity to use activity as a remedy for depression. If you smoke and find yourself mindlessly reaching for a cigarette, listen for your Wheedler voice commanding you to consume. Pick up on this voice and contest it, and you are on your way to quitting. You may hear a defiant voice saying, "You smoke for pleasure. No one can stop you from doing that." You may hear a weepy voice that says, "You need something to calm down. Light up now. You can quit later." Whatever voice you hear, your recognition of this form of addictive thinking is a start on the path to freedom from nicotine addiction.

If you smoke and decide to quit, here are a few cognitive and behavioral tips:

- Do a cost analysis. Put your expenses into perspective. Quitting smoking is clearly going to save you a significant number of dollars. If you have an $8-a-day habit, you can save $2,920 a year. Can you think of a more productive use for those dollars? (Some people put what they save into a jar and deposit the dollars every week. Watching the dollars grow can feel rewarding.)

■ Withdrawal symptoms are temporary. They typically pass in about two weeks. Knowing that this is a time-limited event can help make the process tolerable.

■ Consider using a nicotine patch. This approach tends to ease withdrawal pangs.

■ Exercise regularly. This will boost your endorphin level, and increases in endorphin production can substitute for the effects of nicotine. You can also reduce the feeling of being winded due to a lack of exercise and smoking.

■ Make a plan. The psychological reactions to smoking tend to last longer than the approximately two weeks of physical withdrawal. For a time, you'll continue to associate smoking with certain times of day, time intervals, having a cup of coffee, studying for a test, certain moods, and associated sensory experiences. Plan corrective actions for each of these psychological triggers for cravings. Execute the plan.

## The Reverse Five-Minute System

The reverse five-minute method is where you make an agreement with yourself to delay for five minutes before acting on a destructive urge. This system applies to any potentially mindless act, such as when you gobble one potato chip after another or slug down one beer after another. Here is how it works. When you have an urge to consume, wait five minutes. At the end of that time, decide on waiting another five-minute interval. This strategic delay can buy time for the urge to pass.

# ABCDE METHOD FOR DEFUSING LFT THINKING

You feel frustrated because you missed your plane. You tell yourself that you can't stand it. What is the "it" that you can't stand? Is it missing the plane, believing that you can't stand what you don't like, or the inconvenience? If you tell yourself that you can no longer stand feeling depressed, what is there about depression that is intolerable?

The following ABCDE problem-solving sequence describes how to act against "I can't stand it" LFT distress talk.

| |
|---|
| **Activating event (experience):** "A depressed mood." |
| **Rational beliefs about the event:** "The mood is unpleasant. I'd prefer to live without it. But it is what it is and will pass when it does." |
| **Emotional and behavioral consequences for the rational beliefs:** "Acceptance of the unpleasant mood. An absence of double trouble over the mood." |
| **Irrational LFT beliefs:** "I can't stand it. It's too much." |
| **Emotional and behavioral consequences for the irrational LFT beliefs:** "Preoccupation with the mood. Distress over the mood. Diminished tolerance for frustration." |
| **Disputes for irrational LFT beliefs:** (1) "Why can I not stand what I don't like (the mood)?" Sample answer: "I can stand it because I have stood it. But I still don't like experiencing a depressed mood." (2) "What is the 'it' that is too much?" Sample answer: "My belief that I have suffered too long. However, dwelling upon the unpleasant often extends suffering. I'll work to grimly accept depression as time-limited, debilitating, and unpleasant. I'll do what I can to go about my life with the temporary handicaps that accompany depression." |
| **Effects of the disputes:** "Acceptance of depressive mood and frustration about such tensions. Relief from a secondary mental misery imposed over the basic misery of depression. A clearer mind. A lesser preoccupation with the mood of depression. Optimism that depressive negativity can be overridden by rational reason. A corresponding increase in frustration tolerance." |

When LFT thinking is linked to your depression, you can use the following chart as a guide to map and counteract this thinking.

| |
|---|
| **Activating event (experience):** |
| **Rational beliefs about the event:** |
| **Emotional and behavioral consequences for the rational beliefs:** |
| **Irrational LFT beliefs:** |
| **Emotional and behavioral consequences for the irrational LFT beliefs:** |
| **Disputes for irrational LFT beliefs:** |
| **Effects of the disputes:** |

# END DEPRESSION PLAN

**Key ideas** (What three ideas did you find most helpful in this chapter?):

1.

2.

3.

**Action steps** (What three steps can you take to move closer to your goal of overcoming depression?):

1.

2.

3.

**Execution** (How did you execute the steps?):

1.

2.

3.

**Results** (What did you learn that you can use?):

1.

2.

3.

## PART 4

# Special Strategies to Anchor Positive Changes

Stabilize your life with activity scheduling.

Use rewards that work.

Feel good through exercising.

Eating healthily and stay healthy.

Improve your sleep and improve your life.

Rally your energy with reverse imagery.

Build a solid self-concept.

Break the perfectionism-procrastination-depression connection.

Establish empathic relationships.

Prevent RIPS in your relationship.

Manage intimacy.

Find friendships and avoid loneliness.

Use the famous BASIC-ID method to rid yourself of depression.

Prevent depression with confident composure.

Achieve tolerance, self-acceptance, and peace of mind.

# CHAPTER 17

# Activity Scheduling to Defeat Depression

When you feel depressed, you are likely to withdraw and avoid normally pleasurable activities, such as reading the newspaper or talking to friends. By scheduling pleasurable activities into your daily routine, you can bring about improvement in your thinking, mood, and actions so that you can soon get back to doing what you enjoyed before depression hit.

Psychologist Peter Lewinsohn, with his University of Oregon associates, was among the first to develop behavioral activation methods to help people counter depression by increasing their pleasurable activities and reducing activities that contribute to their depression (Lewinsohn and Graf 1973). This approach involves building rewards into your schedule of activities. It enjoys strong research support (Dimidjian et al. 2006; Cuijpers, van Straten, and Warmerdam 2007; Ekers, Richards, and Gilbody 2008; Mazzucchelli, Kane, and Rees 2009).

This evidence-based method helps relieve symptoms for those suffering from ongoing depression (Sturmey 2009). If you have recurrent depression, following an activity schedule may help you go for longer periods without feeling depressed (Dobson et al. 2008).

## REWARDING YOURSELF

Activity scheduling is a behavioral approach where you schedule antidepression activities for yourself. You follow the activities with a reward that increases the odds that you'll do the antidepression activities. This chapter will cover my version of this approach.

Behavioral approaches commonly use rewards to encourage behavioral change. These rewards are used to boost deficiencies and to reduce excesses. If you look to your future pessimistically, giving yourself no out, this is an example of deficiency thinking. To help eliminate this deficiency, you might consider positive alternatives. Spending your time in isolation could qualify as excessive, so you would want to reduce the amount of time you spend alone. The following chart illustrates how you can use rewards to increase or decrease certain behaviors.

| Behaviors to Increase | Rewards for Progress | Behaviors to Decrease | Rewards for Progress |
|---|---|---|---|
| Resolving disagreements with family members | Drinking a cup of gourmet coffee | Moping and complaining to family members | Watching birds on bird feeder for fifteen minutes for every three hours after keeping complaints to yourself |
| Considering positive alternatives | Watching favorite news show | Spending time in isolation | Obtaining a library book on a favorite topic after spending a set amount of time with others |

Rewards come in positive and negative varieties. These two reward systems work differently.

## Positive Rewards

*Positive rewards* are feel-good experiences. For these rewards to be effective, they need to follow the behavior that you want to increase. For example, if every time you scratched your nose, you got a twenty-dollar bill, the chances are you'd scratch your nose more often. The money functions as a reinforcer. Feeling better after you exercise reinforces exercising.

What you reward is important. If you feel relief after a decision to delay, you are experiencing a *rogue reward* for procrastinating. If you smoke and drink to temporarily dull the pain of depression, and you succeed in dulling it, you've given yourself a rogue reward that reinforces intolerance for tension and that detracts from actions to overcome depression. So it's important to be aware of what behavior you are rewarding. You need to be careful about what you reinforce.

You are not a mindless robot when it comes to rewards. You can resist responding to positive rewards. Moreover, positive rewards may not feel so positive when you feel depressed. However, if constructive activities are remedies for depression, following a reward schedule is an example of a disciplined and constructive activity.

## Negative Rewards

We all have negatives in our lives that we'd like to end. When you remove such negatives from your life and feel better, this is a called a *negative reward*. You feel better because you've eliminated something negative.

Negative rewards are common. If an aspirin ends your headache, you'll likely use aspirin again the next time you get a headache. Turning off the television when you are trying to concentrate on your work is a negative reinforcer if you do more work without the distraction. When you challenge a depressive thought, take away its validity, and feel relief, challenging your thinking is reinforced.

A single negative reward rarely changes the momentum of a mild or major depression. Nevertheless, you may quickly see the emotional and practical benefits of removing negatives from your life. This awareness can motivate you to sustain an effort even when you feel pressure to procrastinate. (Part 2 gives many examples of how to remove negative thinking from your life and to benefit from the effort.)

> By taking proactive steps, followed by rewards, you can establish a momentum for activities that compete with depression.

When you are depressed, new psychological, social, and environmental stresses frequently arise. You may have previously experienced a positive relationship with your mate, and you now experience ongoing friction. You may feel stressed about declining grades. You lose the pay raise that you were going to get before you got depressed. The financial loss adds to your sense of malaise. These stresses distract from sustaining positive activities for getting rewards (Liu et al. 2011).

If added stress further diminishes your capacity to experience normal rewards, then acting to remove or reduce these stresses can open opportunities for you to experience a rewarding sense of relief.

The remainder of this chapter will look at how you can use activity scheduling as a positive reinforcement to increase antidepression behaviors and earn relief from depression. The first step is to create a rewards store where you stock items to reward yourself with whenever you accomplish an antidepression activity.

# BUILDING A REWARDS STORE

Your rewards store is a list of feel-good rewards from which you can choose to reward yourself for completing an antidepression activity. Here are some guidelines:

- Reward items should be readily available, easily dispensed, and emotionally worthwhile.

- Make most of your rewards short term. You are more likely to stimulate your brain-reward circuitry with short-term rewards. However, have rewards available for longer-term accomplishments as well, such as sticking with your activity schedule 80 percent or more of the time over a one-week period.

- Rewards for meeting short-term objectives may be sensory, such as taking a warm bubble bath in winter or a cool dip in a pool on a hot summer day.

Note that rewards can be things that you normally like to do as long as you hold off on doing them until after you've accomplished something. This is the essence of Premack's principle, which is covered next.

## *Premack's Principle*

Psychologist David Premack (1965) found that you can use some of the behaviors that you normally engage in to reward a behavior that you want to increase. To gather this information, you might first record what you tend to do or find satisfying to do, such as reading your favorite newspaper columnist or drinking a glass of chocolate milk. Over the next several days, you can create an activity log and list ongoing items as you experience them.

The idea is to pair antidepression activities with rewards. If you regularly read the newspaper, you can pair this reading with an antidepression activity. For example, you can increase making social contacts by reading your favorite columnist only after you contact a friend.

Suppose you decide to take twenty minutes to write out your depressive thoughts to make them more visible and accessible to self-questioning. You know that this is desirable to do, but you keep putting it off. Suppose that you also enjoy watching the tropical fish in your fish tank. You can use watching your fish as a reward for logging your depressive thoughts.

1. Pick a time to start the depressive-thought log.

2. Record your depressive ideas for a twenty-minute period.

3. At the end of the twenty minutes, watch your fish for ten minutes.

If from this awareness exercise, you experience relief from depressive thinking, then you are getting a double reward for the same activity.

# APPLYING PREMACK'S PRINCIPLE

Use the following chart to plan antidepression activities and to list rewards for executing these activities. Then do your antidepression activities and earn your rewards.

| Counter-depression Activity | Positive Activity That You Ordinarily Do |
| --- | --- |
| Example: Record depressive thoughts in a diary and question them for twenty minutes. | Watch fish in tank for ten minutes. |
| | |
| | |
| | |
| | |

## *Cognitive-Emotive, Sensory, and Material Rewards*

I like to include cognitive-emotive, sensory, and material items in a rewards store. Cognitive-emotive rewards involve thinking and feeling items. As a thinking item, you might imagine yourself in a peaceful place. For example, I have a room of angles in my house. I feel good when I'm in that space and even when I imagine being there. Sensory items are ones that affect one or more of your five senses. They include a whiff of a daisy or the feel of velvet. Material rewards are things that have practical value or hold a special interest. Material rewards need not be expensive. The reward may be as basic as buying a tool or a new crystal for your watch. Here is an example of a cognitive-emotive, sensory, and material rewards store:

| REWARDS | Cognitive-Emotive | Sensory | Material |
|---|---|---|---|
| **Short-term** | Look at a picture of a person whose face you find pleasant.<br><br>When you are by yourself, read a favorite poem aloud. | Take a pleasant bubble bath.<br><br>Take a walk in the park to see something new. | Get a smiley face button and wear it.<br><br>Have lunch at your favorite restaurant. |
| **Long-term** | Read a novel by your favorite author.<br><br>Travel to visit a close relative or friend (an ancient Egyptian activity that is still valid today). | Receive a professional massage.<br><br>Visit a live butterfly exhibit in an enclosed garden setting. | Purchase a new outfit.<br><br>Purchase a flat-screen TV. |

You can use scientifically grounded rewards to relieve depression. For example, massage was effective with a subgroup of people who suffered from depression (Rich 2010; Moyer, Rounds, and Hannum 2004). The process appears to reduce stress hormones and increase the neurochemicals serotonin and dopamine, which are believed to alleviate a depressed mood and accompanying symptoms (Field et al. 2005). Neuroimaging results suggest that looking at aesthetically pleasing faces lights up reward centers in the brain (Aharon et al. 2001). By keeping pictures of pleasant faces in a folder, you can tap into this resource when the time comes for dispensing this type of reward to yourself.

As with items on a Chinese dinner menu, you will find some rewards more appealing than others. Pick those that best fit your situation.

# STOCKING YOUR REWARDS STORE

Use the following chart to list your cognitive-emotive, sensory, and material rewards.

| REWARDS | Cognitive-Emotional | Sensory | Material |
|---|---|---|---|
| Short-term | | | |
| Long-term | | | |

# USING A WEEKLY PLANNER

The idea of using a weekly planner relies on Premack's principle, where you schedule regular behaviors that you enjoy to reward other behaviors that you want to encourage in yourself. You do this to regularize your schedule and to schedule antidepression activities.

Your weekly planner would include basic activities of daily living, such as showering, attending to toiletries, dressing, eating breakfast, and exercising, along with other activities that you plan to do during the week. You can assign a fixed time for each of these activities, such as walking between 8:30 and 9:30 a.m. As you complete the items, check them off. (You can make printouts of this routine so that you have a new list each week.)

# YOUR WEEKLY PLANNER

List your critical daily routines (activities) in the order you plan to do them, followed by a reward for each one. The following planner gives some sample routine activities and rewards in the left-hand column.

| Sample routines | Mon. | Tue. | Wed. | Thur. | Fri. | Sat. | Sun. |
|---|---|---|---|---|---|---|---|
| Shower (reward: massage face). | | | | | | | |
| Dress (reward: read chapter of novel). | | | | | | | |
| Eat breakfast (reward: finish with cup of tea or coffee). | | | | | | | |
| Walk outside 8:30 to 9:30 a.m. (reward: Read the news.) | | | | | | | |
| | | | | | | | |
| | | | | | | | |
| | | | | | | | |

Check the boxes after you complete an activity. To give yourself a visual treat, use a highlighter with your favorite color. This can serve as visual recognition of your accomplishments.

If you are moving slower than you'd like in completing your schedule of activities, or you occasionally skip some, you can encourage yourself with a larger reward at the end of the week for achieving, say, 80 percent of them. Watching a pleasurable movie might be an example of a larger reward.

# MAKING A SPECIAL-RESPONSIBILITY ACTIVITY SCHEDULE

Activity schedules are helpful for reminding you about things you need to do. For example, if you are attending a conference, you may schedule things to do before you depart, with rewards for completing each item.

Keeping your finances in order is an area that many tend to let slide when they are depressed. Some necessary financial activities are infrequent activities, such as ordering new checks. Others may be weekly routines. Note that the following activity schedule for keeping finances in order includes specific times and dates scheduled, as well as rewards for completion.

| Activity | Time and Date Scheduled | Check When Completed | Reward for Completion |
|---|---|---|---|
| Order replacement checks from the bank. | Monday before 1:00 p.m. | | Cultivate flowers in garden. |
| Set up automatic payment schedule at bank. | Monday before 1:00 p.m. | | Relax in the shade. |
| Deposit a minimum of five dollars weekly into savings account. | Friday before 1:00 p.m. | | Purchase favorite magazine. |
| Deposit checks within forty-eight hours of receiving them. | As needed | | E-mail friend to see what's happening. |
| Pay half of monthly mortgage twice a month to reduce your long-term interest expenses. | First and middle of the month | | With each payment, read a poem from the collected works of favorite poet. |

When depressed, you may delay following through on special occasions, such as planning for a parent's, friend's, or child's birthday. You can use a special-responsibilities activity schedule to manage special occasions.

# YOUR SPECIAL-RESPONSIBILITY ACTIVITY SCHEDULE

Use the space provided to list activities to do, times and dates to do them, and rewards for completion of a special or ongoing responsibility. Check off each activity as you complete it. Reward yourself for effort and accomplishment.

| Activity | Time and Date Scheduled | Check When Completed | Reward for Completion |
|---|---|---|---|
|  |  |  |  |
|  |  |  |  |
|  |  |  |  |
|  |  |  |  |
|  |  |  |  |

# AVOIDING OVERSCHEDULING

As you start coming out of depression, you may decide that you need to catch up with what you've fallen behind on doing. You may overschedule yourself.

You don't have to operate like a dynamo to make up for lost time and opportunity. Some activities will be overripe and no longer worth doing, or only worth considering after you have finished your most pressing activities first. The adage "Don't bite off more than you can chew" applies here. Instead of trying to make up for lost time, consider that time spent with depression is like time spent with a broken leg. You wouldn't expect to run a marathon when your leg is just starting to mend. Pick what is most important for you to do now. Emphasize that.

# GETTING REWARDS FROM REVERSE IMAGERY

Nosheen Kahn-Rahman, Ph.D., a former professor/director of the Centre for Clinical Psychology, University of the Punjab, in Lahore, Pakistan, offers her top tip for helping people who suffer from depression. Kahn-Rahman (pers. comm.) suggests the following reverse imagery exercise for daily use by "clients who feel low and depressed, and who have feelings of inadequacy":

Write an answer to the question, "What has brought me pleasure?" Rank these activities from high to low on a happiness scale. Your list may include playing tennis or reading a book. Then make a short-term daily goal that you'll take steps to do daily to change your mood in a positive direction. Follow each step toward your goal with something from your happiness scale that can bring you pleasure. Record what you did to achieve your goal in your journal or diary. Create an image of yourself working toward your goal and doing what you can to feel happy. (You need not feel locked into your original goal. As your life changes, make goal revisions.)

When you use traditional imagery techniques, you start with the image and then move to the behavior. This is a reverse-imagery technique. You start with doing the behavior first and then connect this live experience with positive imagery. Here's how. (1) Start with square breathing, where you breathe in for four seconds, hold your breath for four seconds, breathe out for four seconds, wait four seconds, and then repeat the pattern for two minutes. (2) When you feel relaxed, start the reverse-imagery exercise. Imagine yourself doing what you have already done: take steps toward your goal, followed by experiencing a reward from your happiness scale. If tennis brings you pleasure, imagine yourself playing a match. Imagine yourself reading a book by a favorite author. (3) Now, focus on any positive feelings you experience. (4) Do this exercise for fifteen minutes daily and keep a daily record of your feelings during and immediately following this exercise.

Pace yourself. There is no universal law that says that you must operate like a fury to make up for time losses when you were depressed.

It is important that you keep revising the actions you take and the rewards you give yourself through this reverse-imagery exercise. That gives you fresh imagery materials to think about. Do this exercise for thirty days to build a momentum toward associating positive feelings with positive activities, and see if your mood changes.

As a bonus exercise, write down a negative thought that goes through your mind when you feel depressed. At a separate time of the day, repeat the square-breathing exercise. This time, as you exhale, imagine this negative thought leaving each time you breathe out.

As a second bonus exercise, think about the question: "Who am I?" List what you believe characterizes you when you are not feeling depressed: your behaviors, your emotions, your talent, your values, and your traits. List these qualities from high to low on their value to you. Do your square-breathing exercise. As you do, imagine yourself expressing your top positive characteristics.

I find this reverse-imagery exercise very effective in bringing about positive energy, improving motivation, building a positive self-concept, and identifying the "cognitive" link between a negative and a more favorable mood. Once my clients see the link, they increasingly learn how to use this information to build a positive sense of command and control over themselves.

# END DEPRESSION PLAN

**Key ideas** (What three ideas did you find most helpful in this chapter?):

1.

2.

3.

**Action steps** (What three steps can you take to move closer to your goal of overcoming depression?):

1.

2.

3.

**Execution** (How did you execute the steps?):

1.

2.

3.

**Results** (What did you learn that you can use?):

1.

2.

3.

# CHAPTER 18

# Behavioral Methods to Feel Good Again

In this chapter we'll explore exercise, diet, and sleep techniques to improve your mood and your health. As practically everyone knows, these techniques look good on paper, but translating them into action—even when you are not feeling depressed—is normally challenging.

Beyond a depressed mood and lethargy, procrastination is likely to get in the way, which partially explains the high failure rate in these three areas. Here you'll learn to apply concepts from chapter 5 to overcome health procrastination, or the putting off of activities that are necessary to maintain or advance good physical and psychological health. You can then follow through on these corrective actions for overcoming your depression.

## MODERATE EXERCISE FOR MOOD CONTROL

Exercise is an evidence-based method for overcoming depression that has added health benefits. Rockefeller University Professor Bruce S. McEwen offers two top tips for both overcoming and preventing depression. The first involves a process for gaining psychological and physical benefits from exercising, as McEwen (pers. comm.) explains:

> Being "stressed out" means being overwhelmed and feeling unable to cope with what is going on in your life. This can result in combinations of irritation, anger, and helplessness. It can also produce an unhealthy lifestyle, including sleep loss and harmful behaviors such as smoking, drinking too much alcohol, eating too much "comfort food" and neglecting regular physical activity and interactions with friends and family. All of these factors contribute to you *rallostatic load*, the "wear and tear" on the body resulting from trying to cope with too much stress and a stress-related unhealthy lifestyle (McEwen and Lasley 2002; McEwen 2006).Besides adopting a healthy diet and limiting calorie consumption, regulating alcohol intake, and not smoking, there are two especially valuable actions you can take to lighten your allostatic load.
>
> The first is regular physical activity. This does not mean that you have to become a marathon runner. Walking sixty minutes a day at least five days per week is a minimum program that has been

shown to reduce the incidence of type 2 diabetes and to generate new neurons in the *hippocampus*, a part of the brain involved in memory of daily events, spatial orientation, and mood regulation. Physical activity improves mood and is one of the best antidepressants. You are likely to have improved memory and decision-making ability. However, you won't gain the benefits without pushing yourself to start and sustain the effort.

The second action is social support and integration. Social support is what you get from regular contact with friends and family members, and social integration is feeling that you are part of a community or group and sharing common goals and problems. Both activities have been shown to help people sleep better and improve overall health.

## What Physical Exercise Is Right for You?

You may wonder what exercises to do and how long to do them. As a rule of thumb, follow an exercise program that you are physically able to do without excessive strain. If you have any question about your physical condition concerning exercise, get a physical examination and a stress test before beginning an exercise program.

There are four conditions for designing your exercise plan: type, frequency, location, and intensity.

**Type:** Pick exercises that you have previously found appealing, such as swimming, kayaking, biking, jogging or walking on a treadmill, climbing stairs, rowing, using a Hula Hoop, playing tennis, playing golf, or lifting weights. The idea is to get your heart rate up to a reasonable level and for a reasonable time for your current physical condition, health, and age.

**Frequency:** You are likely to experience improvement in your mood by exercising thirty minutes a day (Barnes et al. 2010). This improvement correlates with an improved attitude and willingness to continue exercising (Kwan and Bryan 2010). If you exercise for thirty minutes a day in five-to-ten minute segments, you can get adequate fitness and health benefits (Hansen, Stevens, and Coast 2001). However, a daily sixty-minute walking routine appears to generate broader health benefits.

**Location:** You can work on your own, combine exercising with group interaction (aerobic exercise or dance class), or do it both ways at a health facility with exercise equipment and professional instruction.

**Intensity:** You are more likely to tolerate low-intensity exercises. You are moderately exercising when you raise and maintain your heart rate twenty to thirty beats above your normal level for about twenty minutes. Both aerobic (walking, swimming, or biking) and anaerobic (weight training and stretching) exercises appear equally effective for improving your mood.

Exercise is an evidence-based remedy for depression and a buffer against future depression. The research is all over the place regarding what is minimum and adequate. This book offers guidelines based on existing research, but you should experiment to find out what works best for you.

Moderate exercise can reduce fatigue, increase your energy level, boost your immune system, mute the pain of a depressed mood, and activate brain regions associated with improved executive functioning and memory. The sooner you get started, the better.

# YOUR EXERCISE PROGRAM

To gain the benefits of regular exercise, define your exercise plan and then do it.

| | |
|---|---|
| **Type of exercise** | |
| **Location** | |
| **Intensity** | |
| **Frequency (days and times)** | |

## SCHEDULE EXERCISING AS AN ACTIVITY

Make exercising a priority and set up an exercise activity schedule. Pick a time each day to exercise. Draw a reward from your rewards store for each day that you stick with the program. Reward yourself quickly after you have finished your exercise routine.

You don't have to do the same exercise every day for the same amount of time. You can exercise for one hour one day, then twenty minutes the next, and repeat the pattern. You may bike on one day and walk on another.

# YOUR EXERCISE ACTIVITY SCHEDULE

Write down the type of exercise you plan to do, when you will do it, and the rewards you will give yourself for following through.

| Exercise | Type | Time | Reward |
|---|---|---|---|
| Mon | | | |
| Tue | | | |
| Wed | | | |
| Thur | | | |
| Fri | | | |
| Sat | | | |
| Sun | | | |

## Overcoming Procrastination

As people living in westernized countries become more sedentary, they increasingly risk depression (Teychenne, Ball, and Salmon 2010). Well-publicized studies about the positive benefits of exercising have done little to reverse this sedentary trend.

When you are depressed, introducing exercise into your routine comes at a time of high pessimism and low energy. But you have an added incentive. You are not only acting to get into better shape—good for general health reasons—but you are also acting to alleviate a distressful depressive state. Exercise also helps prevent a relapse. However, procrastination can interfere with the best of plans.

The cognitive behavioral methods that you've been learning in this book can help you procrastinate less and accomplish more in the way of healthful exercise.

## DO A COST-BENEFIT ANALYSIS

A cost-benefit analysis is simple to do. You compare the potential short- and long-term benefits of procrastination with taking productive actions. Although making this comparison may not be a course changer, it gives you something to think about that may inspire productive action. Here's an example.

| Benefits | Physical Exercise | Procrastination |
|---|---|---|
| **Short-term** | Break inertia from inactivity to physical activity.<br><br>Gain confidence as you shift from a sedentary to a more physically active lifestyle.<br><br>Demonstrate a will to change to a healthy lifestyle.<br><br>Pit realistic optimism against depressive pessimism. | Avoid hassles that naturally come with physical exercise, such as getting to an exercise location, exertion, and no guarantee for gratification. |
| **Long-term** | Look younger.<br><br>Build stress tolerance.<br><br>Improve attention and concentration.<br><br>Aid cardiac functioning.<br><br>Protect against type 2 diabetes.<br><br>Boost endorphins. Feel good.<br><br>Prevent osteoporosis.<br><br>Replace depression with feeling good.<br><br>Enjoy improved productivity.<br><br>Burn calories.<br><br>Develop a slimmer appearance.<br><br>Feel healthier.<br><br>Avoid many hidden effects of a sedentary lifestyle, such as losing your ambition. | Avoid hassles that naturally come with physical exercise, such as getting to an exercise location, exertion, and no guarantee for gratification. As you fall behind, you may experience more stress. Procrastination may result in accumulation of things left undone. This is a formula for feeling overwhelmed. |

Here are two more short-term benefits for exercising. You can normally experience an improved mood for a time following either aerobic or anaerobic exercise (Yeung 1996). Immediately following twenty-five minutes of treadmill walking, women with major depression experienced less automatic depressive thinking and a better mood. Following an exercise routine, people with the greater degree of depression tended to experience the greatest magnitude of positive change (Lash 2000).

## YOUR COST-BENEFIT ANALYSIS FOR EXERCISING

Do your own cost-benefit analysis for exercising. Write down the short- and long-term benefits of doing physical exercise versus the short- and long-term benefits of procrastinating.

| Benefits | Physical Exercise | Procrastination |
|---|---|---|
| Short-term | | |
| Long-term | | |

### ELIMINATE PROCRASTINATION EXCUSES

Your cost-benefit analysis makes moderate physical exercise a logical choice for attacking depression. Nevertheless, you may wait to feel better or inspired before you start. That's a classic procrastination ploy. Here are some sample common reasons for putting off exercising and some examples of corrective thinking that you can use to counter these fictions:

| Reasons for Not Exercising | Corrective Thinking |
|---|---|
| "It's inconvenient." | In the short term, it is inconvenient. But there is a longer-term view. Consider the value of the above benefits you will receive from exercising. Like most things of value in life, benefits are earned. So what's more important? Doing the work and getting the benefits or avoiding the hassle of exercising? |
| "Exercise takes effort." | Exercise does take effort. But so what? If your goal is to live life effortlessly, expect a boomerang effect. If you choose to take a different path and pay for gains through effort, then you are headed in the right direction. |
| "It makes no sense to start something that I won't follow through on." | Feeling defeatist is common when you are depressed. But this foreclosure is only as true as you make it. |
| "It's tough to muster motivation when I am depressed." | True. But it's tougher to stay depressed when you have countermeasures available to tip the balance in the direction of feeling better by doing better. |
| "If I work out at a health club, I'll look bad compared to others." | At one time, practically everyone at the health club was in worse shape. Some may be in worse shape than you now. Most will share a common goal of getting and staying fit. |
| "Since I'm doomed, anything that I do to improve my physical conditioning is a waste of time." | Hopelessness thinking is important to uproot with evidence that comes from doing rather than stewing about the futility of exercising as a corrective and prophylactic action. |

# YOUR CORRECTIVE THINKING EXERCISE

If you hear yourself saying "I'm too busy to exercise. I don't have time to exercise. I wouldn't know where I'd fit this into my schedule," it's time to turn your attention to these reasons and figure out a better alternative. List your reasons for procrastination and correct your thinking.

| Reasons for Not Exercising | Corrective Thinking |
|---|---|
|  |  |
|  |  |
|  |  |
|  |  |
|  |  |

## OVERCOME DISCOMFORT DODGING

Discomfort dodging is a common excuse for putting off exercising. This is where you default to easier or safer activities. Let's say that you like the benefits of exercising. You have good reason to believe that exercising can eventually bring relief from depression. At the same time, you are stewing about how bad you feel. Stewing is a diversion.

You come to a crossroads where you can choose between doing and stewing. Now you face the timeless procrastination double-agenda dilemma. You want the benefits from exercising. You also want to avoid the discomfort of gearing up for exercise and exercising, especially when you already believe that you lack energy. That's the dilemma.

As you face the dilemma, you may experience a struggle of the mind against itself. Exercising takes effort and can be uncomfortable, so you get signals from your lower brain not to do it. You know the long-term benefits of exercise, so your voice of reason says to do it. You now have an opportunity to compromise with yourself. You can accept that exercising is uncomfortable and give your primitive brain its due. Then follow instructions from your enlightened reason.

Here are additional ways to tip the balance in favor of a reasoned approach to exercising:

- Exercise even when you don't feel like it.

- Accept that avoidance urges last only so long. They are not terminal.

- Rather than waiting to feel inspired while lying on the couch, wait out your urge to diverge while riding your bicycle to the gym.

- Refuse to accept the bunk that if you are severely depressed, exercising is impossible for you to do or that it would be worthless even if you could do it. Instead, treat such thinking as hypothetical. Test your hypotheses, even in small measure.

## GRIND IT OUT

I've exercised with reasonable consistency for over forty years. During this time, I can't recall looking forward to working out. While at the gym, I often think of shortening the circuit, but I don't. I don't feel thrilled when I'm finished. However, I know the evidence of the benefits of exercise. I rely on that information as a guide to action. I stoically put myself through the paces.

If I waited until I felt like working out, I'd be in poor physical shape. Instead, I do what I've suggested to others. Resign yourself to the reality that you can't benefit from exercising without exercising.

On July 24, 2011, the American Psychological Association database listed over 15,505 documents in which the words "physical exercise" or "physical activity" appeared. Only nine mentioned "procrastination." Yet procrastination is likely to be the biggest barrier to exercise. But you can learn to get past it.

By grinding it out, you may find that exercise is not as bad as your primitive mind thinks. And even if it is, you've acted to benefit yourself. You've substituted a healthy form of stress for double-trouble stresses that come from finagling and primitive avoidance reasoning. You avoid the lethargy of inactivity. You improve your chances for better mental and physical health.

# A NO-DIET WEIGHT PLAN

Diet is an ancient Greek remedy for depression. If you lived over two thousand years ago, a physician might recommend that you eat well to curb melancholy.

When depressed, you may have lost your appetite, or you may eat too much. You may binge eat to get a temporary mood lift. You can manage any of these diverse problem-eating conditions by following a no-diet plan. The no-diet plan is for regulating your eating routines. By following the no-diet plan, you curb undesired eating excesses and deficiencies, and as a by-product, you can increase or decrease your weight. The no-diet plan is simple. Eat appealing food in proper proportions with the necessary nutrients for a balanced diet. This is a good habit to practice whether or not you are depressed.

The no-diet plan has a special feature. Each day, you roughly consume the number of calories you need to maintain a desired weight. Follow this plan and you'll gradually level off (with adjustments) to around that target weight. Stick with it, and you'll stay within your desired weight zone.

Suppose you are a five foot five, forty-year-old woman who weighs 150 pounds and who, after building exercise into her routine, now exercises moderately. With moderate exercise, it takes about 2,100 calories a day to maintain your weight at 150 pounds. If it were your goal to weigh around 125 pounds, for example, it would take about 1,919 calories to stay around 125 pounds.

You could make a small adjustment in your diet and take in about 1,919 calories a day. For example, drop two slices of enriched bread from your diet, and you've eliminated about 250 calories. You would lose a pound every ten to twelve days or so, but less as you go. If you wanted to gain ten pounds, this same formula would work in reverse. Note that you should pick a weight that is reasonable for you, given your age and bone structure, and that you can attain and maintain.

With this plan, you don't have to go crazy weighing and measuring food to reach a certain calorie count. A basic understanding of calories by food type is a reasonable knowledge to have, and this information is readily obtainable through books or the Internet. However, since weight-loss plans are normally far from perfect, plan on making adjustments as you go.

What you eat doesn't matter as long as it is reasonable. For example, the Mediterranean diet is considered healthy. There is empirical evidence that it is a weight-containment diet that buffers you against coronary heart disease and type 2 diabetes. The key words for any good diet are "balance" and "moderation."

The no-diet plan for reaching and maintaining your goal weight reduces your risk of cycling through diets and weight gains, whether you are depressed or not. Follow this plan with disciplined consistency, and eventually you'll level off at your goal weight. As your physical activity level or health status changes, you will need to make adjustments. Consistency is key if you want to avoid returning to the same old dysfunctional habits.

## *Maintaining Consistency*

Even when you are not depressed, you can forget about performing like a well-maintained machine. The best you can expect is to operate with reasonable consistency, within the time and resources that you have available. That's good enough.

You are thinking like a person who intends to address depression when you prepare yourself as well as you can to operate with reasonable consistency. You'll naturally tend to do less than normal when you are depressed. You'll probably bog down more often. This is your new normal until you get less depressed. However, by progressively mastering the steps to get up from depression, you build consistency, resiliency, and behavioral resources to overcome depression sooner and to slide back less often.

## PLAN AHEAD

Diet is a good opportunity for training yourself to be more consistent. Because of normal urges to devour food, maintaining a consistent diet can be challenging.

You can prepare yourself by gathering the information you'll need about diet and consumption.

- Ferret out the facts and the science of healthy eating.

- Set up a no-diet eating schedule where you use the information you've gained.

- Plan your meals daily or weekly, whichever works best for you, and use an activity schedule to record your plans.

Now put your plan into action.

## REWARD YOURSELF

Rewarding yourself for consistency is one way to help you be consistent.

- Reward yourself after each meal when you stick to your plan. (Exclude eating a giant piece of chocolate cake or other calorie-charged food.)

- Give yourself a bigger reward each time you meet your weekly objectives. When you meet your weight objective, give yourself a still bigger reward.

- For each month that you maintain your objective, reward yourself.

When you have ample evidence that you have established a new lifestyle eating habit, fade out the rewards. Your new rewards are likely to be internal and linked to a sense of confident composure.

## MEASURE THE RESULTS

To increase the odds of positive change, keep close track of what you are doing and what results. For example, weighing yourself every other day is likely to be more productive then measuring your weight monthly. If your no-diet plan calls for dividing your calories into three meals, you can measure your performance on a meal-by-meal basis. Are you sticking with the program?

Doing these things will provide direct feedback. Based on the results you get, you can also make adjustments and thus develop a program that exactly suits your goals and abilities.

## *Stop Dallying with Your Diet*

Scottish poet Robert Burns's oft-quoted adage applies to eating healthily: "The best laid schemes of mice and men go often askew." As with physical exercise, weight control is a major challenge. Because it is easy to revert back to the same patterns that got you into trouble in the first place, the odds are that you'll find weight control challenging. Many factors can interfere with maintaining good habits. You have natural eating urges and cravings. You may feel tempted to quit your no-diet plan when you feel stressed. In each case, you are likely to face the familiar double-agenda procrastination dilemma.

You have an intended weight goal and simultaneously have urges that pull you in a different direction. Satisfying the urge is your second, or implied, agenda. For example, your second agenda is to avoid inconvenience and discomfort. You now face a typical double-agenda dilemma conflict. You can either accept the discomfort that goes with changing a major habit of consumption, or you can duck discomfort and sabotage your goal. Side with the second agenda and you are likely to stay snared in the unhealthy habit of excess eating that got you into trouble in the first place. Stick with the first and you achieve your goal.

Since you won't know when you'll face this dilemma, it's impossible to schedule for it. You can, of course, simulate conditions where you'd have urges and train yourself to buttress yourself against them. I invented a technique I call *rational emotive problem simulation* for this purpose. Here's an example: if you tend to have cookie cravings, set aside a time when you have a bowl of cookies before you. Allow yourself to experience an urge to consume without actually eating them until the urge dissipates. Toss the cookies into the trash. Reward yourself with something you find pleasurable, such as picking flowers from your garden.

# DIETARY SUPPLEMENTS

What you eat matters. For example, depression and coronary heart disease are lower in fish-eating cultures, such as in Okinawa and among the Inuit people of Greenland (Kromhout 2005). There is compelling evidence that consuming fish helps prevent coronary death and relieves depression.

## Omega 3 Fatty Acids and Depression

Fish are a rich source of omega-3 fatty acids, which are an essential nutrient that the body doesn't produce. People with both coronary heart disease and depression appear to have lower omega-3 concentrations in the body (Jiang et al. 2011; Frasure-Amith, Lespérance, and Julien 2004). Maintaining an adequate concentration of omega-3 polyunsaturated fatty acids (PUFAs) appears promising for improving your mood and coronary functioning.

Omega 3 consumption appears effective against major and bipolar depression (Nemets, Stahl, and Belmaker 2002; Lin and Su 2007; Araujo et al. 2010). With adequate omega-3 concentrations, you may see measurable improvements within a three- to four-week period (Osher and Belmaker 2009).

At least 250 milligrams a day of long-chain n-3 PUFA, or two servings per week of oily fish, may be sufficient to confer benefits (Calder 2004; Gebauer 2006). However, this is minimal. Having three or more weekly servings appears to promote better results.

Oily fish, such as sardines, mackerel, and herring, and cold-water fish, such as halibut, are rich sources of the long-string omega-3 polyunsaturated fats. Broiled and baked fish convey greater benefits than fried fish. Fish oil capsules confer similar benefits.

The old saying that fish is brain food, may have merit, especially among the elderly. There is promising research that polyunsaturated fats improve cognitive functioning. There is also contradictory data. We'll have to wait and see how this controversy is settled.

University of Texas Southwest physician Dr. William J. Knaus II notes that fish oil contains two forms of omega-3 that are important for both coronary health and improved mood. He suggests that you do your own research. If you think an omega-3 trial is right for you, and you prefer to use capsules, check with your doctor for guidance on what brands and dosages to consider, given your age, gender, race, and general health.

## St John's Wort and Depression

St. John's wort is a wild-growing yellow-flowered plant that contains the herb *hypericum* and other ingredients that can be effective in addressing depression. Its use as an antidepressant, and for correcting sleep problems, goes back to ancient Greece.

The herb is widely used as an antidepressant in Europe. It appears effective for mild depression (Kasper et al. 2008), moderate to severe depression (Szegedi et al. 2005), major depression (Fava et al. 2005), atypical depression (Mannel et al. 2010), and shorter-term treatment programs for addressing depression (Carpenter 2011).

The herb has similar side effects as inert placebos. It is generally well tolerated (Ernst et al. 1998). There are little downside and potential upside benefits.

European research supports the use of this inexpensive herb. The composition appears standardized and supported by the research. In the United States, when you buy St. John's wort, you may get varied compositions and quality. Some US drug studies of *hypericum* suggest no effect beyond that expected from a placebo (Krishna and the Hypericum Depression Trial Study Group 2002). You may want to do your own research to see if St. John's wort can be of help to you.

If you are currently using a prescription antidepressant, simultaneously using St. John's wort is a bad idea. This combination may contribute to serotonin syndrome, a potentially life-threatening drug interaction. There are other counterindicators for using the herb. Check with your physician about dose, quality, and interaction issues.

# BEHAVIORAL TECHNIQUES FOR INSOMNIA

Insomnia is trouble falling asleep, or waking and having trouble falling back to sleep. These sleep problems are highly common among people with major depression. With atypical depression, you may sleep longer than usual, and there is some evidence that this condition of excessive sleep is associated with weight-gain problems and weight-related health risks. Going to sleep at about 11:00 p.m. and rising about 7:00 a.m. helps with this issue.

The relationship between insomnia and depression is bidirectional. Insomnia increases the risk of depression, and insomnia is a somatic symptom of depression. In a thirty-four-year follow-up study of medical students at Johns Hopkins Medical Center, the risk of developing depression among students who had insomnia during medical school was twice that of those without insomnia. Failure to adequately address insomnia increases the risk of a depression relapse (Chang et al. 1997).

Insomnia is increasing worldwide (Ohayon and Paiva 2005). Restorative sleep correlates with reductions in depressed mood, depressive thinking, and other common symptoms of depression. Addressing insomnia early can lead to quality-of-life improvements and depression prevention (Guazzelli and Gentili 2008).

Stress is a precipitating factor in both depression and insomnia, especially when you have stressful, ruminative cognitions and have trouble sleeping because of them. Defusing the impact of stress cognitions is associated with restful sleep (Brand et al. 2010). Cognitive behavioral therapy is an effective nonpharmacological approach to help promote this sleep (Edinger et al. 2001).

Some sleep medications can prove productive. However, if you've tried medication to restore sleep without significant success or are prone to addiction for some of these prescriptive medications, here are some cognitive and behavioral methods for restoring healthy sleep patterns.

## Cognitive Ways to Get to Sleep

There is a significant scientific literature on the relationship between sleep problems and negative thinking. For example, you may worry over lack of sleep and about performing less well following interrupted sleep. Worry is distracting. The anxiety that can extend from worry creates an unpleasant feeling of arousal that can keep you awake. Here are four cognitive countermeasures.

**Use what you know to defuse negative nighttime chatter.** You can overcome double troubles, such as mulling over past losses. You have the tools to put such matters into perspective with techniques from the first three parts of this book. Use what works best for you, such as keeping perspective without elaborating, magnifying, and generalizing about the target situation.

**Work things out in your mind during the day with a serenity exercise.** Write down the content of your negative thought themes. Without struggling against them, accept their presence. Put them to music. Think of one positive event for each of those that are negative. This change in pace can cause a shift in perspective. Then at night, repeat this serenity exercise.

**Engage the pink elephant dilemma.** As you struggle to rid yourself of an unwanted thought, the harder you try, the higher your level of distress. You are now facing the pink elephant dilemma; that is, when someone tells you not to think of a pink elephant, you are more likely to think of a pink elephant. You may try to distract yourself by thinking of a purple fox, but the pink elephant is likely to remain in the recesses of your mind. When this happens, start with passive volition. Passive volition is an attitude of allowance. It boils down to this: "If I think of a pink elephant, so I think of a pink elephant." By giving up the struggle of trying to control your thoughts (active volition), you are more likely to feel rested.

**Adopt a coping perspective.** If you have trouble sleeping because you reflect on the trials and tribulations of the day, this is a signal that you can profit from resolving daily conflicts as they arise. If you have difficulty falling asleep because you anticipate a negative occurrence tomorrow, flip things around and concentrate on best outcomes.

## Behavioral Ways to Get to Sleep

You'll probably discover what works best for you through experimenting. Fortunately, you can find many evidence-based and commonsense behavioral approaches for this experiment. Here are a number of behavioral techniques for improving your sleeping patterns:

- Follow a regular sleep schedule. Go to bed when you are likely to feel sleepy.

- Give your body cues associated with sleep, such as listening to a favorite soothing song about fifteen minutes before you are scheduled to retire.

- When you are unable to sleep, get out of bed. The idea is to avoid associating the bed with wakefulness. Return when you are ready to sleep.

- If you routinely fall asleep on the couch while watching TV—and then awaken a few hours later and stay awake for the next several hours—change the routine. Do something active that will keep you awake until a regular bedtime.

- Associate your bed with sleeping. Avoid reading or watching television in bed or doing work in bed. If you insist on watching TV in bed, use the sleep timer to shut off the TV within sixty minutes. That way you are less likely to awaken when you are in the lighter phases of sleep.

- Spend about a half hour in direct daylight each day. In the morning, go out in the sun for about fifteen minutes. This can help set your sleep-time clock.

- Do moderate aerobic exercise during the afternoon every day. Most sleep experts suggest avoiding exercise two to four hours before you go to bed. Note: There is some research indicating that mild evening exercise at night aids sleep. Use your experience as a guide.

- Avoid ingesting coffee, cola, tea, or chocolate (or other caffeine-containing substances) seven hours before your regular bedtime.

- If you smoke, refrain from doing so several hours before going to bed. (Because of demonstrated health risks, it is a good idea to stop smoking permanently.)

- Avoid alcohol for three hours before going to bed. A glass of wine in the evening may cause you to feel relaxed, which may make it easier for you to fall asleep; however, as the body breaks down alcohol, your sleep is likely to be disturbed.

- Sleep in a well-ventilated room with a room temperature of sixty-five to sixty-eight degrees Fahrenheit. Sleep is associated with a drop in body temperature.

- Take a warm bath about two hours before sleeping. This can be relaxing, and the two-hour time interval gives your body ample time to cool down before sleeping.

- Massage your feet for ten minutes immediately before going to bed. Use relaxation as a sleep aid. Relaxing your muscles and visualizing relaxing imagery can help dull some of the sharp edges of sleeplessness.

- Reduce controllable external noises that serve as sleep distractions. Try white noise to muffle outside sounds that can't be eliminated. An example of white noise is a low-volume sound from a nonoperating television channel.

- Relax your body during periods of interrupted sleep.

- Some sleep experts advise sleeping with your head facing north. The theory is that the pineal gland responds to magnetic forces with increases in melatonin production. (I'm unconvinced that this makes any difference, but turning your head north can't hurt.)

- If you are inclined to watch a clock to see when you awaken, use one without an illuminated dial or light. You are less likely to preoccupy yourself with how much sleep time you might be losing.

- Count backward from one thousand by threes.

- Play barely audible background music that you associate with restfulness and sleep.

- Plan to rise between 6:00 a.m. and 7:00 a.m. There is some evidence that sleeping late increases the risk of depression (Olders 2003).

- If I have trouble sleeping, I'll sometimes take a small LED flashlight and quickly flash it into my eyes three times. I feel like yawning. I typically fall asleep shortly thereafter. There is no science behind this idea, but it does illustrate how inventing solutions may sometimes prove useful.

## Melatonin and Sleep

Melatonin is a sleep hormone secreted by the small, pine-cone shaped, pea-sized pineal gland located near the center of the brain. Light and darkness presumably cue the gland to produce melatonin. The rise and fall of melatonin production presumably regulates the twenty-four-hour circadian rhythms that relate to sleep. The highest melatonin levels peak at about 2:00 a.m.

Small amounts of melatonin may improve sleep patterns. However, there is no meaningful evidence affirming the effectiveness of melatonin pills sold in health food stores or through mail-order marketing organizations.

Pecans, bananas, turkey, rice, tomatoes, oats, sweet corn, milk, and barley are rich sources of tryptophan, which is thought to boost melatonin levels. Meditation may also boost melatonin levels.

## Procrastination and Sleep

Even when you know what to do to establish healthy sleep patterns, you may not do it. It's easier to lapse back into familiar patterns or to hope for a better day when good sleep will automatically come your way. That's not a gamble worth taking, but millions will take it anyway.

If you are procrastinating on addressing your sleep problems, here is a sample activity schedule with two cognitive antidotes and two behavioral ones.

| Sleep Antidote | Procrastination Interference | Procrastination Antidote | Reward for Executing Antidote |
|---|---|---|---|
| Defeat the pink-elephant double trouble. | Think that it's impossible to stop the thought and thus delay corrective action. | Instead of struggling to stop the thought, accept it without a struggle. | Watch your favorite news show first thing in the morning after you arise from sleep. |
| Address the double trouble of worrying about what tomorrow will bring. | Feel out of control; decide to do nothing except worry. | For each worry thought, think of a positive alternative that works out well. | Put your favorite fruit on your favorite cereal in the morning. |
| When you have trouble falling asleep, get up from bed for five minutes. | Tell yourself that getting up from bed is too tough. | Test the research that says leaving and then returning to bed is more likely to be followed by sleep. Your alternative hypothesis is that continuing to ruminate contributes to staying awake. | Smell a rose first thing in the morning. |
| Follow a regular healthy schedule for going to bed. | Nap earlier and then stay awake later. | Do light exercise when you would ordinarily feel inclined to nap. | Take a warm bubble bath each morning when you follow a healthy schedule for getting to bed. |

# YOUR SLEEP PLAN

Come up with your own sleep plan. Test it.

| Sleep Antidote | Procrastination Interference | Procrastination Antidote | Reward for Executing Antidote |
|---|---|---|---|
|  |  |  |  |
|  |  |  |  |
|  |  |  |  |
|  |  |  |  |

## *Behavioral Techniques for SAD*

Seasonal affective disorder commonly occurs in northern climates at around the time the days grow short. You may start to feel irritable, sad, and anxious. Sleep problems commonly accompany SAD. You can defuse the depressive thinking that ordinarily accompanies this form of depression. Light therapy can also help reduce SAD effects.

The use of light has promise as a general way to curb depression (Tuunainen, Kripke, and Endo 2004). The technique also has promise for reducing depression among pregnant women who are prone to depression (Epperson et al. 2004).

There are specialized lighting systems for treating SAD. Research shows that 10,000-lux florescent light (about twenty times as bright as ordinary inside light) can reduce the intensity of seasonal depression. Sit about thirty inches from the light. Approximately twenty to thirty minutes daily of this higher intensity exposure may yield results in two to three weeks. Dim light filtered through a slightly red-tinted visor worn directly over the eyes may be effective. Going for a walk on a sunny morning may yield similar results, and you will benefit from the exercise.

# END DEPRESSION PLAN

**Key ideas** (What three ideas did you find most helpful in this chapter?):

1.

2.

3.

**Action steps** (What three steps can you take to move closer to your goal of overcoming depression?):

1.

2.

3.

**Execution** (How did you execute the steps?):

1.

2.

3.

**Results** (What did you learn that you can use?):

1.

2.

3.

# CHAPTER 19

# Avoiding the Pitfalls of Perfectionism

Perfectionism can mean many things. It can be stretching for excellence. It can reflect a nitpicky, defect-detecting, and controlling style. More often, we see people afflicted by perfectionism as holding to lofty standards and demanding unyielding compliance from themselves or others, the environment, or everything. This demanding form of perfectionism is about more than being a stickler for details and getting upset when anything falls short of a perfectionist standard. It's an attitude of mind that promotes needless stress and strains.

In this case, perfectionist thoughts bond with negative emotions (anxiety, anger) and psychological states, such as depression. Perfectionism is like a ball of twine with different colored threads that you can label "high expectations," "fear of failure," "dread over rejection," "fear of blame," "anxiety," "procrastination," and more.

It's the combination of demanding self-talk ("should," "must") and alarmist self-talk ("awful," "terrible," "can't stand") that elevates the risk of depression (Cox and Enns 2003). Not surprisingly, a negative perfectionism with multiple strings attached is robustly linked to depression (Graham et al. 2010; Wheeler et al. 2011).

## PERFECTIONISM AND SELF-WORTH

Neoanalyst Karen Horney (1950) was among the first to make the connection between demands, irrational claims, and neurotic misery. Her description of neurotic misery refers to a pattern of demands, anxiety, and depression. However, it was Albert Ellis who took this concept and made it useful to millions.

Early in his career as a rational-emotive therapist, psychologist Albert Ellis (1994) found a pattern of thought in depression that includes perfectionism and a negative self-concept. He saw that perfectionist demands coupled with self-downing contribute to a downward depressive spiral. Even Sigmund Freud (2005), who got hung up on oral-fixation theory as a cause of depression, suggests that self-criticism is partially responsible for melancholia (depression).

If you dread the thought of performing poorly, you may experience anxiety as you anticipate a failing performance. If you believe that because of your imperfections, you have no hope, you can feel as if you are in over your head and sinking fast. This defect-detection process invariably leads to frustrations born of false expectations that can extend into depression.

No one is perfect. Disposition, intelligence, personal characteristics, and behavior vary from person to person. Some have quirks. People's thoughts get muddled. We all make mistakes. We have gaps in our knowledge. Memory is imperfect. Yet with perfectionist thoughts storming through the mind, the fact that human fallibility is normal often gets lost in the shuffle.

## Depression and Contingent-Worth Thinking

If you filter reality through a perfectionistic lens, you'll see your present and future performances as successes or failures and your personal worth according to this same judgmental process. You are a winner or a loser, worthy or worthless, strong or weak, and so the list goes on. For example, you decide that a B+ grade is respectable. You expect this performance from yourself. The goal may be reasonable. The expectation is not. You get a B and feel like a failure. This is contingent-worth thinking, where you value yourself as a person based on meeting perfectionist standards.

You may suffer from an "I am not" pattern. Here, the formula for happiness and success rests with being something you are not. To achieve success, you have to be more beautiful, talented, powerful, or charming in a way that you can never be. For example, your IQ needs to be fifty points higher, or else you won't find the right mate, so you don't try or end up settling rather than selecting. This "I am not" pattern is a prelude to depression. It can seem pretty depressing if your solution for a better life involves meeting standards that you can never meet.

Perfectionism can be absolute. In a psychological world of fixed convictions, it is not enough to do well enough; you have to do perfectly well. It's not enough to have typical performances; they must be off the charts. When attaining perfection becomes a contingency for personal worth, anxiety and depression are predictable emotional consequences.

> Perfectionism can reflect an ideal with a thorny tail that lashes back upon itself.

If you define your worth based on what you can't directly control, you're on a slippery slope. But in the area of self-development, there is a way off this slope. You can adopt a no-failure plan. Here, you look at the challenges you face as experiments in which you try to find out what works and what doesn't. Whatever the results, you've succeeded. In this way, you've philosophically eliminated failure from self-development concerns.

## A Language of Perfection

You tell yourself that you should make a bank deposit before the bank closes at 4:00 p.m. Here you demand nothing. The use of the word "should" is conditional. On the other hand, you could tell yourself something like "I should never look foolish." In this case, "should" takes on a whole new meaning.

"Should," "must," "ought," "require," and "expect" are part of the stress-activating vocabulary of perfectionism. The intent behind these words can be the source of much mental misery. For example, "should," when used as a judgment word, can have a strong emotional impact. If you fail to do what you should, you may condemn yourself for not living up to a demanding standard. Guilt and shame may follow. But since we live in a fluid world, where change is ongoing, it is impossible to anticipate everything and to respond perfectly to what you anticipate.

# A PREFERENTIAL OUTLOOK

When you believe that you must have what you think you need, what happens when you don't get it? What does it mean when you make a mistake and then tell yourself that you should not have erred, or that you should have done something different from what you did? The eighteenth-century English poet Alexander Pope has an answer: "And, spite of pride, in erring reason's spite, one truth is clear, whatever is, is right."

## When Demands Make Sense

Demands and requirements are part of our social communications. They are common in the military, schools, religions, corporations, and governmental agencies. There are many times when requirements are reasonable and realistic. You insist that a long-overdue report get submitted. You require a two-year-old child to stay in your fenced yard to avoid the risk of running into a busy street. You may hold to certain values, such as responsibility and integrity, and these values guide how you choose to live your life. However, some requirements are objectively meaningless. You blame someone for falling short of perfection. Your favorite team loses an important game, and you blame the coach for not acting according to your script. In short, others did not do what you believe they should have done. But how does rearview thinking change anything?

The spirit of the demanding philosophy is: "I should have acted differently," "I must not make mistakes," "People ought to act fairly," "I must have others think well of me." While such outcomes are often desirable, translating them into requirements is like hitting a barrier and telling yourself that it should not exist.

Some perfectionist ideals seem desirable, even when they cannot be permanently attainable. What reasonable person wouldn't want to achieve the ideals of happiness, success, approval, control, comfort, and certainty? Make them into requirements, however, and you can undermine yourself.

## Going for What You Want

A preferential philosophy is radically different from one of irrational requirements or demands. A preferential philosophy involves desires, wishes, and wants. These conditions of mind serve as positive motivators. Going after what you want, experiencing happiness, and gaining approval can each be parts of a preferential philosophy. But such conditions are by-products of doing something else first.

Preferring a result has a different feel from demanding that you must get what you think you need now. From a self-development perspective, a preferential philosophy has these advantages:

- You are likely to experience less self-inflicted misery.

- Perfectionist extension-of-blame thinking will decline.

- You are likely to appear friendlier and more open, agreeable, and approachable.

- You'll have less fear of failure; you'll experiment and learn more.

- You are likely to focus more on problem solving than on helplessness thinking.

- You are likely to think more clearly and creatively.

- You are more likely to follow up on responsibilities and therefore procrastinate less.

- You'll experience a broader range of positive emotions.

The following two lists contrast the language of demanding with the language of preferring. One word list characterizes a demanding outlook, the other a preferential outlook.

| Demanding Outlook | Preferential Outlook |
|---|---|
| expect | would prefer |
| demand | wish |
| require | desire |
| insist | want |
| need | favor |
| have to | care to |
| should | hope to |
| ought | would like |
| must | aspire to |

A demanding outlook can activate anger and anxiety. These emotions can promote positive actions, but it's more likely that the thinker will collapse into a self-absorbing malaise or act impulsively and in a self-defeating way. On the other hand, a preferential outlook normally activates determination.

## Taking a Softer Approach

The idea that a softer approach can lead to more powerful results may sound counterintuitive. It might seem as if you'd get further by driving yourself with demands. While sometimes you might, it comes at a big cost. I suggest that you try both ways, and see what results.

Building preferential resources takes more than substituting a *desire* word for a *demand* word. Saying "desire" when you mean "demand" is rarely helpful. So what about eliminating such words as "should," "ought," "must," "require," "expect," or "demand" from your vocabulary? That's unlikely. Try to eliminate your Social Security number from your memory. The memories of emotionally laden words don't evaporate by decree.

Making a shift from a demanding to a preferential philosophy starts with shifting from a self-absorbing perspective to one that is objectively self-observant. For example, if you demand that you have your way all the time, here is a question to ask yourself: "Why must things be only as I expect them to be?"

You have many ways to avoid negative effects from perfectionist thinking. For example, you can learn to put events on a continuum. Instead of saying "I failed," you might say, "I got 40 percent of what I wanted." You can begin to qualify your thoughts and responses: "I generally approve of the position of X, but differ in this respect...." You can consider perfectionist thinking to be an assumption or opinion. This makes each thought less of an absolute and more accessible to review and reason.

# QUESTIONING IF-THEN LOGIC

All-or-nothing perfectionist thinking commonly involves *if-then* conditional-worth messages: "If I'm not what I think I should be, then I'm worthless." "If you violate my expectations, then you are condemnable." "The world should be fair, and if it is not as it should be, then it should be destroyed." Unfortunately, this extremist thinking is all too common.

If-then perfectionist logic has other twists: "If I don't do what I think you think I ought to do, then I'm unworthy." Charles Horton Cooley (1902) called this a "looking-glass self." Here, you unconsciously project your inner imagery upon someone else and believe that they see you as you see yourself.

Perfectionist if-then logic gets you boxed into a demoralizing system where "then" represents a belief ("Worth is based on perfection"). "If" provides the reason ("Infallible actions, thoughts, and consistency make for perfection"). So if you are perfect, then you are worthy. If you are imperfect, then you are not. This type of contingent-worth reasoning is a version of superstitious thinking.

Perfectionism is a magical solution. By meeting perfectionist conditions for gaining worth and security, you believe you can avoid bad luck, disappointment, and feelings of worthlessness, discomfort, and despair. But this is like thinking you can avoid bad luck if you avoid black cats.

> Perfectionism detours you from discovering what you can do.

# SEEKING SELF-ACCEPTANCE

People will make their worth contingent on meeting perfect standards. But if you are not perfectly infallible in every possible respect, how does it follow that you are worthless?

Albert Ellis (1988) asserts that "worthless" or "worthy" is definitional. If so, you can define worthlessness out of existence by saying that you are worthless only if you have twenty fingers on one hand and claws on the other.

As an alternative to basing your worth on unreasonable standards, Ellis suggests that you give yourself unconditional self-acceptance. This is where you accept your global self, even if you don't like some of the things that you do.

Unconditional self-acceptance doesn't absolve people of responsibility for their actions. Rather it is a means of maintaining perspective and avoiding self-intolerance.

# BREAKING THE BONDS OF SELF-IMPRISONMENT

You can set the stage to switch from a demanding to a preferential view by contrasting a static state of self-imprisonment (perfectionism) with a process of self-development (a preferential approach).

## State of Self-Imprisonment

A state of perfectionism is one of self-imprisonment with these characteristics:

- Attainment of certain "needs" is seen as a solution for perceived inadequacy, incompetence, lack of internal order, or emptiness.

- Failure to attain these needs leads to distress, which is usually perceived as an inability to attain what you want.

- Inner demands and expectations fuel strain and tension. In interpersonal relationships, someone else must fill what you lack.

- Your external efforts are directed toward pressuring, coercing, or manipulating to get your way.

## *A Process of Self-Development*

A self-development process has these positive characteristics:

- You believe goals are attained through individual initiative and innovation. This can occur in collaboration with others or alone.

- Joy and accomplishment are seen as by-products of working to develop skills and competencies.

- Effort is directed toward creating positive results.

- Meeting productive (sometimes creative) objectives can lead to happiness, accomplishment, or friendship.

- Concrete goal attainment opens opportunities for new challenges and goals.

You can, of course, choose to live exclusively with a demanding philosophy or bend to reality with a preferential view. You now have enough information to choose. If you choose the preferential way, here is a direction to follow.

# YOUR COUNTERPERFECTIONISM STRATEGY

Answer the following questions to devise your own counterperfectionism strategy.

What actions can you take to get beyond perfectionist demands that bond with negative emotions? (What ideas can you doubt? What actions that oppose perfectionist thinking can you start to take?) _____

_____

_____

What actions can you take to strengthen a goal-directed problem-solving approach? (What hopes, aspirations, and wishes do you have that you can work to achieve? How can you make yourself accountable for keeping promises that you make to yourself?) _____

_____

_____

Act upon your counterperfectionist strategies to switch from a demanding perfectionist outlook to a softer, goal-directed approach.

═══════════════════════════════════════════════

Granted, if your goal is perfection, there are some ways to achieve it. "Whoa," you say. "After this discussion on the perils of perfectionism, it seems more important to curb than encourage these tendencies. Why give a mixed message?"

In some respects, you are already perfect. You know the alphabet from A to Z. Is that not perfect? You know your multiplication tables. Is that not perfect? It's what you do with this knowledge that makes the difference. In another respect, you are the perfect embodiment of yourself. No one can be a more perfect you than you. You can build on that resource you call your "self" to gain advantages, avoid penalties, and enjoy your life.

# PERFECTIONISM, PROCRASTINATION, AND DEPRESSION

Perfectionism is a risk factor for procrastination and depression. You expect a great performance. You have doubts as to whether you can achieve perfection. You have an urge to diverge and do something less threatening. At the same time you insist to yourself that you must be more accomplished. This is an example of perfectionism-driven depression and procrastination.

There are at least six operations in a perfectionist process where your performance is at stake:

- You hold to lofty standards.

- You have no guarantee you'll do well enough.

- Less than the best is not an option.

- Along with thinking you are not doing well enough, you feel uncomfortable.

- You fear the feelings of discomfort.

- You hide your imperfections from yourself and dodge discomfort by doing something safer, such as playing computer games.

You will repeat this exasperating process until you accept yourself as a fallible person and begin doing the best you can without demanding perfection from yourself.

Perfectionism is addressable by applying cognitive measures. By thinking about your thinking and separating desires to do well from requirements to perform perfectly well, you're on your way to a positive change. If you hear your inner voice telling you that if you are not great, you are a big nothing, you've found a perfectionist belief. Discrediting this thinking can help end perfectionism hassles.

You can effectively dispute perfectionism thinking. For example, you are always more complex than what you produce. You can improve. So you can't be either perfect or imperfect. As a person with many attributes, you can fail but can never be a failure.

# ABCDE METHOD FOR DEFUSING PERFECTIONIST THINKING

The following chart shows how to apply the ABCDE method to perfectionist thinking:

| |
|---|
| **Activating event (experience):** "Imperfect performance." |
| **Rational beliefs about the event:** "I'd prefer to do better next time." |
| **Emotional and behavioral consequences for the rational beliefs:** "Disappointment. Work to improve performance." |
| **Irrational perfectionist beliefs:** "I should have done better. I'm stupid." |
| **Emotional and behavioral consequences for the irrational perfectionist beliefs:** "Distress. Withdrawal." |
| **Disputes for irrational perfectionist beliefs:** (1) "Where is the law in the universe that says I must behave flawlessly?" Sample answer: "There is no such law." (2) "Can I accept myself even when I don't like my performance?" Sample answer: "Acceptance is a choice. However, acting with tolerance and self-acceptance frees my mind for problem solving, and the opportunity to do better." |
| **Effects of the disputes:** "Still disappointed over performance. Renewed efforts to do better. Sense of self-acceptance." |

When perfectionist thinking is linked with your depression, you can use the following chart as a guide to map and counteract this thinking.

Activating event (experience):

Rational beliefs about the event:

Emotional and behavioral consequences for the rational beliefs:

Irrational perfectionist beliefs:

Emotional and behavioral consequences for the irrational perfectionist beliefs:

Disputes for irrational perfectionist beliefs:

Effects of the disputes:

# END DEPRESSION PLAN

**Key ideas** (What three ideas did you find most helpful in this chapter?):

1.

2.

3.

**Action steps** (What three steps can you take to move closer to your goal of overcoming depression?):

1.

2.

3.

**Execution** (How did you execute the steps?):

1.

2.

3.

**Results** (What did you learn that you can use?):

1.

2.

3.

# CHAPTER 20

# Managing Relationships

When you are depressed, your relationships are likely to suffer. It's not because you necessarily want that to happen. Rather, when depressed, you are likely to withdraw into yourself. You may have a short fuse and become easily frustrated when you are around other people. By looking beyond the moment, you may act now to avoid having to rebuild your social bridges later.

## EMPATHY BUILDING

Preliminary research confirms that empathy may go on vacation when depression is on the scene (Cusi et al. 2011; Grynberg et al. 2010; Lee 2009). When depressed, you may experience trouble reading the emotions of others, such as their feelings of sadness, fears, and anger (Papp, Kouros, and Cummings 2010). By training yourself to be more empathetic, you may prevent or resolve relationship rifts before they fester. Restoring your empathic ability is a step on the path to enjoying your relationships once again.

You're empathic when you identify and understand the feelings of others. A mutual empathy creates bridges for communications. When you recount a sad part of your past, you sense that others know how you feel. When you tune in to the feelings of others, you can see yourself walking in their shoes. Acceptance flows from empathy. People who experience acceptance normally think well of those who accept them.

### Using the Five E Factors

Here are five E factors for building empathic bridges.

**Examine** your relationships to identify opportunities where you can create empathic bridges. For example, if someone close to you is frustrated, you may be able to relate to this experience. You probably have this same feeling at times. For example, your depression may be more tenacious than you'd prefer, and you have to accept that it takes time to work your way out of depression. Knowing this can help you be empathic toward someone else who experiences frustration.

**Evaluate** your opportunities to keep paths open between you and those who are normally significant to you. What three people are most important to you? What can you do to reach out constructively? For example, on special occasions send a gift that fits with their hobby or interests. Set a date when lunch is on you. Inquire by e-mail how they are doing.

**Explain** to others that you appreciate their patience during your period of depression. Empathize with others' challenges, such as noting that you may not be so pleasant to be around when you are off-kilter with depression. If you have a support group, acknowledging their contribution in support of your well-being can make it easier for all parties to weather the storm.

**Elicit** feedback from the others as to how you can improve communication with them.

**Evolve** your relationships. Stretch a bit. In time, you may feel socially reconnected.

The following is an example of an empathy-building plan:

| Empathy Plan | Distraction | Empathy Direction |
|---|---|---|
| **Examine** | Ignore others' concerns by focusing too hard on your own worries, troubles, and mood. | Do emotional impact experiments. How will others feel if you distance yourself from those who care about you? |
| **Evaluate** | Feel an impetus to retreat. | Reach out to make contact with others. |
| **Explain** | Blame others for your troubles. | When it's appropriate, talk about depression as a temporary drag on your relationship that will linger and leave in its own time, but note that you are working at speeding up the process. |
| **Elicit** | Provoke conflict by arguing. | Ask for periodic feedback about how to improve your relationship. Follow the activity remedies to support your relationships as you struggle to overcome depression. These remedies may help both with your relationships and in defeating depression. |
| **Evolve** | Get on a downward cycle of faultfinding, arguing, and withdrawing. | Stretch a bit to maintain perspective and to preserve your rights without needlessly interfering with the relationship rights of others. |

# YOUR EMPATHY EXERCISE

Use the following space to structure and practice an empathy building plan:

| Empathy Plan | Distraction | Empathy Direction |
|---|---|---|
| **Examine** | | |
| **Evaluate** | | |
| **Explain** | | |
| **Elicit** | | |
| **Evolve** | | |

Apply empathy toward yourself as well as others. With self-empathy, you understand that a depressed mood is to be expected for as long as it lasts. You, like millions of others, experience a painful mood. You may not like this state, but it is much more tolerable when you can empathize with yourself.

# REPAIRING RELATIONSHIP RIPS

Sooner or later, practically everyone has relationship interference provoking strains (RIPS) for different reasons and in varied degrees. Some are temporary. Others linger. Depression is one of those conditions that can lead to lingering RIPS.

A major depression may follow RIPS in marital relations. These frictions can include hostility and a lack of affection (Gotlib and Hammen 1992). Awareness of these potential RIPS opens an opportunity for you to suppress these urges and try a different, perhaps more empathic, way.

Relationship stresses and depression can also be bidirectional. For example, a client named Danny was in love with his wife. One morning he woke up and hated her. Then he got a divorce. He wondered if he'd made a mistake. Danny was prone to bipolar depression. His history showed a pattern of major life changes when his depression came out of the blue: changing jobs, moving to a new area, divorce. Danny engaged in self-empathy. He accepted that his perceptions and thoughts get distorted when he is depressed. He helped stabilize his routines with activity scheduling. He preserved his current relationships by following the five E factors of empathy building. He broke his dysfunctional pattern by suspending judgments about any major changes when he was depressed.

When one partner in a relationship is significantly depressed, this is likely to stress the other partner. However, interactions before and during depression may be similar. For example, bickering and fighting often characterize the interactions of couples in distressed relationships (Jackman-Cram, Dobson, and Martin 2006). Empathy building interferes with this destructive pattern, but like most significant changes, it normally takes time and effort to tip the balance from discord toward empathy.

> ## Use Empathy in Repairing RIPS
>
> **Examine** the reasons for the RIPS.
>
> **Evaluate** opportunities for making repairs.
>
> **Explain** what you want to accomplish.
>
> **Elicit** cooperation.
>
> **Evolve** the relationship with joint problem solving.

## Common RIPS and Solutions

During periods of depression, it takes an extra effort to do your part to maintain your primary relationships. By making this effort, you help yourself in several ways. You are engaging in a constructive activity as a remedy for depression. You are reducing the risk of additional stress that can accompany withdrawal or friction in your primary relationships. You're also making it easier for others to support you, for providing support is usually easier for others when they understand that their role is important and that you are willing to do your part, even when you feel down.

Here are some countermeasures that you can take to keep some common RIPS factors from interfering with the quality of your relationships.

### CONFRONT YOUR ILLUSIONS

Illusions are something you believe are real and true. They may reflect a partial truth, but are generally self-deceiving. Believing that getting drunk will end depression is an illusion. You are likely to feel worse later.

Believe that your relationships are meaningless, and will always be that way, and this pessimism is a prescription for seclusion, isolation, and more depression. Uncover and act to defuse this and other relationship illusions, and you can cut back on RIPS, avoid needless disappointment, and ground your relationships realistically.

### AVOID NEEDLESS BLAMING

Blame can be a way of assigning accountability and taking responsibility for your actions. That definition of blame has social value. Blame also has extensions, such as when you villainize your mate for making mistakes or for violating your expectations. That's a needless form of blame. Drop this extension of blame, and you eliminate what may be the biggest reason for RIPS.

### STOP ACCUSING AND ESCALATING

Feeling cranky, you may accuse your mate of any fiendish thing that comes to mind. There are food-encrusted dishes in the sink. Your mate is inconsiderate. Your child did poorly on a test. Your mate is too lazy to help. When accusations trump empathy, you can put your mate on the defensive. If your mate tries to rebut your accusation, you have a reason to escalate the conflict: "You never listen. You don't understand me."

How do you stop these RIPS? You can make a positive shift in perspective through working on empathy by doing a PURRRRS exercise. *Pause* and *use* your abilities to shift from a self-absorbing view to a self-observant view. *Reflect* on what's going on. Spontaneous accusations may reflect a partial truth. However, perspectives change with new information. *Reason* it out. Ask yourself, what is the empathic approach in this situation? *Respond* with an expression of empathy and preference. *Review* and *revise* based on the feedback that you get. *Stabilize* by repeating this PURRRRS pattern to prevent RIPS. Give yourself a deserved pat on the back.

## Communicating with Your Partner

When you communicate clearly, you've dropped ambiguity as a source of conflict. Specificity is a vital part of this process. This is the ability to articulate what you want using words and ideas that the other person can understand and act on. Specificity begins with your being clear in your own mind about what you want. "I want you to go for a walk with me" is an example of a specific, achievable, and measurable goal communication. "I want you to make me happy" is a prelude to needless bickering and conflict.

## Intimacy and Empathy

A loss of sexual desire is common among people with mild to severe depression and with masked depression. There are added complications. Fatigue is a factor. Antidepressant medications are often associated with a loss of sexual desire and responsiveness. Performance anxieties may cause withdrawal. You may feel unattractive, and this thinking gets in the way of sexual arousal.

Diminished interest in sexual intimacy often goes with depression. If you experience yourself as barely able to get through the day, having a better love-sex relationship may partially depend on the abatement of depression. If you are among those with depression whose sexual desire has declined, doing and feeling better may be a higher priority than feeling sexy again. Nevertheless, disinterest in sex can lead to a challenging situation for couples when one partner wants an intimate sexual relationship and the other doesn't.

### SENSATE FOCUS

Here is a method that serves a dual purpose as an antidepression strategy and as a possible way to reduce conflicts over sex. Sensate focus is a form of massage used to help people with sexual performance anxieties. There is a dearth of scientific literature on the use of this method when one person is depressed. However, I've prescribed the method with some positive and some neutral results. Perhaps sensate focus will help you.

Sensate focus is primarily used to alleviate anxiety over intercourse. Because the method involves rubbing and massaging nongenital areas of the body, it seems suitable for both the person who feels depressed, who may benefit from massage, and the other partner, who may be more interested in eventual sexual fulfillment. This two-stage nondemanding approach takes twenty to sixty minutes, two to three times a week for six weeks, to complete:

1. For the first two weeks, each partner takes turns massaging the other's body minus erogenous zones of breasts and genitals. Each concentrates on the texture and other qualities of the partner's skin and body. The goal is to experience tactile sensation. Intercourse is disallowed.

2. In weeks three and four, each takes turns massaging the other as before. Then massage can be mutual, and it is okay to touch and stimulate each other's erogenous zones and genitals. Intercourse is also omitted at this stage, but you can manually stimulate each other to orgasm.

3. In weeks five and six, repeat steps 1 and 2. If there is sufficient comfort by both parties, intercourse will naturally follow. If not, continue with massage and mutual stimulation, and work toward a time in the future when you are both ready.

Sensate massage is a nondemanding method because neither party tries to force a conclusion. As this is an experimental method, either partner should feel free to terminate the experiment at any point. It's important to suspend making either critical comments or positive comments in the form of compliments. When you are depressed, you may have a negative reaction to compliments. Instead, the key is to work on empathy.

# TALKING ABOUT DEPRESSION

When you are depressed, you are likely to be difficult for others to deal with. That goes with the territory. This should be nothing to deny. It is something to share.

It's important that you convey information to family and friends about the depression that you experience. If you bring them to an understanding of what is happening, you may be surprised at their supportive response. Most people can accept that escaping the grips of depression normally takes time. Here are some thoughts to share:

■ Although you can have a rapid cessation of symptoms, the concept of a broken leg can sometimes put matters into perspective for you and others. It takes a broken bone time to mend. Depression is like that broken bone, but there is a difference. By exercising your mental, emotional, and behavioral muscles to rid yourself of depression, once you are on the mend, the chances are that you will feel stronger than before.

■ Moping and brooding are common expressions of a depressed mood. Your friends and relations need not take your mood and expressions personally, no more than they would take a broken leg personally. Despondency goes with the territory, much as a cast often goes with a broken leg. You have a part to play in biting your tongue to quell the expression of needless complaints.

■ Words of cheer and encouragement often do more harm than good. In short, for most forms of depression (atypical depression may sometimes be an exception), words of cheer rarely help. Walking with you for an hour is likely to have a positive benefit, especially if your friend also needs the exercise.

Increased reliance on television for entertainment lowers the rate of social contacts, loosens social bonds, promotes a sedentary lifestyle, and this increases the risk of depression.

In addition to talking with your friends and relatives about what to expect from your depression, you should give your friends and relatives permission to remind you if you are acting difficult. If you are struggling with depression, others will tend to be more supportive if they see that you are willing to help yourself than if you are starting arguments, complaining, and expecting others to take up the slack.

If you have recurrent depression, your friends and family are more likely to exhibit tolerance and acceptance if you take the extra step to let them know when to approach you, when this is iffy, and when it is wise to give you space. The following story shows how this can work in a family context.

## ■ Barbara's Story

Barbara was married with three children, ages six, eight, and ten. She suffered from mild ongoing depression that worsened at different points in her menstrual cycle. She reported that this irritability started after her first pregnancy. It worsened over the years. She found no medically effective remedy. She reported that her physician had run "every imaginable test and come up empty." She had been in therapy for three years to address her depression. She and her counselor worked to link her depression to early life experiences. She remained depressed.

Barbara experienced depression at two levels. Her ongoing mild depression erupted into moderately severe depression that occurred every month or two and lasted for a week or more. During this time, she experienced considerable agitation, feelings of being overwhelmed, helplessness, and a sense of being out of control.

*She withdrew at times, and her family had to "fend for themselves." At other times, she felt agitated and erupted into angry outbursts. During these times, her husband reported that nobody in her family was safe from her "blame attacks."*

*To establish control over her responses to her ongoing mild depression and blame attacks, Barbara first recorded information to see if the agitated phase of her depression followed a predictable pattern. She marked days on the calendar when she had an anger attack. She figured that if she could predict when her depression intensified, she could devise a plan to manage herself during these periods.*

*Barbara's intensified depression often started five days before her period, and she practically always recognized some of the early warning signals. She reported, "It was like a wave coming over me. I loved my husband the day before, and suddenly he became a devil. My kids became monsters. I now understand that my feelings have more to do with me than with them."*

*Once Barbara developed awareness of the significance of her "wave," she wondered what she could do to disengage from it. A practical tactic involved, first, to refuse to find fault and blame, and second, to use a button system.*

*The button system involved red, yellow, and green pin-on buttons. When she wore the red button, Barbara was communicating that she had a wave-of-tension condition. Her husband and children knew to back away. When Barbara wore a yellow button, this was a caution. On green-button days, Barbara felt quite resilient and approachable.*

*The button exercise served several purposes. Her family stopped blaming themselves for Barbara's depression. It reminded her to stop blaming them. She saw herself as having control through deciding on what button to wear. The red and yellow buttons reminded her to think about her thinking. This process increased her sense of control.*

*Following successful use of the button system, Barbara obtained a part-time job. She had not worked for ten years. Now that all of her children attended preschool or school, she thought she could handle a part-time job. She joined a dance class. She had previously enjoyed dancing. She soon came to look forward to that routine. Within a few months, her depression diminished. Simultaneously, the frequency and length of red-button times significantly declined.*

The button system worked for Barbara. You may want to try this technique or choose more subtle signals to let your family and friends know when your depression may get in the way of positive interactions. Without mutual cooperation, however, the technique may fall flat.

# LONELINESS AND DEPRESSION

A supportive network can help you live through sadness and, perhaps, avoid succumbing to deeper depression. Your network may include family, friends, or a community of people who face challenges that are similar to yours. Having a social network can help you work through such problems as the loss of a family member or job or illness.

## Using the Buddy System

For many people, it's important to be with others to avert loneliness and to get the support. When you are depressed, a buddy (friend or family member) can encourage you to engage in positive activities, perhaps accompany you to the health club for exercise, help you monitor your progress, or support you if you enter into a contract with yourself to address your depression.

Buddies who believe that it's their job to cheer you up may be barking up the wrong tree. For most forms of depression, this is likely to do more harm than good. You are likely to take praise and encouragement the wrong way.

Suppose you don't want to involve family or close friends in your antidepression program, but you believe you could do better with some form of social support. You may be able to find a helpful support group for people with depression in your community.

## Moving from Isolation to Support

Peer support is effective for a subgroup of people for reducing their symptoms of depression (Pfeiffer et al. 2011). A basic challenge is to identify and engage positive-thinking individuals and groups where this may lead to friendships and eventual mutual support. But how is this to be done when you are depressed and making connections with others looks like climbing a steep cliff?

You may be isolated and feel lonely, and your depression grows from too much time alone. You may be at home after your mate has passed on, you may be in a hospital setting with an illness and no visitors, or you may believe that you are frozen out of the social world because of shyness or petrifying anxieties over rejection that spill over to depression. Whatever your situation, having contact with positive-minded people for everyday activities, such as lunch meetings, book discussions, or political discussions can break a sense of isolation.

### YOU'RE NEVER TOO OLD

If you are in your senior years and alone, loneliness doesn't necessarily lead to depression (Cacioppo, Hawkley, and Thisted 2010). However, when solitude contributes to depression, this can turn into a vicious cycle of feeling depressed over being alone. Senior centers, social clubs, religious groups, and volunteer work provide avenues for experiencing the amount of people contact that you desire. Your greatest hurdle may be yourself. If you tell yourself you are "too old," you're probably procrastinating on establishing meaningful ties and contacts. This excuse making may link to insecurities. What are you too old for? Too old to socialize? Too old to read stories to children? Too old to enjoy a sunset? "Too old" thinking may be more handicapping than aging.

If you are ordinarily shy or have social anxieties and fears, you may feel inhibited, avoid people, experience social isolation, feel lonely, and cycle into depression. If you get in your own way by negatively ruminating about the horrors of rejection, looking like a fool, or being an unwanted intruder in the lives of others, go back to chapter 14 for information on how to address recurring anxieties and fears.

## REHEARSING SMALL TALK

Suppose you lack confidence in your ability to engage in small talk. You avoid contact with new people for this reason. If you tend to get tongue-tied, you may find the following method helpful for rehearsing small talk with someone whom you would like to get to know better:

1. Create a scene in your mind where you want to act friendly using small talk as a social icebreaker. Think of someone with whom you'd like to have a conversation.

2. Imagine a location where you'll engage with the other person: by the water cooler, over a backyard fence, at a local coffee shop.

3. Come up with questions that have easy answers, such as "How is your family?"

4. Imagine an answer. Follow up with another question. Remember that people who ask questions that inspire others to talk are typically viewed as good conversationalists.

You can also imagine making passing comments to friendly-looking strangers at malls, grocery stores, and other places where people gather. This can include asking for the time of day or making a casual comment about something in the surrounding environment, such as an unusual item behind a display window. You can practice by creating a scene in your mind where you encounter someone you'd like to talk with at the grocery store, at a local restaurant or shopping mall, or on a hiking trail. Imagine saying hello and passing the time.

The next step is to practice in a real setting. Practicing with strangers is perhaps less risky than practicing with someone you already know. If you are at a social gathering, for example, you might introduce yourself to five people and see what happens.

Some people are responsive to small talk. You'll find some people who are not. So if the conversation stalls, you have no obligation to carry on.

## ACTIVITY SCHEDULING FOR SMALL TALK

Say you decide to make small talk with a normally friendly neighbor. You rehearse your comment on the weather: "It's a bit humid today." After mentally rehearsing, you can use an activity schedule to convert your small-talk rehearsal into action. The following chart gives some antidotes for cognitive, emotive, and behavioral interferences that you might encounter after deciding to talk with your neighbor. It also shows the rewards on many levels that you would receive from applying these antidotes and executing the task.

# SMALL-TALK GOAL CHART

Social goal: Make small talk with your neighbor—"It's a bit humid today."

|  | Task Interferences | Antidotes | Rewards for Execution |
|---|---|---|---|
| **Cognitive** | Tell yourself that your neighbor will reject your invitation to communicate and say something like, "Who gives a damn about the weather? Don't you have anything better to do with your time than ask silly questions?" Holding the fearsome anxiety thought in mind, you can catastrophize and awfulize to a fever pitch, feel sick to your stomach, and hide in a dark room. | Flip this mental interference around by looking at it as a humorous exaggeration where you blow a remote possibility into a reality. Now, get real. What's the likely response? How would you respond if your neighbor made the same comment? | Testing a false premise can lead to relief when the worst-case scenario doesn't happen. However, this relief can reinforce future social avoidances. Instead, attach relief to your actions for testing the hypothesis. Second, give yourself a reward, such as putting together a puzzle that you enjoy assembling, after you talk with your neighbor. |
| **Emotive** | Feel anxiety over the possibility that your neighbor will reject not just your comment but also you. | Accept the feeling of tension without double-troubling yourself over the feeling and then capsizing your emotional boat by filling it with emotional waters from a mental machination that you can't stand a feeling that you don't like. | Living through the anxiety shows that you can tolerate tension, even the variety that is born from negative-thinking excesses. For not cowering before a concocted emotional strain, read a chapter in the novel you've begun. |
| **Behavioral** | Sidetrack yourself by convincing yourself that it is impossible for you to change. Hide in the corner and play computer solitaire. | Using the mental rehearsal small-talk exercise, imagine putting yourself through the paces with your neighbor and receiving a friendly response in return. Now try this out with your neighbor. | You add to your social skills by engaging in the small-talk exercise. You play computer solitaire as a reward for making small talk with your neighbor. |

Now it's your turn to create an activity schedule, execute it, and review the results, and to then take advantage of what you learned.

# YOUR SMALL-TALK EXERCISE

Use the following space to record your experience with using small talk to make connections with others.

|  | Task Interferences | Antidotes | Rewards for Execution |
|---|---|---|---|
| Cognitive |  |  |  |
| Emotive |  |  |  |
| Behavioral |  |  |  |

# END DEPRESSION PLAN

**Key ideas** (What three ideas did you find most helpful in this chapter?):

1.

2.

3.

**Action steps** (What three steps can you take to move closer to your goal of overcoming depression?):

1.

2.

3.

**Execution** (How did you execute the steps?):

1.

2.

3.

**Results** (What did you learn that you can use?):

1.

2.

3.

# CHAPTER 21

# A Multimodal Approach
# to Defeat Depression

Arnold A. Lazarus (1992) views people as biological beings who think, feel, act, sense, imagine, and interact. Each of these "modalities" is an important part of making positive changes, such as with depression. He developed a BASIC-ID anagram to remind us to explore and correct each of these key modalities when addressing depression and other forms of distress:

B = behavioral

A = affective

S = sensations

I = imagery

C = cognitive

I = interpersonal

D = drugs/biology

Lazarus's BASIC-ID framework gives you a convenient way to organize information covered in his book, but also this modality approach gives you a pithy framework for organizing your actions for making positive changes.

In helping his clients overcome depression, Lazarus looks at the interaction between two or more of these modalities. Depending on the person and situation, some modalities will dominate more than others. For example, you may feel especially burdened by a loss of pleasure, appetite, and sleep. This would fall under Lazarus's drug/biology modality. Your thoughts may feel tied to the ground by cognitions of pessimism, your interpersonal life may be strained by loneliness, and so on. Using this modality is a way to pull it all together when it comes to addressing and overcoming depression.

# HOW BASIC-ID WORKS

Lazarus's goal is to create conditions whereby people with mild to moderate depression can achieve a relatively rapid remission of their depression symptoms and can prevent relapse. Using the BASIC-ID anagram, you can catalogue your depressive symptoms, prioritize their importance (or impact on you), and develop a plan to take positive action to address each one.

The *behavioral* modality would include activities such as avoidance and escapist routines, withdrawal, procrastination, decreased work performance, fidgeting, complaining, and outbursts. Lazarus sees a connection between an increase in positive behavioral activity and a drop in melancholic mood. Thus, action exercises for defeating depression are prescriptive remedies. Even a monotonous activity, such as filling out an insurance form, can temporarily distract you from depressive thinking and a negative mood.

The *affective* modality refers to the emotions you experience, such as joy, happiness, frustration, and love. Depressive affects commonly include sadness, anxiety, anger, shame, and guilt. Lazarus suggests relaxation, meditation, and calming statements to help reduce the tensions associated with negative affect. However, the affective dimension rarely exists in isolation from behavior and cognition. Assertiveness skill development can serve as an inoculation against future depression. Recognizing and questioning depressive thinking can improve mood.

*Sensations* include tension; fatigue; pain; or feeling cold, hot, dull, and so forth. Scheduling pleasant events for positive sensory stimulation can help when you feel dull or lack sensory stimulation. As a remedy, for example, schedule times to view something visually appealing; listen to calming music, an upbeat song, or water tumbling over rocks; smell a scented candle; get a massage or take a warm bath to stimulate tactile sensations; or taste a drop of honey.

*Imagery* includes fantasies, dreams, and self-image. Some depressive images are metaphorical, such as imagining yourself frozen in a block of ice. You can create positive images that clash with depression imagery. Imagine yourself in a block of ice in the warm summer sun. Can you feel the ice melting away? Here are other examples of positive imagery: recall when you met a challenge and felt good. Remember a time when you lived beyond a disappointment. Imagine yourself bathing in a pool of tranquility. Lazarus also suggests time-projection imagery, where you visualize yourself taking positive steps as you approach your future.

*Cognitive* processes involve knowing, memory, reasoning, reflection, imagination, believing, and more. We live our lives primarily through our habits, along with our beliefs, perceptions, and thoughts. In a depressive mind-set, beliefs take the form of schemas, or organized thought patterns. "I am useless" can be part of a depressive schema, or core belief. This schema can have mental tentacles, such as "I'll never change." These gross exaggerations distort perception and perspective. Uprooting them includes Socratic ways of arguing, the PURRRRS system, and the ABCDE method for disputing irrational beliefs.

*Interpersonal* processes include managing relationships at work, home, or elsewhere. Depending on social circumstances, this can involve avoidance of complaining; selecting words and phrases that convey positive messages; initiating small talk with others; resolving conflicts before they fester; developing a pleasant style of speaking; and avoiding criticizing others.

*Drugs/biology* refers to both medications and the biological dimensions of depression. This modality involves an evaluation for antidepressant medication, actions to eliminate the abuse of addictive substances, a physical examination to rule out physical causes of depression, actions to improve appetite and sleep, and physical exercise.

These different modalities give you a way to categorize information within a framework that links symptoms to change techniques. By then creating and following an understandable sequence of steps, you may see encouraging opportunities for taking self-corrective actions.

You may have to get at your depression from several angles to diminish or end your depressed mood. Your path may not always be as clear as a plan on paper, and you may have to improvise along the way. You may also find the following to be true:

- The modalities tend to overlap and interact; the divisions between them are not as conveniently clear-cut as the anagram would indicate.

- The modalities cover much ground. However, you may discover a modality of motivation that includes initiative, inventiveness, and will. People are understandably complex, and other modalities of interest are possible.

- When anger and depression coexist, you may have negative images, misconceptions, dysphoric sensations, and interpersonal conflicts. If you also abuse alcohol, you may have to focus on building tolerance to drinking urges while juggling other challenges. The multimodal system provides frameworks for isolating and addressing each of these conditions. Alcohol abuse, for example, is primarily a drug issue that can have branches and roots in the other six modalities.

All in all, the multimodal framework is designed to help you to take an organized approach to change, and it can be as fluid as necessary or as tightly segmented as you choose to make it.

Lazarus's BASIC-ID anagram is a good memory device. However, you don't have to follow the modalities in succession. The BASIC-ID order is flexible. For example, you can order the modalities according to their impact. If cognitive and drug modalities predictably head the list of problem features in your depression, then you would normally address them first. If you have no depressive imagery, then there is no need to work toward reducing negative imagery. However, you could create positive images where you imagine yourself meeting the challenges of implementing the other modalities.

# APPLYING THE MULTIMODAL SYSTEM: A CASE STUDY

Joan was twenty-five, single, and unemployed. She suffered from a moderately severe depression that had gone on for more than a year. She had previously tried antidepressant medication and had experienced unpleasant side effects.

Prior to the onset of her depression, Joan had socialized with a group of friends from her high-school days and others from work. She said that her job could be stressful at times, but she generally enjoyed her career. Just before the onset of her depression, she had reestablished a relationship with her high-school sweetheart. She said that the relationship had gone well, though she added, "I used to worry if my relationship with Don would last." Joan described herself as a worrier.

Joan started to feel depressed shortly before her company downsized and she lost her job. Thereafter, her depression worsened. Once out of work, she put off writing her résumé. She avoided looking in the newspapers or talking to her friends about jobs.

She gradually stopped answering telephone calls and e-mail messages. Her off-and-on exercise program abruptly ended. She increasingly spent time shopping online to distract herself but stopped when her money ran out. She complained of eating too much junk food, oversleeping, and lacking energy. She felt she was no longer fun to be around. She described spending several hours each day in her bedroom, especially in the morning, when she had trouble getting herself out of bed. Also conspicuous were the omissions in her life. She had previously enjoyed hobbies, such as gardening and golf. She also had considered herself to be organized, but now she rarely addressed what she needed to do. She noted a sense of mental tenseness that she thought caused muscular tension. She described herself as living in a dark pit.

Joan had broken up with Don shortly after her job had ended: "I didn't want to burden him with my troubles." She also felt shame that she'd drained her parents' finances after they began to assume responsibility for her expenses. She described a negative self-concept, great pessimism that she'd ever feel normal again, and a pervasive sense of helplessness. She said she cried a lot, sometimes for no reason. She reported feeling "dull."

Joan agreed to try a multimodal approach to defeat her depression.

## Joan's BASIC-ID Plan

Joan's BASIC-ID plan came from several sources: a depression test (see chapter 2), her self-reflections, and her therapist's observations from her initial screening interview.

Her main themes for change were dealing with basic priorities, staying out of the bedroom during waking hours, reestablishing hobbies, dealing with crying, overcoming shame, managing stress and tension, decreasing her sense of dullness, exiting the dark pit, questioning negative thinking, reestablishing previously valued relationships, and taking actions to reduce the biological symptoms of depression. From this list, she classified her information under the BASIC-ID modalities. She next sketched a plan for addressing each modality issue.

| Modality | Examples | Action Plan |
|---|---|---|
| **Behavior** | "Priority activities go by the wayside."<br><br>"Spend long periods of time in bedroom by myself."<br><br>"Omissions in areas that once brought pleasure, such as golfing, gardening, reading, warm baths, comedies."<br><br>"Neglect personal care and appearance."<br><br>"Crying." | "Make to-do list. Do daily priority.<br><br>"Update résumé."<br><br>"Use bedroom for sleeping only during the time normally set aside for that purpose."<br><br>"Do one thing a day to improve garden."<br><br>"Take warm bath every other day."<br><br>"Add new activity each month."<br><br>"Make extra effort each day to keep up with personal care and appearance."<br><br>"Accept crying as a symptom." |
| **Affect** | "Shame" | "Shame is a self-conscious negative evaluation of global self-worth based on a vacuous idea that a complex self can be only one way. A pluralistic view of self can mute the pangs of shame. Punch holes in a shame belief that the self is one way and worthless." |

| **Sensations** | "Tension, stiff muscles."<br><br>"Fatigue and loss of energy."<br><br>"Sense of dullness." | "Massage, stretching exercises, swimming, and biking."<br><br>"Avoid napping during the day. Do repetitive, low-energy garden weeding (to lift spirits)."<br><br>"Burn favorite scented candles. Open curtains to let in light. Paint on canvas. Listen to relaxing music. Fill an eyedropper with a mix of honey and fresh lemon; put drop on tongue. Use foot massager three times a day." |
| --- | --- | --- |
| **Imagery** | "View self as spiraling deeper into a dark pit." | "Imagine being at the bottom of a spiral staircase with each step marked by activities of daily living (daily shower, brushing hair, changing clothes, putting dishes in dishwasher). Put this saying on refrigerator: 'Climbing the spiral stairs each day prepares me for the challenges that lie ahead.'" |
| **Cognition** | "Pessimism."<br>"Sense of worthlessness."<br>"Sense of helplessness." | "Look at pessimism as a symptom, not a fact."<br>"Inventory positive attributes."<br>"Match each helplessness example against a positive action, such as rising and making breakfast." |
| **Interpersonal** | "Self-isolating." | "Reestablish e-mail contact with friends: send out one new e-mail per day. Attend niece's upcoming birthday party. Plan at least one activity each day where others are present: walking through mall, asking for directions. Record event and what resulted." |
| **Drugs** | "Lethargy; lack of exercise."<br>"Sleep."<br>"Diet." | "Start a moderate exercise program: bicycling to post office box each day. Every other day resume home aerobic program for twenty minutes."<br><br>"Slight decrease in oversleeping (from ten hours per night to eight hours per night). Use two larms to awaken."<br><br>"See if pattern changes as depression lifts."<br><br>"Plan and eat three balanced and nutritious meals a day." |

## Implementing the Plan

Joan constructed her BASIC-ID plan during three therapy sessions. Thereafter, she chiefly worked on her own.

Her exercise program required encouragement. A breakthrough came at week seven, when she agreed to bike with her mother to an aerobics class. She did this consistently thereafter.

When she first began to address her depression, Joan reported feeling mostly depressed and discouraged. At about week eight into her program, this hopelessness and worthlessness thinking started to fade.

## Fear of Relapse

Joan faced a special challenge in week ten. At that time, she developed a morbid fear of relapsing. Now that she no longer felt so depressed, Joan viewed with dread a reawakening of depressive sensations. When she experienced a wave of depression, she felt great fear as she focused on the sensation. Thoughts of hopelessness followed. Because she had made progress, however, she knew that she had already mastered programs that she could use again. That was the good news.

Fear of relapse is common among those coming out of depression. Because it is addressable, fear can be a favorable sign. Normally, when people start to worry about relapsing, they have already gained ground and are nicely positioned to bounce back because they now have new tools to use.

In dealing with her tension magnification, Joan learned to accept the depressive sensations (admittedly challenging to do) and to question and debunk her doomsday prophecy about relapsing. Thereafter, when she experienced a wave of tension and negative thinking, she first labeled the negative thinking "depressive thinking." Then she went for a walk. The labeling exercise was especially helpful. She saw depressive thoughts as reflections, not facts.

## What Happened Next

Joan made a significant breakthrough at week eighteen. She learned about a new job opportunity. Understandably, she was apprehensive about explaining to an interviewer why she had been out of work for over a year. However, her worry went beyond normal apprehension. She entered the realm of anxiety as she contemplated failing the interview. She had heart palpitations, tension headaches, and gastrointestinal symptoms.

Once she settled on a plan for answering questions about her recent unemployment, her strain diminished. Her plan was to say that a down economy made it difficult for her to find work and to emphasize how her work skills could benefit this employer. To Joan's surprise, the interviewer did most of the talking and said nothing about the employment gap. She got the job.

Reflecting on her anxiety, Joan learned that she had received a reward for worry. Although this was not the type of reward that many would want, it was still a reward. When the worst she predicted didn't happen, she felt relief. This relief was Joan's reward for worry. Relief for worry can reinforce worry and make recurrence more likely.

Because of this possible worry-reward connection, Joan made a conscious effort to develop a wait-and-see approach. In situations where she couldn't prove that her fortune-telling was factual, she considered a range of possibilities. These predictions included the worst thing that could happen, the best thing that could happen, and possibilities in between. The wait-and-see approach reduced her worry thinking.

At week twenty, Joan contacted Don. She wanted to see if she could reestablish a relationship with him. In advance of the meeting, she worked to maintain an optimistic perspective, but she primarily worked to minimize worrying about the meeting.

When they met, she found that he was happily involved with another woman. She felt saddened, but she also felt happy that she had tried. Not all things work out as we wish they would.

As Joan's story shows, depression ordinarily takes time to address. In Joan's case, a very brief form of therapy or self-help would be grossly insufficient to resolve core issues, many of which would be masked by depression and therefore invisible until they surfaced. Joan's story also illustrates that comprehensive personal change is a process, not an event.

# YOUR STRUCTURE FOR POSITIVE CHANGE

Using the BASIC-ID framework, write down examples of what you need to address in the key modalities. Then plan actions for positive change.

| Modality | Examples | Action Plan |
|---|---|---|
| **Behavioral** | | |
| **Affective** | | |
| **Sensations** | | |
| **Imagery** | | |

| Cognitive | | |
|---|---|---|
| Interpersonal | | |
| Drugs/biology | | |

As a final step, number each modality according to its importance, or impact. Then, address your first priority. Then move on to the second and so forth. To avoid putting off taking action, set a time to start. Draw a reward from your rewards store for starting on schedule.

By taking steps to curb depression through addressing the applicable modalities, you've started down the yellow brick road to where you become your own wizard.

# TRANSLATING FANTASY INTO ACTION

Jack Shannon, a multimodal therapist and Seton Hall University professor emeritus, sees depression as an understandable but complex process that you can address by following a BASIC-ID approach. For his top tip, Shannon (pers. comm.) gives an example of how to use imagery to help break a depressive cycle:

Fantasies are the tools of visionaries, but they can have a boomerang effect when you draw into a world of fantasy to escape the pangs of depression. In this fantasy world, you can quickly prevail over adversities, write great novels in moments, and swim oceans to set records. Encapsulated in this inner world, you risk becoming increasingly dissatisfied with reality. Gently nudge yourself back to the world of reality, where you can benefit from concrete experiences. Target a wish that is possible for you to do, such as studying origami, where you create paper objects, such as airplanes, flowers, or cranes. Break your vision down into doable steps. Mentally rehearse each: "First I order a book on how to do origami." Then take the next step, third, and so forth. If you get in your own way, listen to your self-talk for thought themes that darken your mood and sidetrack you from achieving your vision. Use imagery again to disentangle yourself from what you may call "vampire thoughts." Imagine opening the blinds and extinguishing these thoughts with light. Then get back to the steps you visualized. Move one foot in front of the other until you have the origami skill you set out to acquire. In the process, you may feel your depression expiring.

# LEAD WITH YOUR FOOT, AND YOUR HEART WILL FOLLOW

Multimodal therapist Clifford N. Lazarus, who is cofounder and clinical director of the Lazarus Institute, takes the position that activity is a remedy for depression. Lazarus (pers. comm.) gives this tip for overcoming depression:

Your head and heart will follow your feet. In other words, how you act (your feet) will often determine how you think (your head) and feel (your heart). Indeed, I often tell my therapy clients, "You can't think your way out of depression, and I can't simply talk you out of it, but I can walk you out it." Hence, how you act can either carry you deeper into depression or lead you out of it.

This is because there are "depressant" actions (that have neurochemically depleting effects on the brain) and "antidepressant" actions (that, like prescription antidepressants, have neurochemically replenishing effects on the brain).

Depressant actions typically include withdrawal, isolation, disconnection, general inactivity, and disengagement. Not surprisingly, antidepressant behavior usually involves participation, engagement, social involvement, physical movement, and reconnecting to activities you used to enjoy.

It might take some time to defeat depression because the idea that "the head and heart follow the feet" means that thoughts and feelings will come into alignment with action patterns but not necessarily right away. Your happier thinking and pleasant mood will lag behind the antidepressant actions just a bit. It takes the slower-learning part of the brain extra time to catch up. So, be patient. Let your feet "walk you out of depression."

Lazarus's popular books, *Don't Believe It for a Minute: Forty Toxic Ideas That Are Driving You Crazy* and *The 60-Second Shrink: 101 Strategies for Staying Sane in a Crazy World*, have been translated into over a dozen languages.

# FIGHTING DEPRESSION THE MULTIMODAL WAY

Multimodal therapist Jeffrey A. Rudolph is a licensed clinical psychologist and a board-certified diplomate in cognitive behavioral therapy. He is in private practice in Manhattan and Ridgewood, New Jersey. Rudolph (pers. comm.) offers this counterdepression tip:

When you are depressed, your efforts tend to become anemic, and your pathways for positive expression and experience get choked off. Your capacity for sensory fulfillment and positive images of self and future becomes impaired. Your behavior is likely to be more defensive and ritualistic. You become less health minded (exercise and nutrition). When tangled in depression, you may experience a loss of identity and motivation, and increase in passivity, helplessness, and unhealthy dependency on others.

Your thinking becomes negative and self-critical. That's an unpleasant picture of what is a common reality for countless millions. The following multimodal tip helps you halt and reverse this process.

You can fight depression by knowing yourself (your resources, problem triggers, tried-and-true coping strategies), and by knowing how to build and employ strategies that work to prevent, minimize, or eliminate depression from your life. Start by scanning your BASIC-ID to examine and review your core personality dimensions: B (behavior), A (affect-emotions), S (sensations), I (imagery-visualization), C (cognition-thoughts and beliefs), I (interpersonal-relationships), D (drugs, health, biological/medical state). If you are a doer and/or more of a relationship-oriented person, you can prevent a depressive episode, and minimize its intensity or duration by systematically increasing your productivity, set and achieve short-term goals, and make a deliberate effort to connect with people whom you know, care for, and trust. Physical exercise helps, too, but choose a particular activity that feels least difficult or most interesting, such as a walk in the park or a bike ride.

Alternatively, if you are more of an imagery and sensory-based individual, you may want to visit a local garden, take photographs, cook a flavorful meal, or listen to meditational or relaxation music. Similarly, if you are more of a thinker, depression is likely to weigh you down with negative and obsessive thoughts.

By routinely taking your emotional temperature—scanning your BASIC-ID profile to keep tabs on how you are doing—you can assess and address modality deficiencies before they grab hold. By inoculating yourself against depression, you improve your resiliency to stress and protect yourself against having future depression. Similarly, when you are actually feeling depressed, you can target your key modalities with modality-specific strategies to address your emotional needs, style, and natural talents. At any time, you can simultaneously build on your key modalities to strengthen your sense of emotional balance and health. The multimodal approach enables you to honor who you are and employ your best resources to not only prevail over depression but to fulfill your life as you choose.

# A TOP TIP FOR DEPRESSION PREVENTION

Finally, Arnold Lazarus (pers. comm.) recommends the following multimodal method to prevent relapse:

Relapse prevention of depression, from the multimodal perspective, calls for vigilance in checking one's BASIC-ID every few weeks. Thus, depression can creep up on one, but a BASIC-ID checklist may discover, say, negative images, more than unusual untoward sensations (for example, tension), and pessimistic cognitions. It may be advisable to return (to a counselor) for a therapeutic tune-up, or assuage these negative events by systematically going through the BASIC-ID process and taking specific steps to remedy problems.

# END DEPRESSION PLAN

**Key ideas** (What three ideas did you find most helpful in this chapter?):

1.

2.

3.

**Action steps** (What three steps can you take to move closer to your goal of overcoming depression?):

1.

2.

3.

**Execution** (How did you execute the steps?):

1.

2.

3.

**Results** (What did you learn that you can use?):

1.

2.

3.

# CHAPTER 22

# Your Relapse Prevention Program

After your first major bout with depression, you have a 50 percent chance of avoiding a second. Using cognitive, emotive, and behavioral methods to overcome depression, you've already given yourself an edge in avoiding a recurrence. However, there are no guarantees. By maintaining predictable routines, keeping negative thinking and affect in check, and using coping skills at the start of a potential recurrence, you are taking preventive actions to keep from getting sucked back into the darkness of depression.

Some forms of depression are more likely to come around again. If you are a veteran of many bouts of depression, you have a unique advantage. You know that depression comes and goes. You know you can survive depression. Additionally, by not dreading a recurrence, you eliminate a big negative-thinking factor that can be an accelerant for a depressive cycle.

The key ideas and action steps that you recorded for each chapter give you choices among prescribed techniques to apply to your situation. They are psychological tune-up tools for reducing your risk of a recurrence and for shortening the duration of a depression, should it happen again.

## INVESTING IN PREVENTION

Drug companies like to call their antidepressant pills the first line of defense against depression. The use of antidepressants has more than tripled over the past thirty years. At the same time, the prevalence of depression is significantly on the rise. Although a medication approach is a useful tool for some, it is also overdone and beginning to look more and more like the famous French Maginot Line.

The numbers on relapse prevention favor a cognitive approach with a 30.8 percent relapse rate compared to the 76.2 percent relapse rate following the use of antidepressant medications (Hollon et al. 2005). A cognitive, emotive, and behavioral approach has clear advantages.

While it may be too late to prevent a first depression, you can adapt many of the techniques from the book to prevent a recurrence. It is never too late to reduce general health risks that may come about from stresses and an unhealthy lifestyle. The same lifestyle habits that may put you at risk for diseases such as lung cancer, coronary heart disease, or diabetes can also put you at risk for health-related depression. Activating a healthier lifestyle includes doing things that you'd ordinarily do to intervene with depression. These activities include eating healthily, exercising, getting adequate sleep, and dealing with stress.

## Secondary Prevention

Secondary prevention is for averting the onset of another depression by applying psychological self-help tactics. Your awareness of the antecedents of depression is normally not enough to avert the next bout of depression. But when you are aware of general conditions that can spur your depression, you are in a position to make a course change before depression takes hold.

Assume the role of a depression detective. Under what conditions is depression likely to strike? What are your clues? Note: If you are in a physically or mentally abusive relationship, all the antidepression actions you try on yourself won't change your partner's contribution to an adverse situation. When you need to protect yourself, leaving is an option. That's a form of secondary prevention.

Fortunately, you don't have to reinvent the wheel to practice secondary prevention. Most methods in this book are both interventions and preventive measures for depression.

### REVIEW KEY IDEAS AND ACTION STEPS

Review your key ideas and action steps at the end of each chapter. Highlight the key ideas and actions that both address depression and can help you reduce future risk. For example, you can attack anxiety at its inception using key idea and action methods that you've already used and found effective.

### PRACTICE WITH SIMULATIONS

List depressive thought themes and antidepression themes, and then countermand them. If helplessness thinking dominates, then show yourself that you can avert the pain this thinking brings, by generating a perspective where you imagine yourself confronting negative thinking and then thinking constructively. Follow your constructive thoughts.

## Tertiary Prevention

You can act at the onset of any new depression to avert a worse condition. The idea behind tertiary prevention is to detect depression early on and nip it in the bud before it grows into a full-blown episode. For example, if you tend to dwell a lot on worries and troubles before depression comes on, plan to address worry at the onset, before depressive worries get out of hand. Ideally, if you can catch depression before it gains traction, you've done yourself a big favor.

Tertiary prevention affords little latitude for procrastination, where you hope that if you wait, things will not get worse. The potentially devastating effects of depression are too great to delay corrective actions when you feel depression coming on.

It's not what you think about the horrors of depression that counts as much as what you know you can do to curb the double troubles of depression.

## HALT EARLY-ONSET DOUBLE TROUBLES

Double troubles are common cognitive signatures of depression. For example, you catastrophize over real or imagined problems, lament over the horrors of feeling depressed, and tell yourself that you can't stand feeling depressed. Now you have multiple problems instead of one.

If you pay too much attention to how depressed you feel, as many people do, then depression can swell into double trouble. Often multiple negative thoughts and feelings coalesce into a grand convection of jarring ruminations. By shifting to objective self-observation, you intervene before double troubles snowball.

Here are three key forms of double trouble, accompanying self-absorbing views, and self-observant prevention remedies that you can take:

| Double Trouble | Self-Absorbing View | Objective Self-Observant Prevention Remedies |
|---|---|---|
| Magnification (concentrating too much on a dreaded situation and your feelings about it) | "Depression is so awful I can't stand feeling this way." | "Depression is unpleasant, but I am standing what I don't like. This is a resilience solution to the early-onset phase of depression." |
| Overgeneralization (going beyond what is warranted by either facts or plausibility) | "I'll never feel good again." | "I may think that depression will go on forever, but I know differently. Depression has a life span of about six months to two years if I do nothing, and an abbreviated life span if I take early corrective action. This is the acceptance solution to the early-onset phase of depression." |
| Circularity (going round in circles where a false premise feeds a feeling that falsely verifies the premise) | "I can't change. My depression will go on forever." | "Each circular-thinking chain has weak links. The first lies in the assumption that I can't change. Change the idea from, 'I can't change' to 'I assume that I can't change,' and I've made a change." |

## HALT CIRCULAR THINKING

Practically every recurring human disturbance includes circular thinking. This thinking contains a non sequitur, or a conclusion that doesn't logically follow from the preceding premise: "My depression will last forever. Because I feel depressed, this will go on forever."

You can recognize the logical gaps in your own circular thinking and label the non sequiturs. As you do this, you will be less likely to grow dizzy running round in a depressive circle of thought. You'll have taken an important step in blunting a full-blown recurrence.

## EXERCISE YOUR PROBABILITY-THINKING ABILITIES

When you feel depressed, you are prone to tell yourself absurd and ridiculous things, such as "I have no life." Are such vague but emotionally potent thoughts true just because you say so? Teach yourself to think two-sidedly. For every negative prediction, make a positive one.

You may believe that your depression will go on forever because you can't prove that it will come to an end. That's a depressive-thinking trap that is worth halting at the earliest opportunity.

One intervention is to remember that the absence of personal experiences to disprove this view doesn't make the belief true. In examining negative arguments, psychologist Albert Ellis is famous for this question: "Where is the evidence?" You argue that the proof that your depression will last forever is that you feel depressed now. But where is the evidence for this? You may advance your belief that depression must be terminal in your case because you can't change. But where is the evidence? You may argue that you must stay depressed because you don't feel positive. But where is the evidence? With regard to depressive thinking, it boils down to this: arguing from negatives proves nothing other than that you are arguing from negatives.

> One false argument doesn't logically support another false argument.

When you have no factual evidence to rely upon, teach yourself to think using probabilities, thereby preventing yourself from falling into the common arguing-from-the-negative fallacy trap. For example, what does the scientific literature say about the average duration of depression? What's the probability that you'll find yourself within those boundaries? Probabilities are like hypotheses. They are something to test. Let the results determine the answer.

## ACHIEVE TOLERANCE AND ACCEPTANCE

The three dimensions of acceptance refer to unconditional acceptance of self, others, and life (Ellis 2003). This amounts to viewing reality as it is, not as you might expect it to be. Making demands—that you should be different, others must change, and the world must be as you expect—is a formula for distress. The dimensions of acceptance are the antidotes.

The dimensions of acceptance are discretionary, of course. You can choose to debase yourself, debase others, and debase your environment and world, but this is ordinarily counterproductive. Here's a comparison to consider:

| Dimensions of Acceptance | Demands | Acceptance |
|---|---|---|
| Self | "I should be happy. I should be perfect." | "There is no law to say that I must be an ideal me. I am as I should be, a person who can choose, adjust, and act constructively." |
| Others | "People should do as I expect, look the way I expect, be fair to me, and act perfectly wonderful toward me." | "People vary considerably in their values, beliefs, attitudes, abilities, and behaviors. I may influence some people, some of the time, but never all people, all of the time." |
| Life | "The world should be as I expect. Natural disasters are outlawed, there should be no illnesses, and pleasant serendipity is the rule of the day, week, and year, forever." | "I can control very little outside of myself, and I can choose to control what I can, including my perspective on events that are out of my control that, nevertheless, influence me directly." |

With a demanding philosophy, you are going to think categorically and make yourself more prone to feeling upset. With an enlightened outlook, you accept a higher level of responsibility for your thoughts, feelings, and actions. You realize that you are not responsible for your human fallibilities. Nevertheless, you are responsible for taking self-correcting actions if you want to do and feel better. You are not responsible for others' destabilizing ways. But you are responsible for protecting yourself against unwelcome or unjust intrusions into your life.

Enlightened acceptance involves asserting your rights and interests without needlessly trampling on the legitimate rights and interests of others.

# PREVENTING DEPRESSION WITH CONFIDENT COMPOSURE

Confident composure is an alternative to depressive ways of knowing, feeling, and doing. This cognitive, emotive, and behavioral state applies to personal growth as much as it does to preventing depression.

Confident composure means recognizing that you can directly command only yourself, and you choose to do so. You don't demand that others and the world change for you; you don't need them to change. With this softer but more resilient view, you can better influence the controllable events that take place around you. When you feel confident and composed, you are likely to come across as sincere and capable.

> Confident composure is forged from facing the fires of adversity, such as meeting the challenge of finding and using ways to curb depression.

Confident composure arises from your belief that you can respond effectively to situations to accomplish a favorable result. With an emerging sense of confident composure, you replace depressive habits with productive efforts.

You will practically always have opportunities to steer yourself onto a steady life course with confident composure. Here are some sample concepts and applications for confident composure:

| Concepts for Confident Composure | Actions for Confident Composure |
|---|---|
| **Perspective** | Some realities are relatively constant while others are in flux. You can recognize and examine assumptions that routinely appear under either set of conditions. You can examine the direction you expect to take by following your assumptions. You can consider different assumptions and possible outcomes. As you gain distance from assumptions about reality, you get less ego-involved in proving you're right and more involved in exploring reality. |
| **Pluralistic self** | As a pluralistic self, you recognize and accept that you are a composite of your traits, abilities, experiences, and beliefs. Your self-concept is one of self-acceptance and the ability to initiate effective actions. You can and should rate your actions but never your entire self. Correct what you don't like or what doesn't work well for you. |
| **Stress tolerance** | Accept stress, but the right kind. Tension that arises from overcoming obstacles is a propellant, healthy stress. Hand-wringing is distressful. Each stress represents a proclivity and a choice. The distress choice may not be easy to recognize. Think about your thinking when you feel distressed. You may hear yourself talking to yourself using language of distress. Stress tolerance is earned through agreeing with yourself to live through necessary tensions to get to the other side of the tension. |
| **Personal mission** | You know where you are going and where you stand. That simplifies life. A sample mission is to advance your work skills to contribute, improve, and prosper. Your actions become more directed when you do something (take specific actions) for achieving your long-range mission. |
| **Priority thinking** | Focus on healthy priorities and objectives. Schedule a fixed amount of time each day to prepare for what comes next. It's normally easier to continue something you started than to begin from scratch. You'll get further attending to what you can control. |
| **Adapt** | Plan on making adjustments that align with emerging realities. It's easier to adapt when you don't glue yourself to fixed assumptions. Support your ideas with facts and plausible alternatives. |

# YOUR CONFIDENT-COMPOSURE PLAN

Compose a confident-composure plan that is right for you.

| Concepts for Confident Composure | Actions for Confident Composure |
|---|---|
| Perspective | |
| Pluralistic self | |
| Stress tolerance | |
| Personal mission | |
| Priority thinking | |
| Adapt | |

# COGNITIVE-EMOTIVE-BEHAVIORAL PREVENTION

Participating in a one-on-one cognitive-behavioral form of therapy substantially reduces your risk of recurrence of depression (Minami et al. 2008; Fava et al. 2004). This book can serve a similar purpose, but there is an obvious difference. You are your own coach.

Based on your prior experience with depression, you can identify cognitive, emotive, and behavioral themes that are likely to be present at the onset of a new depressive episode. You can prepare for this occurrence. If you never have to draw on this work, great! If you catch yourself slipping into depression, however, you will have some tested techniques to use to contain depression.

Throughout, this book has looked at how to conquer depression using cognitive, emotive, and behavioral ways of knowing and doing. You strive toward confident composure using these strategies. With intellect, ingenuity, and will, you can take this process one step further.

Your *intellect* enables you to understand and solve problems. Your *ingenuity* is your ability to find novel ways to meet challenges. Your *will* reflects your faith in your ability to impel and to control the directions of your actions. You can use the following motivational framework to buffer yourself against relapsing into a new depression:

| Prevention Factors | Cognitive | Emotive | Behavioral |
|---|---|---|---|
| **Intellect** | Identify, in advance, depressive thoughts that most seriously affect how you feel and what you do. Outline an early intervention plan to address these thoughts before they gain a foothold. This plan may include creating a wallet-sized card that lists your most likely depressive thought themes and their cognitive and behavioral antidotes. | Identify fears of depression that lead you to feel depressed over feeling depressed. Explore if this fear of the feeling loops back to your thinking. Think about your thinking and separate facts from fallacies. It's a fact that you think what you think. Ask, how does that thinking veer from reality? Accept only plausible or factual answers. | Identify depressive behaviors, such as withdrawing or acting irritable with others. Draw up an activity-scheduling plan where you reward yourself for increasing contacts when you'd be inclined to withdraw. Take a timeout by walking when you are prone to jump down someone's throat. |

| | | | |
|---|---|---|---|
| **Ingenuity** | Maintain a healthy perspective by recognizing the incongruities in depression, such as when you tell yourself that depression is your entire fault while telling yourself that you are helpless. If you are helpless, how are you blameworthy over what you can't control? | Experiment with emotive imaging. When you experience a down mood, imagine accepting it without questioning the sensations that go with it. As an alternative, play with adverse imagery. Write a script for escalating the mood, such as writing about how you have a mood that you can't stand and that must not be. This contrivance can have a paradoxical effect. | Take creative actions. If you view yourself as a wilted leaf when you feel depressed, write a poem on the virtues of being a wilted leaf that suddenly feels infused with water and nutrients. Memorize the poem. Use it when you need to. |
| **Will** | You may be able to will your will into existence to counter the pull of any future depression. Otherwise, you can act as if you had the will to act. By acting as if you had the will, you've conjured up the will that you may have thought you lacked. | The will to succumb to depression may be stronger than the will to resist through executing coping actions. Imagine experiencing a new emotion called *forcefulness*. Pit a will of forcefulness against a will to enter a depressive vortex. Imagine yourself asserting force to translate coping ideas and techniques into action. | To the degree that you are able, assert your will to change actions to counter the magnetic pull of depressive behaviors. Consider these suggestions from three great men: Ben Franklin advised picking qualities you want to develop. Practice using them, and you strengthen them. Role construct psychologist George Kelly (1955) advised practicing productive roles that compete with negative patterns. Try a role. Retain what works. Discard the rest. French educator and philosopher Jules Payot (1909) advised asserting your will to engage in strenuous activities. Look at this effort as a means of developing mental and emotional muscle. |

# YOUR COGNITIVE, EMOTIVE, AND BEHAVIORAL PREVENTION PLAN

Now it is your turn to generate a cognitive, emotive, and behavioral prevention plan that you believe will work for you.

| Prevention Factors | Cognitive | Emotive | Behavioral |
|---|---|---|---|
| Intellect | | | |
| Ingenuity | | | |
| Will | | | |

# PREVENTING PROCRASTINATION

You can have the best depression prevention ideas available, and tell yourself that you have all the time in the world to think about them and use them to avoid a recurrence of depression. That's procrastination, not prevention.

You may convince yourself that the other guy will have a relapse but not you. Besides, there is reasonable evidence that the cognitive skills developed in defeating depression tend to retain their strength and possibly get stronger. There's no need to go into overkill. That's procrastination.

Intellectualized assertions that result in delaying prevention action typically do more harm than good. It is normally wise to get on top of a problem before it gets on top of you. The risk of a second depression is so high that it's silly to put off preparation for preventing or addressing another bout. If you've had more than one bout of depression, the odds are about 70 percent that you'll have a major bout again.

# ELLIS'S APPROACH TO PREVENTING RELAPSE

The beginning of this book noted the contributions of the great rational therapist Albert Ellis. It's only fitting that he should have the last word. Here are some of his thoughts on preventing a recurrence of depression that are based on principles that he applied to himself.

Albert Ellis (pers. comm.) suggested doing the following if you have had a depression and want to prevent recurrence:

1. Assume that depression is partly caused by your damning yourself for your poor behavior and/or damning the world as an awful place.

2. Use the principles of rational emotive behavior therapy (REBT) to give up this kind of damnation and to achieve unconditional self-acceptance (USA), unconditional other-acceptance (UOA), and unconditional life-acceptance (ULA).

3. Strongly, powerfully, and emotionally work at achieving USA, UOA, and ULA.

4. Persistently act against your self-downing and life downing.

5. Each day, fill out at least one REBT self-help form.

By following Ellis's advice, you can strengthen your abilities to build a reasonable perspective, emotional resiliency, and behavioral capabilities, as you buffer yourself against future depression. You roll the dice in favor of experiencing peace of mind more often. A big part of peace of mind is to stop demanding that you, others, and life conform to your demands and expectations and, instead, accept that you, others, and life are what they are. You will then be better able to roll with the punches and create conditions favorable to your existence.

# END DEPRESSION PLAN

**Key ideas** (What three ideas did you find most helpful in this chapter?):

1.

2.

3.

**Action steps** (What three steps can you take to move closer to your goal of overcoming depression?):

1.

2.

3.

**Execution** (How did you execute the steps?):

1.

2.

3.

**Results** (What did you learn that you can use?):

1.

2.

3.

# References

Adamson, K. 2002. *Kate's Journey: Triumph over Adversity*. New York: Insight Publishing.

Agüera-Ortiz, L., I. Failde, J. A. Mico, J. Cervilla, and J. J. López-Ibor. 2010. Pain as a symptom of depression: Prevalence and clinical correlates in patients attending psychiatric clinics. *Journal of Affective Disorders* 130 (1–2): 106–112.

Aharon, I., N. Etcoff, D. Ariely, C. F. Chabris, E. O'Connor, and H. C. Breiter. 2001. Beautiful faces have variable reward value: fMRI and behavioral evidence. *Neuron* 32: 537–551.

Allport, G. W., and H. S. Odbert. 1936. Trait names: A psycho-lexical study. *Psychological Monographs* 47 (211).

Allen, L. A., R. L. Woolfolk, J. I. Escobar, M. A. Gara, and R. M. Hamer. 2006. Cognitive-behavioral therapy for somatization disorder: A randomized controlled trial. *Archives of Internal Medicine* 166(14):1512–1518.

American Psychiatric Association. 2000. *Diagnostic and Statistical Manual of Mental Disorders*. 4th ed. Text rev. Washington, DC: American Psychiatric Association.

American Psychiatric Association. 2010. Stress in America survey. Washington DC: American Psychological Association.

American Sunday School Union. 1848. *The Folly of Procrastination*. Philadelphia: American Sunday School Union.

Araujo, D., R. Marano, M. M. Vilarim, and A. E. Nardi. 2010. What is the effectiveness of the use of polyunsaturated fatty acid omega-3 in the treatment of depression? *Expert Review of Neurotherapeutics* 10 (7): 1117–1129.

Balfour, D. J. K. 1991. The influence of stress on psychopharmacological responses to nicotine. *British Journal of Addiction* 86: 489–493.

Barnes, R. T., S. A. Coombes, N. B. Armstrong, T. J. Higgins, and C. M. Janelle. 2010. Evaluating attentional and affective changes following an acute exercise bout using a modified dot-probe protocol. *Journal of Sports Science* 28 (10): 1065–1076.

Barr, J. T. 1857. *Too Late: The Fatal Effects of Procrastination*. New York: Carlton and Porter.

Beck, A. T. 1987. Cognitive models of depression. *Journal of Cognitive Psychotherapy: An International Quarterly* 1: 5–37.

Beers, C. 1908. *A Mind That Found Itself*. New York: Longmans and Green.

Benazzi, F. 2003. Anger in bipolar depression. *Journal of Clinical Psychiatry* 64: 480–481.

Bradley, R., J. Greene, E. Russ, L. Dutra, and D. Westen. 2005. A multidimensional meta-analysis of psychotherapy for PTSD. *American Journal of Psychiatry* 162 (2): 214–227.

Brand, S., M. Gerber, U. Pühse, and E. Holsboer-Trachsler. 2010. Depression, hypomania, and dysfunctional sleep-related cognitions as mediators between stress and insomnia: The best advice is not always found on the pillow! *International Journal of Stress Management* 17 (2): 114–134.

Brief, A. P., A. H. Butcher, J. M. George, and K. Link. 1993. Integrating bottom-up and top-down theories of subjective well-being: The case of health. *Journal of Personality and Social Psychology* 64 (4): 646–653.

Brown, R. J. 2004. Psychological mechanisms of medically unexplained symptoms: An integrative conceptual model. *Psychological Bulletin* 130 (5): 793–781.

Bulmash, E., K. L. Harkness, J. G. Stewart, and R. M. Bagby. 2009. Personality, stressful life events, and treatment response in major depression. *Journal of Consulting and Clinical Psychology* 77 (6): 1067–1077.

Burns, D. D. 1999. *Feeling Good*. New York: Avon Books.

Burns, D. D., and S. Nolen-Hoeksema. 1991. Coping styles, homework compliance, and the effectiveness of cognitive-behavioral therapy. *Journal of Consulting and Clinical Psychology* 59: 305–311.

Burton, R. 2001. *The Anatomy of Melancholy*. New York: Review Books Classic.

Butler, A. C., J. E. Chapman, E. M. Forman, and A. T. Beck. 2006. The empirical status of cognitive-behavioral therapy: A review of meta-analyses. *Clinical Psychology Review* 26 (1): 17–31.

Cacioppo, J. T., L. C. Hawkley, and R. A. Thisted. 2010. Perceived social isolation makes me sad: Five-year cross-lagged analyses of loneliness and depressive symptomatology in the Chicago Health, Aging, and Social Relations Study. *Psychology and Aging* 25 (2): 453–463.

Calder, P. C. 2004. n-3 Fatty acids and cardiovascular disease: Evidence explained and mechanisms explored. *Clinical Science* 107: 1–11.

Carpenter, D. J. 2011. St. John's wort and S-adenosyl methionine as "natural" alternatives to conventional antidepressants in the era of the suicidality boxed warning: What is the evidence for clinically relevant benefit? *Alternative Medical Review* 16 (1): 17–39.

Chang, P. P., D. E. Ford, L. A. Mead, L. Cooper-Patrick, and M. J. Klag. 1997. Insomnia in young men and subsequent depression: The Johns Hopkins Precursors Study. *American Journal of Epidemiology* 146 (2): 105–14.

Chiesa, A., and A. Serretti. 2011. Mindfulness based cognitive therapy for psychiatric disorders: A systematic review and meta-analysis. *Psychiatry Research* 187 (3): 441–453.

Cohen, E. 2011. *The Dutiful Worrier: How to Stop Compulsive Worry without Feeling Guilty*. Oakland, CA: New Harbinger Publications.

Collishaw, S., B. Maughan, L. Natarajan, and A. Pickles. 2010. Trends in adolescent emotional problems in England: A comparison of two national cohorts twenty years apart. *Journal of Child Psychology and Psychiatry* 51 (8): 885–894.

Compton, W. M., K. P. Conway, F. S. Stinson, and B. F. Grant. 2006. Changes in the prevalence of major depression and comorbid substance use disorders in the United States between 1991–1992 and 2001–2002. *American Journal of Psychiatry* 163 (12): 2141–2147.

Cooley, C. H. 1902. *Human Nature and the Social Order*. New York: Scribner.

Cox, B. J., and M. W. Enns. 2003. Relative stability of perfection in depression. *Canadian Journal of Behavioral Science* 35 (2): 124–132.

Cox, D. L., S. D. Stabb, and J. F. Hulgus. 2000. Anger and depression in girls and boys: A study of gender differences. *Psychology of Women Quarterly* 24: 110–112.

Cuijpers, P. 1998. A psychoeducational approach to the treatment of depression: A meta-analysis of Lewinsohn's "coping with depression" course. *Behavior Therapy* 29: 521–533.

Cuijpers, P., A. van Straten, and L. Warmerdam. 2007. Behavioral activation treatments of depression: A meta-analysis. *Clinical Psychology Review* 27 (3): 318–326.

Cusi, A. M., G. M. MacQueen, R. N. Spreng, and M. C. McKinnon. 2011. Altered empathic responding in major depressive disorder: Relation to symptom severity, illness burden, and psychosocial outcome. *Psychiatry Research* 188 (2): 231–236.

Dalai Lama. 2002. *A Simple Path*. London: Thorsons.

Dalgleish, T., E. Hill, A. J. Golden, N. Morant, and D. Barnaby. 2011. The structure of past and future lives in depression. *Journal of Abnormal Psychology* 120 (1): 1–15.

Das-Munshi, J., D. Goldberg, P. E. Bebbington, D. K. Bhugra, T. S. Brugha, M. E. Dewey, R. Jenkins, R. Stewart, and M. Prince. 2008. Public health significance of mixed anxiety and depression: Beyond current classification. *British Journal of Psychiatry* 192 (3): 171–177.

Davis, L. A. Uezato, J. M. Newell, and E. Frazier. 2008. Major depression and comorbid substance use disorders. *Current Opinion in Psychiatry* 21 (1): 14-18.

Davydov, D. M., R. Stewart, K. Ritchie, and I. Chaudieu. 2010. Resilience and mental health. *Clinical Psychology Review* 30 (5): 479–495.

Deacon, B. J., and G. L. Baird. 2009. The chemical imbalance explanation of depression: Reducing blame at what cost? *Journal of Social and Clinical Psychology* 28 (4): 415–435.

Deffenbacher, J. L. 2011. Cognitive-behavioral conceptualization and treatment of anger. *Cognitive and Behavioral Practice* 18 (2): 212–221.

Deldin, P. J., and P. Chiu. 2005. Cognitive restructuring and EEG in major depression. *Biological Psychology* 70: 141–151.

Diefenbach, G. J., M. E. McCarthy-Larzelere, D. A. Williamson, A. Mathews, G. M. Manguno-Mire, and B. G. Bentz. 2001. Anxiety, depression, and the content of worries. *Depression and Anxiety* 14 (40): 247–250.

Dimidjian, S., S. D. Hollon, K. S. Dobson, K. B. Schmaling, R. J. Kohlenberg, M. E. Addis, R. Gallop, J. B. McGlinchey, D. K. Markley, J. K. Gollan, D. C. Atkins, D. L. Dunner, and N. S. Jacobson. 2006. Randomized trial of behavioral activation, cognitive therapy, and antidepressant medication in the acute treatment of adults with major depression. *Journal of Consulting and Clinical Psychology* 74 (4): 658–670.

Dobson, K. S., S. D. Hollon, S. Dimidjian, K. B. Schmaling, R. J. Kohlenberg, R. Gallop, S. L. Rizvi, J. K. Gollan, D. L. Dunner, and N. S. Jacobson. 2008. Randomized trial of behavioral activation, cognitive therapy, and antidepressant medication in the prevention of relapse and recurrence in major depression. *Journal of Consulting and Clinical Psychology* 76 (3): 468–477.

Dollard, J. 1942. *Victory Over Fear*. New York: Renyal and Hitchcock.

Driessen, E., P. Cuijpers, S. D. Hollon, and J. J. M. Dekker. 2010. Does pretreatment severity moderate the efficacy of psychological treatment of adult outpatient depression? A meta-analysis. *Journal of Consulting and Clinical Psychology* 78(5): 668–680.

Dubois, P. 1909. *The Psychic Treatment of Mental Disorders*. New York: Funk and Wagnalls.

Edinger, J. D., W. K. Wohlgemuth, R. A. Radtke, G. R. Marsh, and R. E. Quillian. 2001. Cognitive behavioral therapy for treatment of chronic primary insomnia: A randomized controlled trial. *Journal of the American Medical Association* 285 (14): 1856–1864.

Edwards, A. C., and K. S. Kendler. 2011. Nicotine withdrawal-induced negative affect is a function of nicotine dependence and not liability to depression or anxiety. *Nicotine and Tobacco Research* 13 (8): 677–685.

Ekers, D., D. Richards, and S. Gilbody. 2008. A meta-analysis of randomized trials of behavioural treatment of depression. *Psychological Medicine: A Journal of Research in Psychiatry and the Allied Sciences* 38 (5): 611–623.

Ellis, A. 1971. *Growth through Reason*. Palo Alto, CA: Science and Behavior Books.

———. 1988. *How to Stubbornly Refuse to Make Yourself Miserable*. New York: Kensington.

———. 1994. *Reason and Emotion in Psychotherapy*. Rev. ed. New York: Kensington.

———. 2003. *Ask Albert Ellis*. Atascadero, CA: Impact.

Epperson, C. N., M. Terman, J. S. Terman, B. H. Hanusa, D. A. Oren, K. S. Peindl, and K. L. Wisner. 2004. Randomized clinical trial of bright light therapy for antepartum depression: Preliminary findings. *Journal of Clinical Psychiatry* 65: 421–425.

Ernst E., J. I. Rand, J. Barnes, and C. Stevinson. 1998. Adverse effects profile of the herbal antidepressant St. John's wort (*Hypericum perforatum L.*). *European Journal of Clinical Pharmacology* 54 (8): 589–594.

Fava, G. A., C. Ruini, C. Rafanelli, L. Finos, S. Conti, and S. Grandi. 2004. Six-year outcome of cognitive behavior therapy for prevention of recurrent depression. *American Journal of Psychiatry* 161: 1872–1876.

Fava, M., J. Alpert, A. A. Nierenberg, D. Mischoulon, M. W. Otto, J. Zajecka, H. Murck, and J. F. Rosenbaum. 2005. A double-blind, randomized trial of St John's wort, fluoxetine, and placebo in major depressive disorder. *Journal of Clinical Psychopharmacology* 25 (5): 441–447.

Felmingham, K., A. Kemp, L. Williams, P. Das, G. Hughes, A. Peduto, and R. Bryant. 2007. Changes in anterior cingulate and amygdala after cognitive behavior therapy of post-traumatic stress disorder. *Psychological Science* 18: 127–129.

Field, T., M. Hernandez-Reif, M. Diego, S. Schanberg, and C. Kuhn. 2005. Cortisol decreases and serotonin and dopamine increase following massage therapy. *International Journal of Neuroscience* 115 (10): 1397–1413.

Fischer, A. G., C. H. D. Bau, E. H. Grevet, C. A. I. Salgado, M. M. Victor, K. L. Kalil, N. O. Sousa, C. R. Garcia, and P. Belmonte-de-Abreu. 2007. The role of comorbid major depressive disorder in the clinical presentation of adult ADHD. *Journal of Psychiatric Research* 41 (12): 991–996.

Flavell, J. H. 1979. Metacognition and cognitive monitoring. *American Psychologist* 34: 906–911.

Frankl, V. 1963. *Man's Search for Meaning*. New York: Washington Square Press.

Frasure-Amith, N., F. Lespérance, and P. Julien. 2004. Major depression is associated with lower omega-3 fatty acid levels in patients with recent acute coronary syndromes. *Biological Psychiatry* 55 (9): 891–896.

Freud, S. 1950. *The Ego and the Id*. Translated by J. Riveriere. London: Hogarth Press.

———. 2005. *On Murder, Mourning, and Melancholia*. London: Penguin.

Gebauer, S. K., T. L. Psota, W. S. Harris, and P. M. Kris-Etherton. 2006. n-3 fatty acid dietary recommendations and food sources to achieve essentiality and cardiovascular benefits. *American Journal of Clinical Nutrition* 83 (Suppl. 6): 1526S–1535S.

Gilbert, D. G., and C. D. Spielberger. 1987. Effects of smoking on heart rate, anxiety, and feelings of success during social interaction. *Journal of Behavioral Medicine* 10: 629–638.

Glassman, A. H. 1997. Cigarette smoking and its comorbidity. In *National Institute on Drug Abuse: Treatment of Drug-Dependent Individuals with Comorbid Mental Disorders,* NIDA research monograph no. 172, edited by L. S. Onken, J. D. Blaine, S. Genser, and A. M. Horton, Jr. Rockville, MD: U.S. Department of Health and Human Services.

Goldapple, K., Z. Segal, C. Garson, M. Lau, P. Bieling, S. Kennedy, and H. Mayberg. 2004. Modulation of cortical-limbic pathways in major depression: Treatment-specific effects of cognitive behavior therapy. *Archives of General Psychiatry* 61: 34–41.

Gollwitzer, P. M. 1999. Implementation intentions: Strong effects of simple plans. *American Psychologist* 54: 493–503.

Gollwitzer, P. M., and G. Oettingen. 2011. Planning promotes goal striving. In *Handbook of Self-Regulation: Research, Theory, and Applications*, edited by K. D. Vohs and R. F. Baumeister. 2nd ed. New York: Guilford Press.

Goossens, L. S., R. Sunaert, E. J. Peeters, L. Griez, and K. R. J. Schruers. 2007. Amygdala hyperfunction in phobic fear normalizes after exposure. *Biological Psychiatry* 62: 1119–1125.

Gotlib, I. H., and C. L. Hammen. 1992. *Psychological Aspects of Depression: Toward a Cognitive-Interpersonal Integration*. Oxford, England: John Wiley and Sons.

Gould, R. A., and G. Clum. 1993. A meta-analysis of self-help treatment approaches. *Clinical Psychology Review* 13 (2): 169–186.

Graham, A. R., S. B. Sherry, S. H. Sherry, H. Sherry, D. L. Sherry, D. S. McGrath, K. M. Fossum, and S. L. Allen. 2010. The existential model of perfectionism and depressive symptoms: A short-term, four-wave longitudinal study. *Journal of Counseling Psychology* 57 (4): 423–438.

Gregory, R. J., C. S. Schwer, T. W. Lee, and J. C. Wise. 2004. Cognitive bibliotherapy for depression: A meta-analysis. *Professional Psychology: Research and Practice* 35: 275–280.

Grynberg, D., O. Luminet, O. Corneille, J. Grèzes, and S. Berthoz. 2010. Alexithymia in the interpersonal domain: A general deficit of empathy? *Personality and Individual Differences* 49 (8): 845–850.

Guazzelli, M., and C. Gentili. 2008. Some reflections on the issue of insomnia and depressive disorders. *Italian Journal of Psychopathology* 14 (4) 389–395.

Guilford, J. P. 1967. *The Nature of Human Intelligence*. New York: McGraw-Hill.

Hansen, C. J., L. C. Stevens, and J. R. Coast. 2001. Exercise duration and mood state: How much is enough to feel better? *Health Psychology* 20 (4): 267–275.

Harvey, A. G., R. A. Bryant, and N. Tarrier. 2003. Cognitive behavior therapy for post-traumatic stress disorder. *Clinical Psychology Review* 23: 501–522.

Hasin, D. S., R. D. Goodwin, F. S. Stinson, and B. F. Grant. 2005. Epidemiology of major depressive disorder: Results from the National Epidemiologic Survey on Alcoholism and Related Conditions. *Archives of General Psychiatry* 62: 1097–1110.

Hawkins, K. A., and J. R. Cougle. 2011. Anger problems across the anxiety disorders: Findings from a population-based study. *Depression and Anxiety* 28 (2): 145–152.

Heller, W., and J. B. Nitschke. 1997. Regional brain activity in emotion: A framework for understanding cognition in depression. *Cognition and Emotion* 11: 637–661.

Hellerstein, D. J., V. Agosti, M. Bosi, and S. R. Black. 2010. Impairment in psychosocial functioning associated with dysthymic disorder in the NESARC study. *Journal of Affective Disorders* 127 (1–3): 84–88.

Hewitt, P. L., G. L. Flett, E. Ediger, G. R. Norton, and C. A. Flynn. 1998. Perfectionism in chronic and state symptoms of depression. *Canadian Journal of Behavioral Science* 30 (4): 234–242.

Hofmann, S. G., A. T. Sawyer, A. A. Witt, and D. Oh. 2010. The effect of mindfulness-based therapy on anxiety and depression: A meta-analytic review. *Journal of Consulting and Clinical Psychology* 78 (2): 169–183.

Hollon S. D., R. J. DeRubeis, R. C. Shelton, J. D. Amsterdam, R. M. Salomon, J. P. O'Reardon M. L. Lovett, P. R. Young, K. L. Haman, B. B. Freeman, and R. Gallop. 2005. Prevention of relapse following cognitive therapy vs. medications in moderate to severe depression. *Archives of General Psychiatry* 62 (4): 417–422.

Horney, K. 1950. *Neurosis and Human Growth*. New York: Norton.

Howren, M. B., and J. Suls. 2011. The symptom perception hypothesis revised: Depression and anxiety play different roles in concurrent and retrospective physical symptom reporting. *Journal of Personality and Social Psychology* 100 (1): 182–195.

Hume, D. 2008. *An Enquiry Concerning Human Understanding*. Charleston, SC: Forgotten Books.

Jackman-Cram, S., K. S. Dobson, and R. Martin. 2006. Marital problem-solving behavior in depression and marital distress. *Journal of Abnormal Psychology* 115 (2): 380–384.

Janet, P. 1913. *Major Symptoms of Hysteria*. London: McMillan.

Jiang W., H. Oken, M. Fiuzat, L. K. Shaw, C. Martsberger, M. Kuchibhatla, R. Kaddurah-Daouk, D. C. Steffens, R. Baillie, M. Cuffe, R. Krishnan, and C. O'Connor. 2011. Plasma omega-3 polyunsaturated fatty acids and survival in patients with chronic heart failure and major depressive disorder. *Journal of Cardiovascular Translational Research* November 1. doi: 10.1007/s12265-011-9325-8.

John, U., C. Meyer, H. J. Rumpf, and U. Hapke. 2004. Depressive disorders are related to nicotine dependence in the population but do not necessarily hamper smoking cessation. *Journal of Clinical Psychiatry* 65: 169–176.

Joiner, T. E., L. R. Wingate, T. Gencoz, and F. Gencoz. 2005. Stress generation in depression: Three studies on its resilience, possible mechanism, and symptom specificity. *Journal of Social and Clinical Psychology* 24 (2): 236–253.

Judd, L. L., R. C. Kessler, M. P. Paulus, H. U. Wittchen, and J. L. Kunovac. 1998. Comorbidity as a fundamental feature of generalized anxiety disorder. Results from the National Comorbidity Study. *Acta Psychiatrica Scandinavica* 98 (Suppl. 393): 6–11.

Kasper, S., M. Gastpar, W. E. Müller, H. P. Volz, A. Dienel, M. Kieser, and H. J. Möller. 2008. Efficacy of St. John's wort extract WS® 5570 in acute treatment of mild depression: A reanalysis of data from controlled clinical trials. *European Archives of Psychiatry and Clinical Neuroscience* 258 (1): 59–63.

Kassel, J. D., L. R. Stroud, and C. A. Paronis. 2003. Smoking, stress, and negative affect: Correlation, causation, and context across stages of smoking. *Psychological Bulletin* 129 (2): 270–304.

Keightley, M. L., G. Winocur, S. J. Graham, H. S. Mayberg, S. J. Hevenor, and C. L. Grady. 2003. An fMRI study investigating cognitive modulation of brain regions associated with emotional processing of visual stimuli. *Neuropsychologia* 41: 585–589.

Kelly, G. 1955. *The Psychology of Personal Constructs*. Vol. 2. New York: Norton.

Kennedy, S. H. 2008. Core symptoms of major depressive disorder: Relevance to diagnosis and treatment. *Dialogues in Clinical Neuroscience* 10 (3): 271–277.

Kessler, R. C., P. Berglund, O. Demler, R. Jin, D. Koretz, K. R. Merikangas, A. J. Rush, E. E. Walters, and P. S. Wang. 2003. The epidemiology of major depressive disorder: Results from the National Comorbidity Survey Replication (NCS-R). *Journal of the American Medical Association* 289 (23): 3095-3105.

Kessler, R. C., P. Berglund, O. Demler, R. Jin, K. R. Merikangas, and E. E. Walters. 2005. Lifetime prevalence and age-of-onset distributions of DSM-IV disorders in the National Comorbidity Survey replication. *Archives of General Psychiatry* 62: 593–60.

Kessler, R. C., E. F. Coccaro, M. Fava, S. Jaeger, R. Jin, and E. Walters. 2006. The prevalence and correlates of DSM-IV intermittent explosive disorder in the National Comorbidity Survey replication. *Archives of General Psychiatry* 63 (6): 669–678.

Kessler, R. C., B. J. Cox, J. G. Green, J. Ormel, K. A. McLaughlin , K. R. Merikangas, M. Petukhova, D. S. Pine , L. J. Russo, J. Swendsen, H. U. Wittchen, and A. M. Zaslavsky. 2011. The effects of latent variables in the development of comorbidity among common mental disorders. *Depression and Anxiety* 28 (1): 29–39.

Kessler, R. C., C. G. Davis, and K. S. Kendler. 1997. Childhood adversity and adult psychiatric disorder in the US National Comorbidity Survey. *Psychological Medicine* 27: 1101–1119.

Kessler, R. C., S. Zhao, D. G. Blazer, and M. Swartz. 1997. Prevalence, correlates, and course of minor depression and major depression in the National Comorbidity Survey. *Journal of Affective Disorders* 45: 19–30.

Kim, S., R. Thibodeau, and R. S. Jorgensen. 2011. Shame, guilt, and depressive symptoms: A meta-analytic review. *Psychological Bulletin* 137 (1): 68–96.

Klassen, L. J., M. A. Katzman, and P. Chokka. 2010. Adult ADHD and its comorbidities, with a focus on bipolar disorder. *Journal of Affective Disorders* 124 (1-2): 1–8.

Klein, D. N., J. E. Schwartz, S. Rose, and J. B. Leader. 2000. Five-year course and outcome of dysthymic disorder: A prospective, naturalistic follow-up study. *American Journal of Psychiatry* 157: 931–939.

Knaus, W. J. 1982. *How to Get Out of a Rut*. New York: John Wiley and Sons.

Koestner, R., N. Lekes, T. A. Powers, and E. Chicoine. 2002. Attaining personal goals: Self-concordance plus implementation intentions equals success. *Journal of Personality and Social Psychology* 83 (1): 231–244.

Koh, K. B., C. H. Kim, and J. K. Park. 2002. Predominance of anger in depressive disorders compared with anxiety disorders and somatoform disorders. *Journal of Clinical Psychiatry* 63 (6): 486–492.

Krampen, G. 1999. Long-term evaluation of the effectiveness of additional autogenic training in the psychotherapy of depressive disorders. *European Psychologist* 4 (1): 11–18.

Krishna, R. M., and the Hypericum Depression Trial Study Group. 2002. Effect of *Hypericum perforatum* (St. John's wort) in major depressive disorder: A randomized controlled trial. *Journal of the American Medical Association* 287 (14): 1807–1814.

Kromhout, H. 2005. Fish consumption, n-3 fatty acids, and coronary heart disease. In *Coronary Heart Disease Epidemiology: From Aetiology to Public Health*, edited by M. G. Marmot and P. Elliott. 2nd ed. Oxford: Oxford University Press.

Kupfer, D. J., E. Frank, V. J. Grochocinski, P. A. Cluss, P. R. Houck, and D. A. Stapf. 2002. Demographic and clinical characteristics of individuals in a bipolar disorder case registry. *Journal of Clinical Psychiatry* 63: 120–125.

Kuyken, W. 2004. Cognitive therapy outcome: The effects of hopelessness in a naturalistic outcome study. *Behaviour Research and Therapy* 42 (6): 631–646.

Kwan, B. M., and A. D. Bryan. 2010. Affective response to exercise as a component of exercise motivation: Attitudes, norms, self-efficacy, and temporal stability of intentions. *Psychology of Sport and Exercise* 11 (1): 71–79.

Lash, J. M. 2000. The effects of acute exercise on cognitions related to depression. *Dissertation Abstracts International, Section B: The Sciences and Engineering* 60 (12-B): 6371.

Lazarus, A. A. 1992. The multimodal approach to the treatment of depression. *American Journal of Psychotherapy* 62: 50–57.

LeDoux, J. 1998. Fear and the brain: Where have we been and where are we going? *Biological Psychiatry* 44: 1128–1138.

Lee, S. A. 2009. Does empathy mediate the relationship between neuroticism and depressive symptomatology among college students? *Personality and Individual Differences* 47 (5): 429–433.

Lewinsohn, P. M., and M. Graf. 1973. Pleasant activities and depression. *Journal of Consulting and Clinical Psychology* 41 (2): 261–268.

Lin, P. Y., and K. P. Su. 2007. A meta-analytic review of double-blind, placebo-controlled trials of antidepressant efficacy of omega-3 fatty acids. *Journal of Clinical Psychiatry* 68 (7): 1056–1061.

Liu, R. T., and L. B. Alloy. 2010. Stress generation in depression: A systematic review of the empirical literature and recommendations for future study. *Clinical Psychology Review* 30 (5): 582–593.

Liu, W. H., R. C. K. Chan, L. Wang, J. Huang, E. F. C. Cheung, Q. Gong, and J. K. Gollan. 2011. Deficits in sustaining reward responses in subsyndromal and syndromal major depression. *Progress in Neuro-Psychopharmacology and Biological Psychiatry* 35 (4): 1045–1052.

Lowenstein, K. G. 2002. Meditation and self-regulatory techniques. In *Handbook of Complementary and Alternative Therapies in Mental Health*, edited by S. Shannon 159–230. San Diego, CA: Academic Press.

Mahalik, J. R., and D. M. Kivlighan. 1988. Self-help treatment for depression: Who succeeds? *Journal of Counseling Psychology* 35: 237–242.

Mannel, M., U. Kuhn, U. Schmidt, M. Ploch, and H. Murck. 2010. St. John's wort extract LI160 for the treatment of depression with atypical features: A double-blind, randomized, and placebo-controlled trial. *Journal of Psychiatric Research* 44 (12): 760–767.

Margaret. 1852. *Thoughtless Little Fanny or the Unhappy Results of Procrastination*. London: Milner.

Masten, A. S. 2009. Ordinary magic: Lessons from research on resilience in human development. *Education Canada* 49 (3): 28–32.

Mazzucchelli, T., R. Kane, and C. Rees. 2009. Behavioral activation treatments for depression in adults: A meta-analysis and review. *Clinical Psychology: Science and Practice* 16 (4): 383–411.

McCloskey, M. S., K. L. Noblett, J. L. Deffenbacher, J. K. Gollan, and E. F. Coccaro. 2008. Cognitive-behavioral therapy for intermittent explosive disorder: A pilot randomized clinical trial. *Journal of Consulting and Clinical Psychology* 76 (5): 876–886.

McEwen, B. S. 2006. Protective and damaging effects of stress mediators: Central role of the brain. *Dialogues in Clinical Neuroscience* 8: 367–381.

McEwen, B. S., and E. N. Lasley. 2002. *The End of Stress as We Know It*. Washington, DC: Joseph Henry Press.

McFarlane, A. C., N. Ellis, C. Barton, D. Browne, and M. Van Hooff. 2008. The conundrum of medically unexplained symptoms: Questions to consider. *Psychosomatics: Journal of Consultation Liaison Psychiatry* 49 (5): 369–377.

McQuaid, J. R., M. B. Stein, C. Laffaye, and M. E. McCahill. 1999. Depression in a primary care clinic: The prevalence and impact of an unrecognized disorder. *Journal of Affective Disorders* 55 (1): 1–10.

Merton, R. K. 1936. The unanticipated consequences of purposive social action. *American Sociological Review* 1 (6): 894–904.

Middeldorp, C. M., A. J. Birley, D. C. Cath, N. A. Gillespie, G. Willemsen, D. J. Statham, E. J. de Geus, J. G. Andrews, R. van Dyck, A. L. Beem, P. F. Sullivan, N. G. Martin, and D. L. Boomsma. 2005. Familial clustering of major depression and anxiety disorders in Australian and Dutch twins and siblings. *Twin Research and Human Genetics* 8 (6): 609–615.

Minami, T., B. E. Wampold, R. C. Serlin, E. G. Hamilton, G. S. Brown, and J. C. Kircher. 2008. Benchmarking the effectiveness of psychotherapy treatment for adult depression in a managed care environment: A preliminary study. *Journal of Consulting and Clinical Psychology* 76: 116–124.

Moyer, C. A., J. Rounds, and J. W. Hannum. 2004. A meta-analysis of massage therapy research. *Psychological Bulletin* 130 (1): 3–18.

Murray, C. J. L., and A. D. Lopez, eds. 1996. *The Global Burden of Disease: A Comprehensive Assessment of Mortality and Disability from Diseases, Injuries, and Risk Factors in 1990 and Projected to 2020.* Cambridge: Harvard University Press.

Mykletun, A., O. Bjerkeset, S. Overland, M. Prince, M. Dewey, and R. Stewart. 2009. Levels of anxiety and depression are predictors of mortality: The HUNT study. *British Journal of Psychiatry* 195: 118–125.

National Institute of Mental Health. 1999. Depression research at the National Institute of Mental Health. National Institutes of Health. U.S. Department of Health and Human Services. http://www.nimh.nih.gov/publicat/depres-fact.cfm.

Nemets, B., Z. Stahl, and R. H. Belmaker. 2002. Addition of omega-3 fatty acid to maintenance medication treatment for recurrent unipolar depressive disorder. *American Journal of Psychiatry* 159 (3): 477–479.

Newman, M. G., L. E. Szkodny, S. J. Llera, and A. Przeworski. 2011. A review of technology-assisted self-help and minimal contact therapies for anxiety and depression: Is human contact necessary for therapeutic efficacy? *Clinical Psychology Review* 31 (1): 89–103.

Nezu, A. M. 1985. Differences in psychological distress between effective and ineffective problem solvers. *Journal of Counseling Psychology* 32: 135–138.

Nezu, A. M., and C. M. Nezu. 2010. Problem-solving therapy for relapse prevention in depression. In *Relapse for Depression*, edited by S. C. Richards and M. G. Perri. Washington, DC: American Psychological Association.

Nunes, E. V., and F. R. Levin. 2004. Treatment of depression in patients with alcohol or other drug dependence: A meta-analysis. *Journal of the American Medical Association* 291 (15): 1887-1896.)

O'Hara, M. W., and A. M. Swain. 1996. Rates and risk of postpartum depression: A meta-analysis. *International Review of Psychiatry* 8: 37–54.

Ohayon, M. M., and T. Paiva. 2005. Global sleep dissatisfaction for the assessment of insomnia severity in the general population of Portugal. *Sleep Medicine* 6: 435–441.

Okasha, A. 2001. History of mental health in the Arab world. In *Images in Psychiatry: An Arab Perspective*, edited by A. Okasha and M. Maj. Cairo. Egypt: Scientific Book House.

Okasha, A., and T. Okasha. 2000. Notes on mental disorder in pharaonic Egypt. *History of Psychiatry* 11 (44, pt. 4): 413–424.

Olders, H. 2003. Average sunrise time predicts depression prevalence. *Journal of Psychosomatic Research* 55 (2): 99–105.

Osher, Y., and R. H. Belmaker. 2009. Omega-3 fatty acids in depression: A review of three studies. *CNS Neuroscience and Therapeutics* 15 (2): 128–133.

Ota, Y, F. Majima, M. Shimura, and T. Ishikawa. 2007. Applicability of autogenic training for psychosomatic patients with depression. *Japanese Journal of Autogenic Therapy* 27 (1): 45–52.

Painuly, N. P., S. Grover, N. Gupta, and S. K. Mattoo. 2011. Prevalence of anger attacks in depressive and anxiety disorders: Implications for their construct? *Psychiatry and Clinical Neurosciences* 65 (2): 165–174.

Papageorgiou, C. 2006. Worry and rumination: Styles of persistent negative thinking in anxiety and depression. In *Worry and Its Psychological Disorders: Theory, Assessment, and Treatment*, edited by G. C. L. Davey and A. Wells 21–40. Chichester, UK: Wiley Publishing.

Papp, L. M., C. D. Kouros, and E. M. Cummings. 2010. Emotions in marital conflict interactions: Empathic accuracy, assumed similarity, and the moderating context of depressive symptoms. *Journal of Social and Personal Relationships* 27 (3): 367–387.

Patten, S. B. 2009.Accumulation of major depressive episodes over time in a prospective study indicates that retrospectively assessed lifetime prevalence estimates are too low. *BMC Psychiatry* 8: 9–19.

Paul, R. 1990. *Critical Thinking: What Every Person Needs to Survive in a Rapidly Changing World*. Rohnert Park, CA: Center for Critical Thinking and Moral Critique.

Payot, J. 1909. *The Education of Will*. New York: Funk and Wagnalls.

Pelusi, N. 2003. Evolutionary psychology and REBT. In *REBT Theoretical Developments*, edited by W. Dryden. New York: Brunner-Routledge.

Penava, S. J., M. W. Otto, K. M. Maki, and M. H. Pollack. 1998. Rate of improvement during cognitive behavioral group treatment for panic disorder. *Behaviour Research and Therapy* 36 (7–8): 665–673.

Perlis, R. H., J. W. Smoller, M. Fava, J. F. Rosenbaum, A. A. Nierenberg, and G. S. Sachs. 2004. The prevalence and clinical correlates of anger attacks during depressive episodes in bipolar disorder. *Journal of Affective Disorders* 79 (1-3): 291–295.

Perugi, G., P. L. Canonico, P. Carbonato, C. Mencacci, G. Muscettola, L. Pani, R. Torta, C. Vampini, M. Fornaro, F. Parazzini, and A. Dumitriu. 2011. Unexplained somatic symptoms during major depression: Prevalence and clinical impact in a national sample of Italian psychiatric outpatients. *Psychopathology* 44 (2): 116–124.

Peters, E. N., L. M. Fucito, C. Novosad, B. A. Toll, and S .S. O'Malley. 2011 Effect of night smoking, sleep disturbance, and their co-occurrence on smoking outcomes. *Psychology of Addictive Behaviors* 25 (2): 312–319.

Petrides, K. V., and A. Furnham. 2003. Trait emotional intelligence: Behavioural validation in two studies of emotion recognition and reactivity to mood induction. *European Journal of Personality* 17: 39–57.

Pfeiffer, P. N., M. Heisler, J. D. Piette, M. A. M. Rogers and M. Valenstein. 2011. Efficacy of peer support interventions for depression: A meta-analysis. *General Hospital Psychiatry* 33 (1): 29–36.

Piet, J., and E. Hougaard. 2011.The effect of mindfulness-based cognitive therapy for prevention of relapse in recurrent major depressive disorder: A systematic review and meta-analysis. *Clinical Psychology Review* 31 (60): 1032–1040.

Plath, S. 1972. *The Bell Jar*. New York: Bantam Books.

Pomerleau, C. S., A. N. Zucker, and A. J. Stewart. 2003. Patterns of depressive symptomatology in women smokers, ex-smokers, and never-smokers. *Addictive Behaviors* 28: 575–582.

Premack, D. 1965. Reinforcement theory. In *Nebraska Symposium on Motivation*, edited by D. Levine. Lincoln, NE: University of Nebraska Press.

Prince, M., V. Patel, S. Saxena, M. Maj, J. Maselko, M. R. Phillips, and A. Rahman. 2007. No health without mental health. *Lancet* 370 (9590): 859–877.

Rabin, L. A., J. Fogel, and K. E. Nutter-Upham. 2011. Academic procrastination in college students: The role of self-reported executive function. *Journal of Clinical and Experimental Neuropsychology* 33 (3): 344–357.

Radden, J. 2000. *The Nature of Melancholy from Aristotle to Krivsteva*. New York: Oxford University Press.

Redding, R. E., J. D. Herbert, E. M. Forman, and B. A. Gaudiano. 2008. Popular self-help books for anxiety, depression, and trauma: How scientifically grounded and useful are they? *Professional Psychology: Research and Practice* 39 (5): 537–545.

Reinach, J. 1977. *Goose Goofs Off*. New York: Holt, Reinhart, and Winston.

Renouvier, C. 1842. *Manuel de philosophie moderne*. Paris, Paulin, S.l., Un Volume.

Rich, G. J. 2010. Massage therapy: Significance and relevance to professional practice. *Professional Psychology: Research and Practice* 41 (4): 325–332.

Ruhmland, M. M. J. 2001. Efficacy of psychological treatments for panic and agoraphobia. Abstract. *Verhaltenstherapie* 11 (1): 41–53.

Salter, A. 1949. *Conditioned Reflex Therapy.* New York: Creative Edge Press.

Sartorius, N., T. B. Üstün, Y. Lecrubier, and H. Wittchen. 1996. Depression comorbid with anxiety: Results from the WHO study on psychological disorders in primary health care. *British Journal of Psychiatry* 168 (Suppl. 30): 29–34.

Schartau, P. E., S. T. Dalgleish, and B. D. Dunn. 2009. Seeing the bigger picture: Training in perspective broadening reduces self-reported affect and psychophysiological response to distressing films and autobiographical memories. *Journal of Abnormal Psychology* 118 (1): 15–27.

Schlamann, M., R. Naglatzki, A. de Greiff, M. Forsting, and E. R. Gizewski 2010. Autogenic training alters cerebral activation patterns in fMRI. *International Journal of Clinical and Experimental Hypnosis* 58 (4): 444–456.

Schultz, J. H., and W. Luthe. 1969. *Autogenic Training.* New York: Grune and Stratton.

Seligman, M., E. P., T. A. Steen, N. Park, and C. Peterson. 2005. Positive psychology progress: Empirical validation of interventions. *American Psychologist* 60: 410–421.

Shin, L. M., and I. Liberzon. 2010. The neurocircuitry of fear, stress, and anxiety disorders. *Neuropsychopharmacology* 35: 169–191.

Shinozaki, M., M. Kanazawa, M. Kano, Y. Endo, N. Nakaya, M. Hongo, and S. Fukudo. 2010. Effect of autogenic training on general improvement in patients with irritable bowel syndrome: A randomized controlled trial. *Applied Psychophysiology and Biofeedback* 35 (3): 189–198.

Simon, B. 1978. *Mind and Madness in Ancient Greece.* Ithica, NY: Cornell University Press.

Smith, G. R. 2001. Somatization disorder and undifferentiated somatoform disorder. In *Treatments of Psychiatric Disorders*, 3rd ed., edited by G.O. Gabbard 2166–2182. Washington, DC: American Psychiatric Publishing.

Stage, K. B., A. H. Glassman, and L. S. Covey. 1996. Depression after smoking cessation: Case reports. *Journal of Clinical Psychiatry* 57: 467–469.

Stein, M. B., J. R. McQuaid, C. Laffaye, and M. E. McCahill. 1999. Social phobia in the primary care medical setting. *Journal of Family Practice* 48: 514–519.

Steinbrecher, N., and W. Hiller. 2011. Course and prediction of somatoform disorder and medically unexplained symptoms in primary care. *General Hospital Psychiatry* 33 (4): 318–326.

Stetter, F., and S. Kupper 2002. Autogenic training: A meta-analysis of clinical outcome studies. *Applied Psychophysiology and Biofeedback*: 27 (1): 45–98.

Sturmey, P. 2009. Behavioral activation is an evidence-based treatment for depression. *Behavior Modification* 33 (6): 818–829.

Sullivan, P. F., M. C. Nealee, and K. S. Kendler. 2000. Genetic epidemiology of major depression: Review and meta-analysis. *American Journal of Psychiatry* 157: 1552–1562.

Szegedi, A., R. Kohnen, A. Dienel, and M. Kieser, 2005. Acute treatment of moderate to severe depression with *Hypericum* extract WS 5570 (St John's wort): Randomised controlled double blind non-inferiority trial versus paroxetine. *British Medical Journal* 330 (7490): 503.

Tang, T. Z., R. J. DeRubeis, S. D. Hollon, J. Amsterdam, and R. Shelton. 2007. Sudden gains in cognitive therapy of depression and depression relapse/recurrence. *Journal of Consulting and Clinical Psychology* 75 (3): 404–408.

Teychenne, M., K. Ball, and J. Salmon. 2010. Sedentary behavior and depression among adults: A review. *International Journal of Behavioral Medicine* (4): 246–254 .

Tsao, J. C., M. R. Lewin, and M. G. Craske. 1998. The effects of cognitive behavioral therapy for panic disorder on comorbid conditions. *Journal of Anxiety Disorders* 12: 357–371.

Turner, J. A., S. Holtzman, and L. Mancl. 2007. Mediators, moderators, and predictors of therapeutic change in cognitive-behavioral therapy for chronic pain. *Pain* 127 (3): 276–286.

Tuunainen, A., D. Kripke, and T. Endo. 2004. Light therapy for non-seasonal depression. *Cochrane Database System Review* 2: CD004050.

Twenge, J. M., L. Zhang, and C. Im. 2004. It's beyond my control: A cross-temporal meta-analysis of increasing externality in locus of control, 1960–2002. *Personality and Social Psychology Review* 8 (3): 308–319.

Ustun, T. B., J. L. Ayuso-Mateos, J. S. Chatter, C. Mathers, and C. J. L. Murray. 2004. Global burden of depressive disorders in the year 2000. *British Journal of Psychiatry* 184: 386–392.

Van Dyck, R., F. G. Zitman, C. A. Linssen, P. Spinhoven. 1991. Autogenic training and future oriented hypnotic imagery in the treatment of tension headache: Outcome and process. *International Journal of Clinical and Experimental Hypnosis* 39 (1): 6–23.

van Gool, C.H., G. I. Kempen, B.W.Penninx, D. J. Deeg, A.T. Beekman, and J. T. van Eijk. 2003. Relationship between changes in depressive symptoms and unhealthy lifestyles in late middle aged and older persons: Results from the Longitudinal Aging Study, Amsterdam. *Age and Ageing* 32: 81–87.

Veltro, F., N. I. Vendittelli, F. Oricchio, C. Addona, G. Avino, G. Figliolia, and P. I. Morosini. 2008. Effectiveness and efficiency of cognitive-behavioral group therapy for inpatients: Four-year follow-up study. *Journal of Psychiatric Practice* 14 (5): 281–288.

von Clausewitz, C. 1968. *On War*. New York: Penguin.

Wampold, B. E., T. Minami, T. W. Baskin, and S. C. Tierney. 2002. A meta-(re)analysis of the effects of cognitive therapy versus "other therapies" for depression. *Journal of Affective Disorders* 69: 159–165.

Watkins, E. R. 2008. Constructive and unconstructive repetitive thought. *Psychological Bulletin* 134 (2): 163–206.

Webb, T. L., and P. Sheeran. 2008. Mechanisms of implementation intention effects: The role of goal intentions, self-efficacy, and accessibility of plan components. *British Journal of Social Psychology* 47 (3): 373–395.

Westrin A., and R. W. Lam 2007. Seasonal affective disorder: A clinical update. *Annals of Clinical Psychiatry* 19 (4): 239–246.

Wheeler, H. A., K. R. Blankstein, M. M. Antony, R. E. McCabe, and P. J. Bieling. 2011. Perfectionism in anxiety and depression: Comparisons across disorders, relations with symptom severity, and role of comorbidity. *International Journal of Cognitive Therapy* 4 (1): 66–91.

Williams, T. A. 1914. A contrast in psychoanalysis: Three cases. *Journal of Abnormal Psychology* 9 (2–3): 73–86.

———. 1923. *Dreads and Besetting Fears*. Boston: Little, Brown and Company.

Wolitzky-Taylor, K. B., J. D. Horowitz, M. B. Powers, and M. J. Telch. 2008. Psychological approaches in the treatment of specific phobias: A meta-analysis. *Clinical Psychology Review* 28: 1021–1037.

World Health Organization. 2001. Cross-national comparisons of the prevalences and correlates of mental disorders. WHO International Consortium in Psychiatric Epidemiology. *Bulletin of the World Health Organization* 78: 413–426.

Yeung, R. R. 1996. The acute effects of exercise on mood states. *Journal of Psychosomatic Research* 40: 123–141.

Young, A. S., R. Klap, R. Shoai, and K. B. Wells. 2008. Persistent depression and anxiety in the United States: Prevalence and quality of care. *Psychiatric Services* 59 (12): 1391–1398.

Zettle, R. D. 2007. *Act for Depression: A Clinician's Guide to Using Acceptance and Commitment Therapy in Treating Depression*. Oakland CA: New Harbinger Publications.

William J. Knaus, EdD, is a licensed psychologist with more than forty years of clinical experience in working with people suffering from anxiety and depression. He has appeared on numerous regional and national television shows including the *Today Show*, and more than 100 radio shows. His ideas have appeared in national magazines such as *U.S. News and World Report* and *Good Housekeeping*, and major newspapers such as the *Washington Post* and the *Chicago Tribune*. He is one of the original directors of training in rational emotive behavior therapy. Knaus is author of twenty books, including *The Cognitive Behavioral Workbook for Anxiety* and *The Procrastination Workbook*.

Foreword writer **Albert Ellis, PhD**, was a pioneering theorist of cognitive behavioral therapy and the founder of rational emotive behavior therapy (REBT). He is author of many books, including *A Guide to Rational Living* and *Reason and Emotion in Psychotherapy*.

# Albert Ellis Tribute Book
# Series Advisory Board

## GENERAL EDITORS

**Bill Knaus**, EdD, founder of rational emotive education; former director of training, Institute for Advanced Study in Rational Emotive Therapy; author of seminal books on procrastination.

**Jon Carlson**, PsyD, EdD, ABPP, Distinguished Professor, Governors State University; proponent of Adlerian psychotherapy.

**Elliot D. Cohen**, PhD, professor, Indian River State College; adjunct professor, Florida State University College of Medicine; founder of logic-based therapy.

## TRIBUTE BOOK EDITORIAL BOARD

**Irwin Altrows**, PhD, associate fellow and training faculty, REBT; adjunct assistant professor (psychiatry) and clinical supervisor (psychology), Queens University.

**Guy Azoula**, PhD, French representative for rational emotive education; supervisor, REBT; teacher at the French cognitive behavior association.

**Aaron T. Beck**, MD, university professor of psychiatry, University of Pennsylvania; president, Beck Institute for Cognitive Therapy and Research.

**Judith S. Beck**, PhD, director, Beck Institute for Cognitive Therapy and Research; clinical associate professor of psychology in psychiatry, University of Pennsylvania; founding fellow and former president of the Academy of Cognitive Therapy.

**Joel Block**, PhD, ABPP, assistant clinical professor of psychiatry, Einstein College of Medicine; author of books on improving relationships.

**Walter Block**, PhD, Harold E. Wirth Eminent Scholar Endowed Chair in Economics at Loyola University; author of a dozen books and over two hundred scholarly articles.

**Giulo Bortolozzo**, MS, Australian representative for rational emotive education; author of *People and Emotions* and *Have a Go Spaghettio!*

**Chuck Carins**, PhD, professor emeritus, linguistics, City College, New York.

**Nick Cummings**, PhD, former president, American Psychological Association; president, Cummings Foundation.

**Rene F. W. Diekstra**, PhD, professor of psychology, Roosevelt Academy International Honors College, University of Utrecht, The Netherlands.

**Rev. Thomas A. Downes**, PhD, Long Island College Hospital chaplain; master chaplain, Academy of Certified Chaplains.

**Michael R. Edelstein**, PhD, fellow and supervisor, REBT; author of *Three Minute Therapy* and *Stage Fright*; past president of the Association for Behavioral and Cognitive Therapy.

**David Ellis**, JD, intellectual property and patent attorney; former adjunct professor, University of Florida and Stetson University.

**Debbie Joffe Ellis**, licensed psychologist (Australia); licensed mental health counselor (New York); REBT fellow, supervisor, and presenter; wife of Albert Ellis; private practice, New York City.

**Susan Ellis**, PhD, licensed psychologist; certified family mediator; author of *Make Sense of Your Dreams* and *Make Sense of Your Feelings*.

**Frank Farley**, PhD, former president, American Psychological Association; Laura H. Carnell Professor at Temple University.

**Pam Garcey**, PhD, adjunct psychology professor, Argosy University-Dallas; clinical supervisor, University of Texas Southwestern Medical Center.

**Edward Garcia**, MA, former director of training, Institute for Advanced Study in Rational Emotive Therapy; coauthor of *Building Emotional Muscle* and *Homer the Homely Hound Dog*.

**H. Jon Geis**, PhD, original director of training, Institute for Advanced Study in Rational Emotive Therapy; taught at New York University, Columbia University, and Yeshiva University.

**Joe Gerstein**, MD, founding president, SMART Recovery Self-Help Network; Harvard Medical School faculty (retired).

**Russ Grieger**, PhD, REBT supervisor; adjunct professor, University of Virginia; author of six books and over fifty professional papers and chapters on REBT.

**Nancy Haberstroh**, MBA, PhD, primary US representative of rational emotive education; director of psychological services, Monson Developmental Center.

**Steven C. Hayes**, PhD, Foundation Professor of Psychology, University of Nevada, Reno.

**Howard Kassinove**, PhD, ABPP, professor of psychology and director, Institute for the Study and Treatment of Anger and Aggression at Hofstra University.

**Tony Kidman**, PhD, director of the Health Psychology Unit, University of Technology, Sidney Australia; member of the Order of Australia.

**Sam Klarreich**, PhD, president, Berkeley Centre for Effectiveness, Toronto, Canada.

**Gerald Koocher**, PhD, ABPP, former president, American Psychological Association; dean and professor, School of Health and Sciences, Simmons College.

**Paul Kurtz**, PhD, professor emeritus, philosophy, State University of New York at Buffalo; founding president, Center for Inquiry; author of fifty books.

**Arnie Lazarus**, PhD, ABPP, professor emeritus, Rutgers University; founder, multimodal psychotherapy.

**Barry Lubetkin**, PhD, founding copresident Behavioral Therapy Center, New York; author of books on resolving marital and social anxieties.

**John Minor**, PhD, associate fellow and training faculty member, REBT; adjunct professor, University of California.

**John C. Norcross**, PhD, professor of psychology and Distinguished University Fellow, University of Scranton.

**Christine A. Padesky**, PhD, Distinguished Founding Fellow, Academy of Cognitive Therapy; cofounder, Center for Cognitive Therapy; author of best-selling book, *Mind Over Mood.*

**Vince Parr**, PhD, president, Rational Living Foundation, Tampa, Florida.

**Leon Pomeroy**, PhD, adjunct professor, George Mason University; president of the Robert S. Hartman Institute; author of *The New Science of Axiological Psychology.*

**Aldo R. Pucci**, PsyD, president, National Association of Cognitive-Behavioral Therapists.

**Nosheen K. Rahman**, PhD, professor/director of Centre for Clinical Psychology, University of the Punjab, Lahore, Pakistan.

**Roberta Richardson**, PhD, vice chair of Association of REBT, United Kingdom.

**Gayle Rosellini**, MS, specialist in 501(-c)(-3) private nonprofit agencies; specialist in treatment of addictions and criminality; author of *Of Course, You're Angry.*

**Will Ross**, webmaster, Rebt.network.org; author and publisher of online REBT self-help materials.

**Richard S. Schneiman**, PhD, codirector of Intermountain Center for REBT, Salt Lake City.

**Sanjay Singh**, MD, DNB, PhD, REBT and REE representative in India; associate professor, Department of Dermatology, Institute of Medical Sciences, Banaras Hindu University, Varanasi, India.

**Deborah Steinberg**, MSW, fellow and supervisor, REBT; child specialty in character development and moral education; author of *How to Stick with a Diet.*

**Thomas Szasz**, MD, professor of psychiatry emeritus, SUNY Upstate Medical University, Syracuse, New York.

**Danny Wedding**, PhD, MPH, professor of psychiatry, University of Missouri, Columbia; director, Missouri Institute of Mental Health.

**Richard Wessler**, PhD, former director of training, Institute for Advanced Study of Rational Emotive Therapy; professor emeritus, Pace University; cofounder of cognitive appraisal therapy.

**Janet L. Wolfe**, PhD, former executive director, Albert Ellis Institute; adjunct professor, New York University; private practice, New York City.

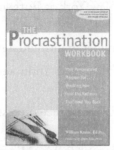
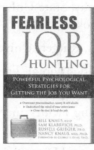
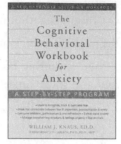
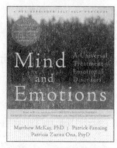
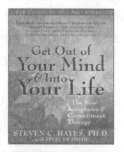
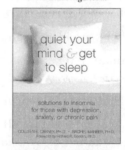

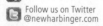